Total Hip Arthroplasty

Karl Knahr

Editor

Total Hip Arthroplasty

Tribological Considerations
and Clinical Consequences

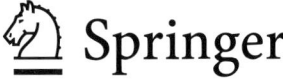 Springer

Editor
Karl Knahr
Orthopaedic Hospital Vienna-Speising
Vienna
Austria

ISBN 978-3-642-35652-0   ISBN 978-3-642-35653-7   (eBook)
DOI 10.1007/978-3-642-35653-7
Springer Heidelberg New York Dordrecht London

Library of Congress Control Number: 2013940609

Printed on acid-free paper

Springer is part of Springer Science+Business Media (www.springer.com)

Preface

Successful long-term results of total hip arthroplasty are mainly due to two facts: long-term stability of the implant and minimal wear of the articulating surfaces. Currently, wear of the articulating components remains the most challenging problem.

The first part of the book includes articles on ceramic technology and clinical implications. The major advantage of ceramic-on-ceramic is the very low wear rate. Nevertheless, there is still concern because of squeaking and possible fracture of the ceramic components. During the last decades ceramic technology has improved dramatically. At the moment we talk about fracture risks of only 0.002 %. Currently ceramic-on-ceramic articulations offer the best option for young and active patients, especially when using large-diameter heads.

For metal-on-metal articulations, concerns have arisen due to the systemic metal ion level elevation and metal allergy resulting sometimes in a local lymphocytic response. Recent reports of increasing failure rates using this material in re-surfacing arthroplasty, as well as in large-diameter head implants, have resulted in official warnings from some State authorities.

Conventional polyethylene-on-metal articulations are complicated in the long-term by wear debris and subsequent osteolysis and loosening. During the last decade cross-linked polyethylene has been shown to have improved wear characteristics compared with conventional polyethylene. Recent reports suggest further improvement by adding vitamin E to polyethylene for prevention of oxidation.

Dislocation of the hip joint ranks number two in reasons for failure of total hip arthroplasty. This problem has been improved by introducing larger femoral heads to improve stability. Several benefits and drawbacks of this approach to hip arthroplasty are discussed within Part IV of this book.

The other contributions are concerned with articles dealing with clinical aspects related to revision surgery and modifications of implants to improve the long-term results of total hip arthroplasty.

The Tribology Day of the 13th EFORT Congress in Berlin was another step forward to communicate between experts and participants the recent knowledge on aspects of tribology in total hip arthroplasty and their important clinical relevance in practice. The authors of this book and myself as editor are looking forward further tribology days at EFORT's annual congresses. We invite you to contribute or participate in this most important topic in total hip arthroplasty.

As in the past years also in Istanbul at the EFORT Meeting from June 5–8, 2013, a full day will be dedicated to the problems of wear and osteolysis in total hip and knee arthroplasty. This tribology day has turned out to be a real highlight within the excellent program of the EFORT Congresses and we invite everyone to be part of this scientific topic.

I would like to acknowledge my secretary Mrs. Susanne Bauer for her dedicated support and assistance in preparing the books on Tribology in Total Hip Arthroplasty.

K. Knahr

Contents

Contents ix

Part I

Ceramic-on-Ceramic Articulations

Technology and Handling of Ceramic Implants

1

Michael M. Morlock, Gerd Huber, and Nick Bishop

1.1 Ceramic Implants for Joint Arthroplasty: Where Do We Stand?

Ceramic bearing articulations were introduced in the 1970s by Boutin and Mittelmeier with the goal of minimizing wear particles and preventing aseptic osteolysis – to fight "the particle disease" caused by polyethylene (PE) wear (Kobayashi et al. 1997), especially in the younger and more active patient (Mittelmeier 1984). Since their introduction, ceramic materials have been greatly improved by reducing grain size and increasing density and by the successive introduction of composite ceramics (Fig. 1.1). With these improvements, the resistance of the materials to crack growth and uncontrolled phase transition was greatly improved (Stewart et al. 2003; Oberbach et al. 2007; Affatato et al. 2012), which is reflected by the material properties (Table 1.1). Controlled phase transition is now even used to limit crack growth (Fig. 1.2).

Considering these material improvements in conjunction with the undoubtedly superior wear characteristics of ceramics and the good biocompatibility of ceramic wear products, the question why ceramic components are not used all the time arises (Mehmood et al. 2008). This can probably be attributed to three issues: fractures, noises, and revision difficulties.

1.1.1 Fractures

Fracture rates in the literature vary quite substantially around a low value. They range from 0.004 % of revisions (Willmann 2000) to 0.1 % (Santavirta et al. 2003) and up to 1.7 % in an Asian study (Park et al. 2006). The most reliable numbers are

M.M. Morlock (✉) • G. Huber • N. Bishop
Institute of Biomechanics, TUHH Hamburg University of Technology,
Denickestrasse 15, Hamburg 21073, Germany
e-mail: morlock@tuhh.de

K. Knahr (ed.), *Total Hip Arthroplasty*,
DOI 10.1007/978-3-642-35653-7_1, © EFORT 2013

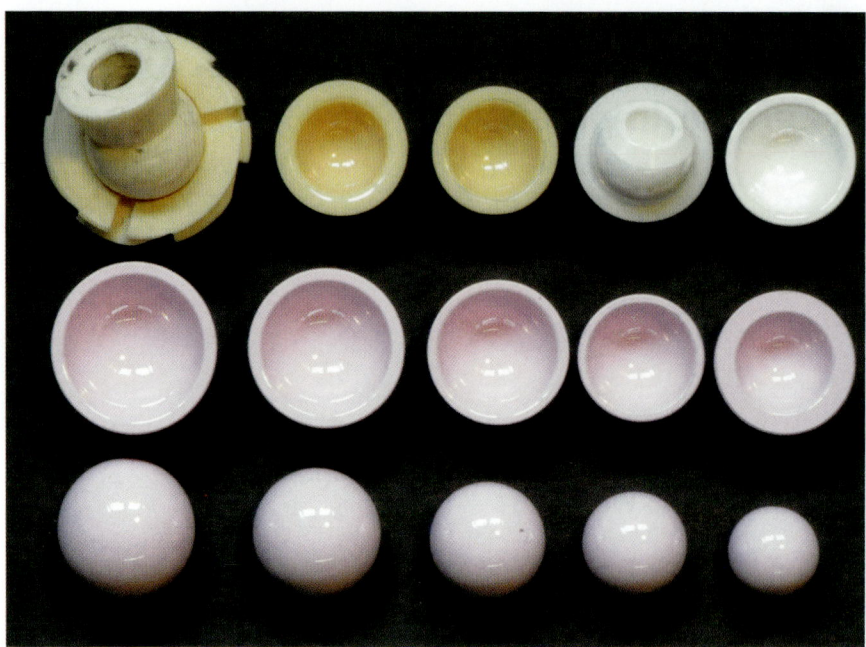

Fig. 1.1 The three generations of ceramics used in hip arthroplasty as bearing materials: (*top left* to *bottom right*) first-generation BIOLOX® threaded cup Ø 38 mm, second-generation BIOLOX®*forte* Ø 28 mm (*thick* and *thin inlay*), third-generation ceramys® Ø 28 mm (*thick* and *thin inlay*), BIOLOX®*delta* Ø 44, 40, 36, 32, 28 mm

Table 1.1 Properties of different ceramic materials used for bearing components in THA

Name	Manufacturer	Generation	Four-point bending strength [MPa]	Biaxial bending strength [MPa]	Toughness [MPa*m$^{1/2}$]
BIOLOX	Ceramtec	First	500		3.0
BIOLOX® forte	Ceramtec	Second	631		3.2
BIOLOX® delta	Ceramtec	Third	1,384		6.5
Bionit	Mathys	Second	–	438	3.4
ceramys	Mathys	Third	–	1,160	7.4
Al$_2$O$_3$ Bio-Hip	Metoxit	Second	550		4.0
ATZ Bio-Hip[a]	Metoxit	Third	1,600		8.0

Values are determined according to ISO6474 (where applicable). Values from different manufacturers cannot be compared directly since they were acquired with different tests
[a]Not commercially available

probably those reported in the annual publications of the national joint replacement registries. The Australian registry attributes 0.4 % of all revisions to head fracture and 0.6–0.9 % to insert fractures (Australian Orthopaedic Association 2012). These include all ceramics (old and new materials) as well as PE components. The registry of the UK and Wales reports slightly higher values (respectively <1 % and 1 %;

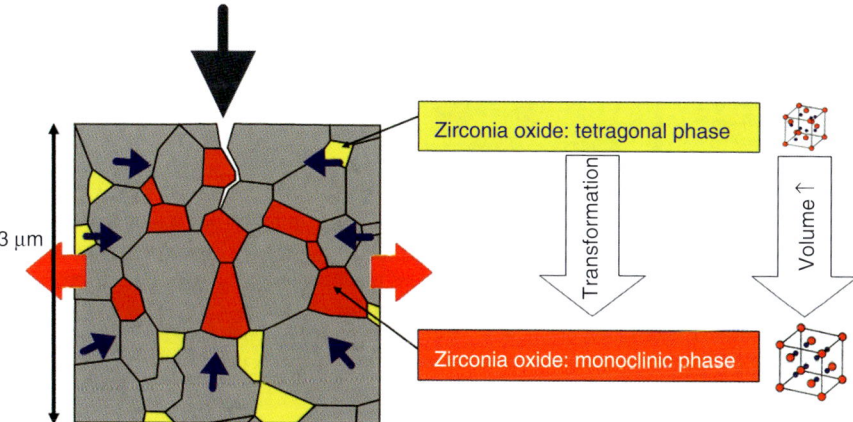

Fig. 1.2 Stress-induced phase transformation of zirconium oxide ceramic grains stopping or slowing down crack growth by volume increase (Adapted from Kuntz et al. 2009). Phase transformation of zirconia from the tetragonal to the monoclinic phase is an undesired event in pure zirconia ceramic components since it is combined with this volume increase and roughening (If it occurs on the surface; Morlock et al. 2001)

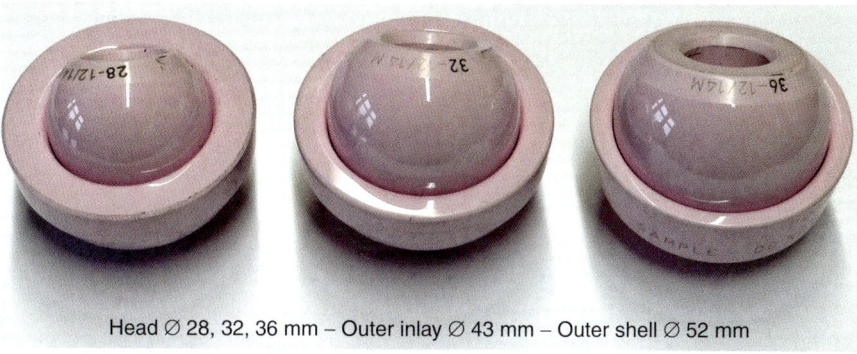

Head Ø 28, 32, 36 mm – Outer inlay Ø 43 mm – Outer shell Ø 52 mm

Fig. 1.3 The thickness of the insert depends on the size of the head. For a given outside diameter Ø of the inlay at the entry plane of 43 mm, liner wall thickness varies between 7.5 and 3.5 mm for 28 and 36 mm heads, respectively (*left* to *right*)

(National Joint Registry 2011)). Considering the material improvements over the years, it can be expected that these failure rates will further decline. However, due to the improved material characteristics, inlay components are made increasingly thinner to accommodate larger heads, possibly partly offsetting the improvement (Fig. 1.3).

Reasons for failure are multiple and include impingement, subluxation, rim loading, or loosening of the head on the stem taper (Nassutt et al. 2006; Park et al. 2006; Poggie et al. 2007; Schlegel et al. 2011). Very few problems are reported for ceramic heads against PE cups. Trauma can be associated with ceramic fractures if

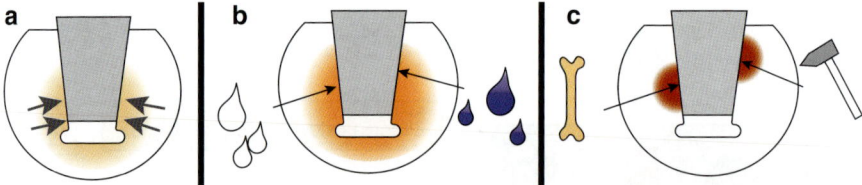

Fig. 1.4 Situation at the taper interface between stem and ball head taper during assembly. (**a**) Clean metal taper: stresses (indicated in *red*) are distributed equally and close to the tip of the stem taper deep within the ball head (area of desired stress transfer indicated by *arrows*); (**b**) wet metal taper (water, blood, fat): stresses in the ball head are higher due to lower friction during assembly resulting in deeper penetration of the stem taper; (**c**) point loads (bone particles)/damaged taper (scratches, wear): stresses in the ceramic ball head are strongly increased locally

the ceramic head becomes subluxated or the cup is rim loaded (Salih et al. 2009; Fard-Aghaie et al. 2012). If the head remains inside the cup, failure is not observed despite high external forces (Salih et al. 2009). Material issues are rarely the reason for fractures with exception of a unique recall by the manufacturer St. Gobain Desmarquest in 1998, when, due to a change in manufacturing procedure, the material properties were altered, which caused a high fracture rate and caused a recall by the company.

The majority of ceramic head or insert failures can be linked to handling (assembly) issues or component positioning.

1.1.1.1 Assembly

The assembly of ceramic heads and inserts onto metal tapers dictates the stress direction and distribution at the interface. Ceramic materials have excellent properties under compression but rather poor properties under tension. A sudden stress increase in tension can lead to critical crack growth, causing the component to fail rapidly ("my hip exploded"). It has to be appreciated that every ceramic has cracks, which do not cause any problems, as long as they are prevented from critical growth (compression is desirable). If due to the assembly a local stress increase occurs, a dramatic decrease in the overall strength of the component (up to 90 % reduction) can result (Weisse et al. 2008). This stress rise can be caused by all situations that prevent a clean circular contact between the ceramic head (or insert) and the taper: contamination (water, blood, fat, bone debris) or taper surface damage (scratches, wear; Fig. 1.4). When the head is removed, the metal transfer from the stem on the female ceramic taper gives an indication of the status of the connection between the ceramic component and the metal taper (Fig. 1.5). It is of crucial importance to clean and dry the metal taper as much as possible before assembling the ceramic components to it.

Following the assembly, the ceramic head (or insert) must be impacted onto (into) the mating metal taper in order to achieve a mechanically stable connection between the two components. Turning the head onto the taper prior to impaction prevents tilting. Inserts should only be assembled using appropriate tools and additional care should be taken to ensure that they are flush with the entrance plane

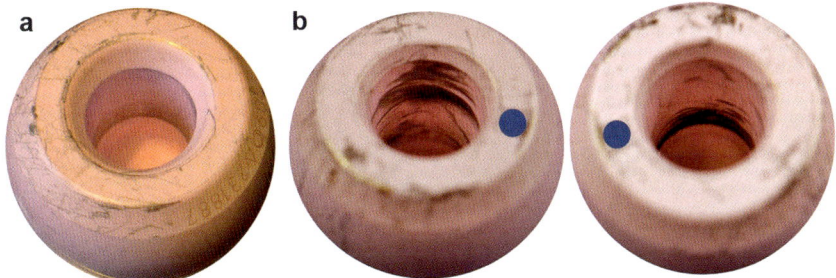

Fig. 1.5 Metal transfer on the female taper of explanted ceramic heads. (**a**) Circular light metal transfer close to the undercut as indication for proper assembly (Fig. 1.4); (**b**) heavy local metal transfer at different depths of the female taper, noncircular but opponent at different levels, indicating a poorly assembled head with toggling during loading and wear of the stem taper (*blue dot* for reference of orientation)

of the metal shell. Once tilting has been ruled out, a firm stroke (~4,000 N peak force) using the appropriate impaction tool should be applied to the ceramic component in order to "lock" it onto (into) the taper (Rehmer et al. 2012).

Assembly of ceramic inserts can be difficult if the metal shell was implanted with a high interference press fit, i.e., excessively underreamed (Langdown et al. 2007). Due to the inhomogeneity of the acetabular stiffness, the metal shell deforms into a noncircular shape (Fig. 1.6a). This makes it difficult to center the insert prior to impaction. If the insert is impacted in a tilted position or not properly impacted (which can lead to tilting of the implant during reduction of the joint; Fig. 1.6b), chipping of the insert rim is to be expected (Fig. 1.6c).

Mismatch between taper and ceramic component must be prevented under all circumstances since this will lead to stress concentrations, which can result in failure of the component (Hohman et al. 2011). The "don't mix and match" precept is crucial. Since the exact taper dimensions cannot be visually identified and labeling can differ between manufacturers, ceramic components should always be obtained from the manufacturer of the metal components. Mismatch between the ceramic components themselves is always an indication for a failed quality assurance during surgery and can have other similarly dramatic consequences (Fig. 1.10). It is hard to believe that as many as 1 % of revision procedures are due to such a size mismatch (National Joint Registry 2011).

1.1.1.2 Positioning/Impingement

Component positioning is a further critical factor for proper operating conditions for ceramic bearings in THA. If the positioning of cup and stem leads to implant-implant impingement or subluxation due to bone-implant impingement, permanent damage can be caused to the ceramic and/or the metal components (Fig. 1.7). Furthermore, if significant forces are exerted on the hip while the head is in rim contact, dramatic stress rises are the consequence, possibly exceeding the fracture strength of ceramic, especially the liner side (Elkins et al. 2012). Fracture risk can

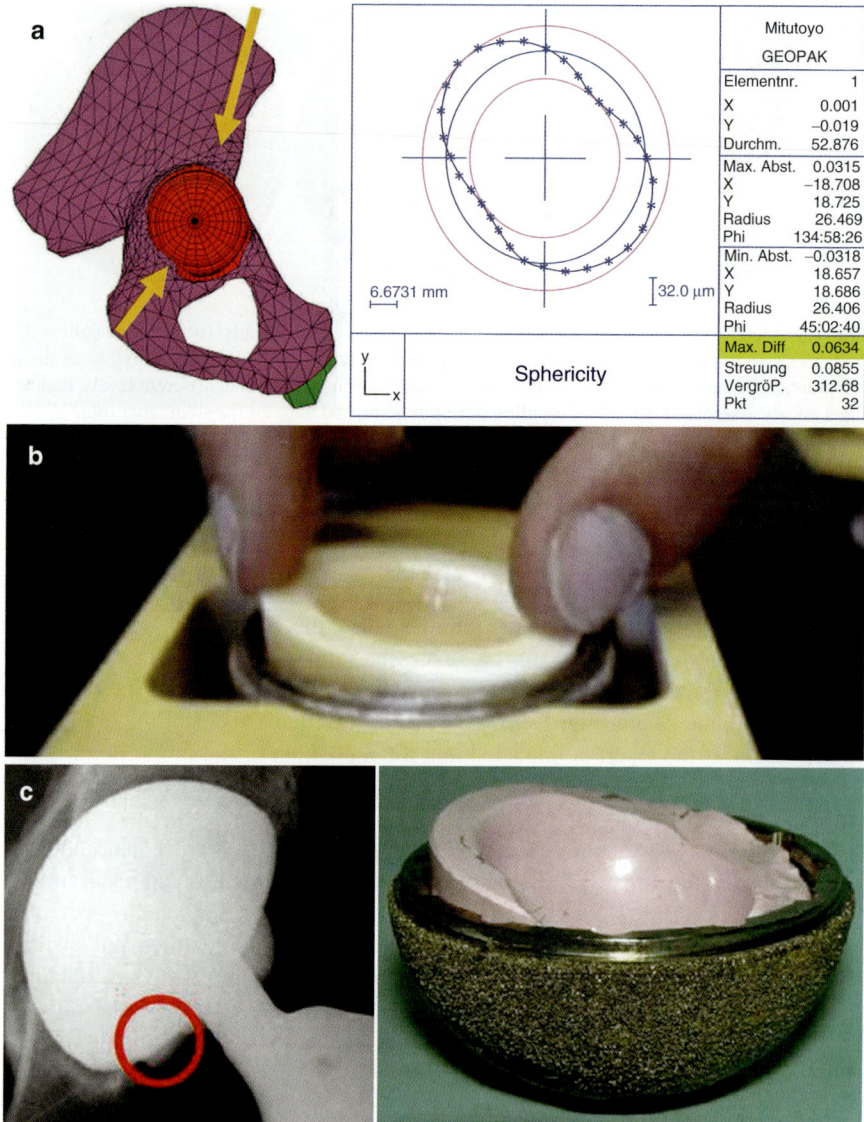

The following tabular data appears in panel (a):

Mitutoyo	
GEOPAK	
Elementnr.	1
X	0.001
Y	−0.019
Durchm.	52.876
Max. Abst.	0.0315
X	−18.708
Y	18.725
Radius	26.469
Phi	134:58:26
Min. Abst.	−0.0318
X	18.657
Y	18.686
Radius	26.406
Phi	45:02:40
Max. Diff	0.0634
Streuung	0.0855
VergröP.	312.68
Pkt	32

6.6731 mm   32.0 µm

Sphericity

Fig. 1.6 (**a**) Elliptical deformation of metal shells during press-fit implantation due to the inhomo-geneous bone stiffness at the acetabulum (Hothan et al. 2011a); (**b**) problem of ceramic liner seating due to excessive underreaming; (**c**) not fully seated insert resulting in chipping of the rim (same implant)

be reduced by surgeons decreasing cup abduction and by patients avoiding specific activities (Elkins et al. 2013).

Another issue related to component positioning is metal transfer from the cup to the ceramic head (Fig. 1.8). Insert designs with an elevated rim, or ceramic insert

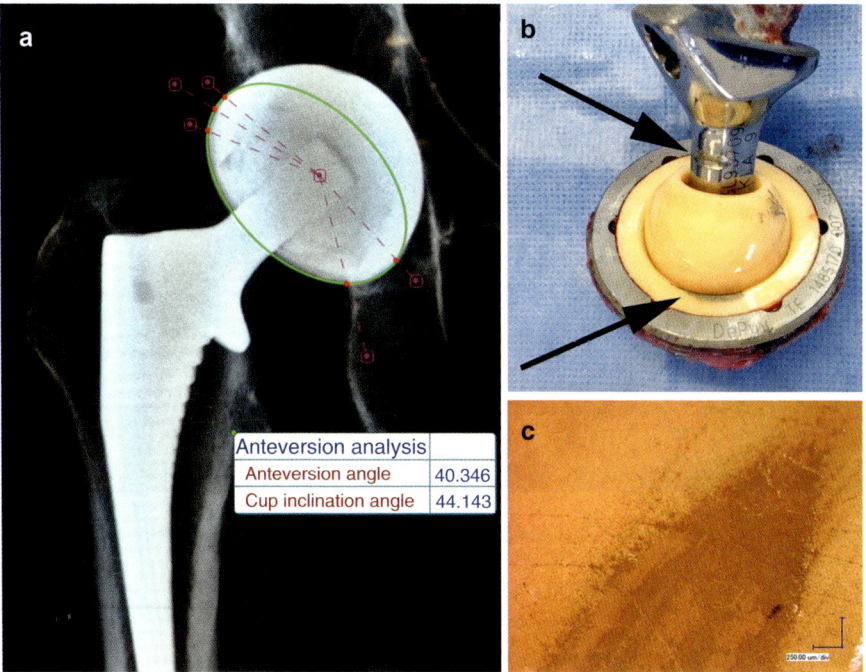

Fig. 1.7 Impingement situation. (**a**) The X-ray shows a large cup anteversion (estimated with the IMATRI.org software). (**b**) Due to the large anteversion of the cup, the neck of the prosthesis stem impinges on the inferior edge of the ceramic inlay during full extension. This causes metal transfer to the insert (*bottom arrow*) and damage to the stem (*top arrow*). (**c**) Stripe wear (grain breakout on the bearing surface) on the top of the ceramic head caused by the subluxation due to the impingement between stem and cup (Courtesy of Tarik Aït Si Selmi)

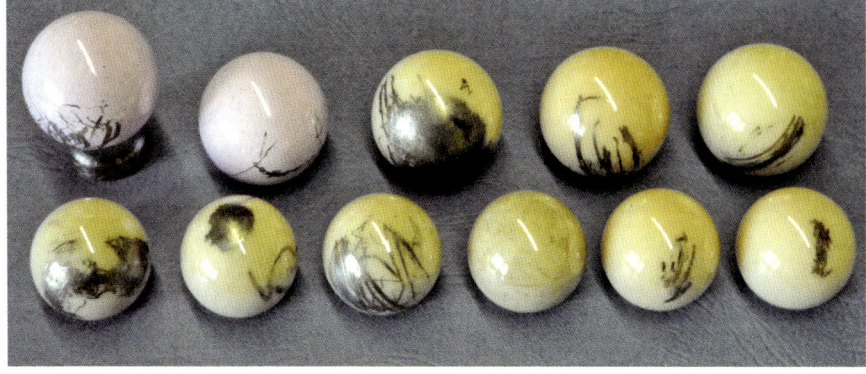

Fig. 1.8 Examples for metal transfer to ceramic heads (Courtesy of Hartmut Kiefer)

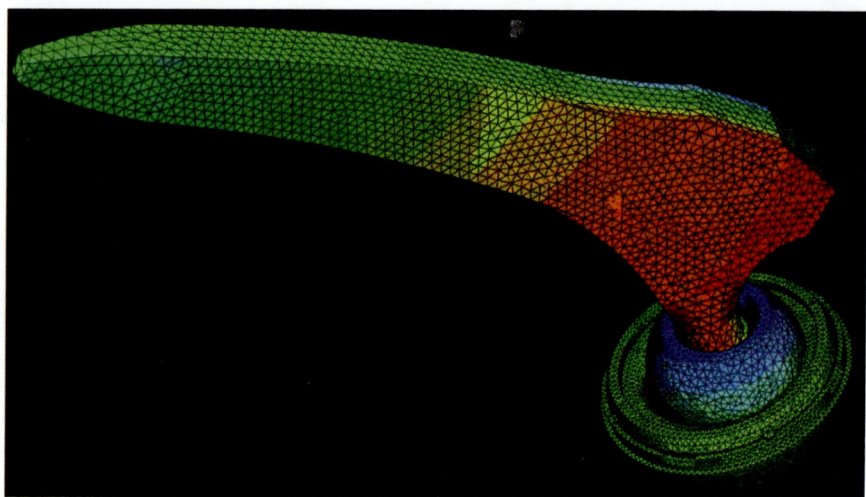

Fig. 1.9 Finite element model of a vibrating THA system. Different colors correspond to different movement magnitudes; warmer colors represent larger movements (Weiss et al. 2010). The frequency of the noise is determined by the natural frequency of the stem (Hothan et al. 2011b)

fracture, or contact of the head and the rim during reduction can partly explain such transfers. The wide variety of patterns observed is not yet fully understood. It is important to note that metal transfer always contaminates the ceramic surface and increases friction (Bal et al. 2007). This is suspected to be the reason for the frequent association of that metal transfer with the occurrence of joint noises in vivo.

1.1.2   Noises

Several different kinds of noises have been reported in the literature since squeaking of artificial hip joints suddenly received intense attention in the USA and Australia. The noises are referred to as popping, snapping, knocking, clunking, clicking, grinding, scraping, crunching, grating, cracking, squeaking, rolling, or even as "the sound of a rusty door hinge" (Glaser et al. 2008). From a technical point of view, two types of noises should be differentiated since they arise from two different mechanisms: squeaking (tonal sounds) and clicking (transient noise). All the different terms used can (and should) be assigned to one of these two types. Squeaking noises are caused by friction-induced vibrations of the whole prosthesis system (Fig. 1.9). A prerequisite for this to occur is high friction in the joint articulation. The frequency of the resulting sound is influenced heavily by the natural frequency of the stem (Hothan et al. 2011b). Clicking noises result from short and "hard" contact events occurring after subluxation when the head locates back into the cup or during impingement.

Theoretically, any bearing couple can be involved, when either the friction in the articulation is high enough or two hard components of the prosthesis system come into "hard" contact. Practically, however, noises are observed nearly exclusively in

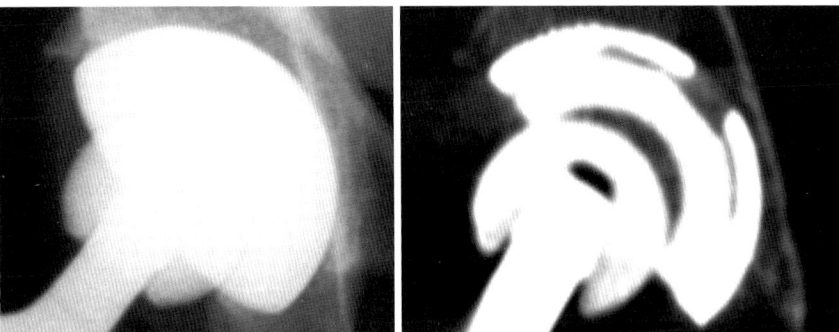

Fig. 1.10 Mismatched ceramic head and ceramic insert. Patient complained about loud squeaking which led to a CT scan (*right*) since mismatch is not easily recognized from the X-ray (Courtesy of Dr. Tarik Aït Si Selmi)

hard-on-hard articulations, namely, metal-on-metal or ceramic-on-ceramic bearings. The superior wear characteristics of these bearing materials are due to their ability to achieve fluid film or mixed lubrication during movement, effectively separating the bearing surfaces and, as such, reducing wear and friction. If the fluid film breaks down, the advantage of hydrodynamic lubrication is completely lost and high friction and wear result. This can be easily imagined by thinking of a car engine without oil. Hard-on-soft bearings with polyethylene always operate in the boundary lubrication mode (the surfaces are in contact) due to the poor wettability of the material. This makes them rather insensitive to the presence or absence of fluid.

The patient himself or herself has nearly no influence on the occurrence of the noise phenomenon. High ranges of joint motion and/or high body weight can be minor factors due to their association with cup edge loading or higher wear (Walter et al. 2007). The major factors, however, are prosthesis design and the surgical procedure, especially those aspects that have the potential to increase friction (Walter et al. 2007; Hothan et al. 2011b; Weiss et al. 2010). Friction is increased mostly due to edge loading, metal transfer (probably caused by impingement or subluxation; Fig. 1.2), mismatched materials (Morlock et al. 2001), the combination of wrong sizes (Fig. 1.10), or by third-body particles. Edge loading and metal transfer can cause a breakdown of the fluid film with the consequences mentioned. Both are related to component positioning, which is probably the most important single factor for the incidence of noises in THA. In some designs the positioning of the components is particularly critical due to certain design features (Chevillotte et al. 2012b). The majority of squeaking events have been reported for one particular THA design using a titanium alloy with a lower stiffness than usual (Stanat and Capozzi 2011). Furthermore, in this system the rim of the ceramic liner is protected by a metal sleeve, facilitating metal transfer to the head, which causes a higher incidence of squeaking occurrence than in other designs.

Interestingly, the rate of noise observations depends on the heritage of the type of bearing materials used. In countries in which ceramic articulations are well established (e.g., France, Germany, Italy), squeaking of THA is rather an anecdotal event, probably since the surgeons are aware of the overwhelming importance of component positioning. In countries, in which ceramics have been introduced more recently, where more forgiving hard-soft bearings were used previously, the squeaking rates reported are higher. This may in part be due to the use of the particular THA system mentioned. Furthermore, the local legal situation might also influence the situation. Realistically, the squeaking frequency of ceramic-on-ceramic articulations in these regions probably lies between 1 and 3 %. Squeaking of metal-on-metal articulations has also been frequently reported. However, this squeaking subsides as the articulation has the ability to wear, such that the increase in contact surface improves lubrication and decrease friction. The substantial metal debris resulting from "bedding in," however, can lead to biological reactions. Since ceramic does not wear easily, the noise phenomenon is usually persistent.

Joint noises should be interpreted as a diagnostic flag since they are an indication of a high-friction situation in the joint, which might otherwise remain unidentified. The surgeon should carefully evaluate the joint functionally and radiologically in order to identify the source of the problem such as extensive cup anteversion, joint laxity, or impingement. In this context it should also be carefully determined how frequently this complication occurs. If the occurrence is rather rare (e.g., "only after 3 h of walking uphill"), the phenomenon might not have a prognostic significance (Chevillotte et al. 2012a). If the phenomenon occurs regularly during daily activities (e.g., stair climbing, lifting objects), the surgeon should use the opportunity to closely examine the mechanical situation in the joint. Repetitive clicking noises are a particular indication for hard contact in small areas resulting in high stresses in the material and potential failure.

1.1.3   Revision

For the revision after failure of a ceramic bearing, it is imperative that certain precautions are observed meticulously (Traina et al. 2011). Three aspects have to be considered: (1) the metal tapers of cup or stem could be damaged due to wear with the ceramic components or fragments; (2) some ceramic particles will always remain in situ after a ceramic fracture; and (3) identify the reason for the failure.

1.1.3.1 Taper Damage
If, prior to fracture, the ceramic head component loosens on the taper (heavy metal transfer can be an indication, Fig. 1.5) or if the patient loads the joint after fracture has occurred, damage to the metal taper interface is to be expected (Affatato et al. 2000). Whether a new ceramic component can be placed onto or into the remaining metal taper depends on the severity of the damage. If the contact area for the new ceramic component is reduced or uneven (Fig. 1.4), stress concentrations might lead to failure once more. In order to prevent the necessity of removing well-ingrown components, titanium adapter sleeves with a 16/18 taper on the outside and a taper matching that of the stem in situ (most of the time also a titanium alloy) were developed (Fig. 1.11). These sleeves are just only in combination with special ceramic

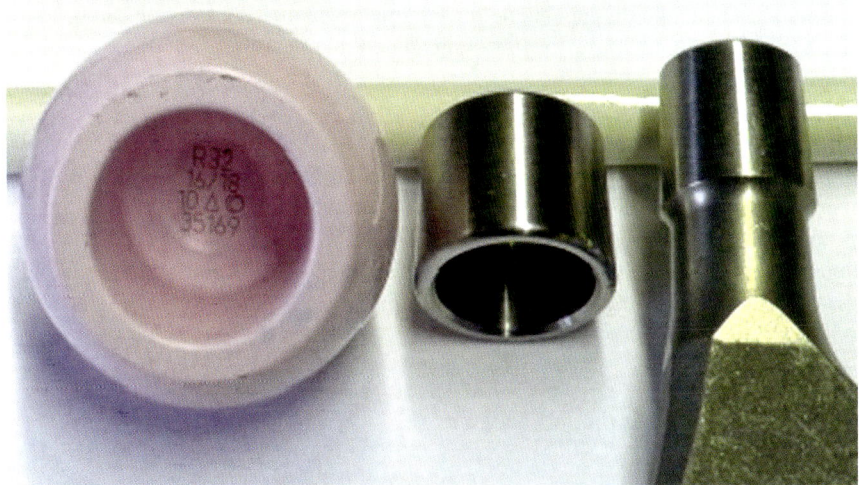

Fig. 1.11 Adapter sleeve for revision of slightly damaged tapers (*middle*). The sleeve has a taper matching the stem taper (e.g., 12/14) on the inside and a 16/18 taper on the outside, which is used in combination with an appropriate ceramic head

heads with a 16/18 taper. This solution creates one more modular junction in the system, which is highly undesirable but cannot be omitted, if the existing stem is to be retained. If damage to the stem taper is too extensive, these adapter sleeves should not be used but the stem revised (Traina et al. 2011).

The question of how to deal with taper damage on the acetabular shell is unanswered. Some designs with ceramic inserts encased into a thin titanium shell are available. These designs allow a new inlay to be inserted into a slightly damaged shell taper. However, these designs are also related to the highest incidence of joint noises (metal transfer) in the patient and the "ease of revision" should not be the dominant factor for the choice of a specific design. The manufacturers do not support replacement of the ceramic insert into a used metal shell, especially after fracture of the insert. If the surgeon is convinced that the shell taper is undamaged, he can keep the shell but under his own responsibility. This is a highly unsatisfactory situation. However, ceramic components do not fail without reason (see 1.3.3).

1.1.3.2 Ceramic Particles

After fracture of a ceramic component, a ceramic-on-ceramic bearing articulation is the bearing of choice from a tribological point of view. The use of a metal-on-PE bearing is contraindicated since any remaining ceramic particles will embed into the PE and rapidly wear the metal head with possibly catastrophic sensorineural consequences including loss of hearing, sight, metallosis, pseudotumors, massive weight loss, and several others (Gallinaro and Piolatto 2009; Pelclova et al. 2012; Kohn and Pape 2007; Hasegawa et al. 2006; Kempf and Semlitsch 1990). In a ceramic-on-ceramic articulation, the remaining particles will be reduced to smaller particles without greatly damaging the bearing surfaces. In a ceramic-on-PE articulation, the ceramic particles will also embed into the PE and increase the wear rate of the ceramic head and the PE cup, but not in a dramatic manner. This option can be used, if other factors do not allow the use of an all ceramic bearing.

1.1.3.3 The Real Problem

Ceramic component fractures are always due to a major stress rise out of whatever reason. Replacing the ceramic component without removing the source of this stress increase (impingement, rim loading, taper contamination or damage, etc.) will most probably result in a very frustrating situation with a renewed fracture event. This applies especially to problems related to component position. Exchange of a ceramic-bearing component alone should, therefore, be the exception, since this will not fully solve the problem.

1.1.4 Final Remarks

Some surgeons call total hip arthroplasty the most successful surgery in the history of orthopedics. This certainly seems justified looking at the growing number of surgeries performed every year and the success rates in the registries. From a bio-mechanical point of view, the problem of THA is under control, as long as patient and surgeon act carefully and responsibly. Established implants and bearing materials have clinically been shown to be successful in the vast majority of patients over periods in excess of 15 years.

The registries do not show great differences between any bearing materials presently used (Australian Orthopaedic Association 2012). The proven advantage of all ceramic THA bearings with respect to wear does not manifest in a reduced revision rate after 8–10 years. It might be that handling and positioning errors counterbalance the wear and biocompatibility advantages. It might also be that 10 years are insufficient to draw a final conclusion.

The ceramic materials used in joint replacement today are high-performance materials, quite comparable to the materials used in Formula I motor racing. Highest performance comes at the price of reduced tolerance to errors. The engineers will try to develop materials that are more forgiving to suboptimal handling and positioning but probably will only be successful within limits. The general rule "high performance comes with little error tolerance" will remain in the foreseeable future. This association clearly demonstrates how the situation for the patient can be improved: better education for involved parties and centers of excellence for challenging surgeries or designs.

References

Affatato S, Ghisolfi E, Cacciari GL, Toni A (2000) Alumina femoral head fracture: an in vitro study. Int J Artif Organs 23:256–260
Affatato S, Modena E, Toni A, Taddei P (2012) Retrieval analysis of three generations of Biolox((R)) femoral heads: Spectroscopic and SEM characterisation. J Mech Behav Biomed Mater 13C:118–128

Australian Orthopaedic Association (2012) National joint replacement registry annual report 2012 Adelaide, AOA

Bal BS, Rahaman MN, Aleto T, Miller FS, Traina F, Toni A (2007) The significance of metal staining on alumina femoral heads in total hip arthroplasty. J Arthroplasty 22:14–19

Chevillotte C, Pibarot V, Carret JP, Bejui-Hugues J, Guyen O (2012a) Hip squeaking: a 10-year follow-up study. J Arthroplasty 27:1008–1013

Chevillotte C, Trousdale RT, An KN, Padgett D, Wright T (2012b) Retrieval analysis of squeaking ceramic implants: are there related specific features? Orthop Traumatol Surg Res 98:281–287

Elkins JM, Pedersen DR, Callaghan JJ, Brown TD (2012) Fracture propagation propensity of ceramic liners during impingement-subluxation: a finite element exploration. J Arthroplasty 27:520–526

Elkins JM, Pedersen DR, Callaghan JJ, Brown TD (2013) Do obesity and/or stripe wear increase ceramic liner fracture risk? An XFEM analysis. Clin Orthop Relat Res 471:527–536

Fard-Aghaie MH, Citak M, Correia J, Haasper C, Gehrke T, Kendoff D (2012) Traumatic ceramic femoral head fracture: an initial misdiagnosis. Open Orthop J 6:362–365

Gallinaro P, Piolatto G (2009) Blind and deaf after total hip replacement? Lancet 373:1944–1945

Glaser D, Komistek RD, Cates HE, Mahfouz MR (2008) Clicking and squeaking: in vivo correlation of sound and separation for different bearing surfaces. J Bone Joint Surg Am 90(Suppl 4): 112–120

Hasegawa M, Sudo A, Uchida A (2006) Cobalt-chromium head wear following revision hip arthroplasty performed after ceramic fracture–a case report. Acta Orthop 77:833–835

Hohman DW, Affonso J, Anders M (2011) Ceramic-on-ceramic failure secondary to head-neck taper mismatch. Am J Orthop (Belle Mead NJ) 40:571–573

Hothan A, Huber G, Weiss C, Hoffmann N, Morlock M (2011a) Deformation characteristics and eigenfrequencies of press-fit acetabular cups. Clin Biomech (Bristol, Avon) 26:46–51

Hothan A, Huber G, Weiss C, Hoffmann N, Morlock M (2011b) The influence of component design, bearing clearance and axial load on the squeaking characteristics of ceramic hip articulations. J Biomech 44:837–841

Kempf I, Semlitsch M (1990) Massive wear of a steel ball head by ceramic fragments in the polyethylene acetabular cup after revision of a total hip prosthesis with fractured ceramic ball. Arch Orthop Trauma Surg 109:284–287

Kobayashi A, Freeman MA, Bonfield W, Kadoya Y, Yamac T, Al-Saffar N, Scott G, Revell PA (1997) Number of polyethylene particles and osteolysis in total joint replacements. A quantitative study using a tissue-digestion method. J Bone Joint Surg Br 79:844–848

Kohn D, Pape D (2007) Extensive intrapelvic granuloma formation caused by ceramic fragments after revision total hip arthroplasty. J Arthroplasty 22:293–296

Kuntz M, Masson B, Pandorf TH (2009) Current state of the art of the ceramic composite material Biolox(R)Delta. In: Mendes G, Lago B (eds) Strength of materials. Nova Science Publishers, New York, pp 133–155

Langdown AJ, Pickard RJ, Hobbs CM, Clarke HJ, Dalton DJ, Grover ML (2007) Incomplete seating of the liner with the Trident acetabular system: a cause for concern? J Bone Joint Surg Br 89:291–295

Mehmood S, Jinnah RH, Pandit H (2008) Review on ceramic-on-ceramic total hip arthroplasty. J Surg Orthop Adv 17:45–50

Mittelmeier H (1984) Hip joint replacement in young patients. Z Orthop Ihre Grenzgeb 122:20–26

Morlock M, Nassutt R, Janssen R, Willmann G, Honl M (2001) Mismatched wear couple zirconium oxide and aluminum oxide in total hip arthroplasty. J Arthroplasty 16:1071–1074

Nassutt R, Mollenhauer I, Klingbeil K, Henning O, Grundei H (2006) Relevance of the insertion force for the taper lock reliability of a hip stem and a ceramic femoral head. Biomed Tech (Berl) 51:103–109

National Joint Registry (2011) 8th annual report for England and Wales

Oberbach T, Begand S, Glien W (2007) In-vitro wear of different ceramic couplings. Key Eng Mater 330–332:1231–1234

Park YS, Hwang SK, Choy WS, Kim YS, Moon YW, Lim SJ (2006) Ceramic failure after total hip arthroplasty with an alumina-on-alumina bearing. J Bone Joint Surg Am 88:780–787

Pelclova D, Sklensky P, Janicek P, lach K (2012) Severe cobalt intoxication following hip replacement revision: clinical features and outcome. Clin Toxicol 50:262–265

Poggie RA, Turgeon TR, Coutts RD (2007) Failure analysis of a ceramic bearing acetabular component. J Bone Joint Surg Am 89:367–375

Rehmer A, Bishop NE, Morlock MM (2012) Influence of assembly procedure and material combination on the strength of the taper connection at the head-neck junction of modular hip endoprostheses. Clin Biomech (Bristol, Avon) 27:77–83

Salih S, Currall VA, Ward AJ, Chesser TJ (2009) Survival of ceramic bearings in total hip replacement after high-energy trauma and periprosthetic acetabular fracture. J Bone Joint Surg Br 91:1533–1535

Santavirta S, Bohler M, Harris WH, Konttinen YT, Lappalainen R, Muratoglu O, Rieker C, Salzer M (2003) Alternative materials to improve total hip replacement tribology. Acta Orthop Scand 74:380–388

Schlegel UJ, Bishop N, Sobottke R, Perka C, Eysel P, Morlock MM (2011) Squeaking as a cause for revision of a composite ceramic cup. Orthopade 40:812–816

Stanat SJ, Capozzi JD (2011) Squeaking in third- and fourth-generation ceramic-on-ceramic total hip arthroplasty meta-analysis and systematic review. J Arthroplasty 27(3):445–453

Stewart TD, Tipper JL, Insley G, Streicher RM, Ingham E, Fisher J (2003) Long-term wear of ceramic matrix composite materials for hip prostheses under severe swing phase microseparation. J Biomed Mater Res B Appl Biomater 66:567–573

Traina F, Tassinari E, De FM, Bordini B, Toni A (2011) Revision of ceramic hip replacements for fracture of a ceramic component: AAOS exhibit selection. J Bone Joint Surg Am 93:e147

Walter WL, O'toole GC, Walter WK, Ellis A, Zicat BA (2007) Squeaking in ceramic-on-ceramic hips: the importance of acetabular component orientation. J Arthroplasty 22:496–503

Weiss C, Gdaniec P, Hoffmann NP, Hothan A, Huber G, Morlock MM (2010) Squeak in hip endoprosthesis systems: An experimental study and a numerical technique to analyze design variants. Med Eng Phys 32:604–609

Weisse B, Affolter C, Stutz A, Terrasi GP, Kobel S, Weber W (2008) Influence of contaminants in the stem-ball interface on the static fracture load of ceramic hip joint ball heads. Proc Inst Mech Eng H 222:829–835

Willmann G (2000) Ceramic femoral head retrieval data. Clin Orthop Relat Res 379:22–28

Long-Term Stability of Ceramic Composite in Total Hip Arthroplasty

2

Bernard Masson and Meinhard Kuntz

2.1 Introduction

Since the year 2000, more than 1.6 million ceramic ball heads and 800,000 ceramic inserts of the new high-performance ceramic composite BIOLOX®*delta* have been successfully implanted. Due to the unique strength and toughness of this material, the risk of fracture has been substantially reduced when compared to conventional ceramic materials.

The outstanding properties of BIOLOX®*delta* rely on complex reinforcing mechanisms. Therefore, it is necessary to assess if reinforcement is maintained throughout the lifetime of the artificial joint, which is anticipated to exceed more than 20 years.

Like any other material which is intended for surgical applications, the suitability must be evaluated based on multiple approaches, like intrinsic mechanical material properties, biocompatibility, system compatibility and finally in vivo scoring of the surgical outcome

The basis of all progress in material development for surgical applications is the intrinsic material properties. When the surgeon decides to replace a known material by a new one, there must be sufficient indication for a substantial benefit. The most challenging question is to predict the reliability of the material after many years of service life.

Within the scope of this chapter, the intrinsic material properties of the composite ceramic BIOLOX®*delta* are analysed. Lifetime can be traced back to basic principles,

B. Masson (✉)
Medical Products Division, CeramTec GmbH,
CeramTec Platz 1-9, Plochingen 73207, Germany
e-mail: b.masson@ceramtec.de

M. Kuntz
Service Center Development, CeramTec GmbH,
CeramTec Platz 1-9, Plochingen 73207, Germany
e-mail: m.kuntz@ceramtec.de

K. Knahr (ed.), *Total Hip Arthroplasty*,
DOI 10.1007/978-3-642-35653-7_2, © EFORT 2013

17

i.e. how can a material be damaged after many years of service. Every material degrades after many years loading in an aggressive environment. It is the challenge to create a material that preserves sufficient residual reliability even under worst-case conditions for many years.

Due to the chemical stability, ceramics obviously provide an intrinsic advantage in comparison to other materials like metals and polymers. Ceramics are produced in the state of a fully saturated chemical bonding. There is no driving power left for further chemical interaction with the environment. Thus, typical lifetime-limiting problems like corrosion or water adsorption are not relevant for high-performance and high-purity ceramics.

It must be considered if there are other mechanisms that may limit the lifetime of ceramics. It is well known that like all other materials ceramics also may suffer degradation from the following distinguished events:

Fatigue	Resistance against long-time static and alternating load
Aging	Resistance against hydrothermal or other chemical attack
Wear	Durability under abrasive conditions

In this chapter, the lifetime-limiting mechanisms and the relevance for the application as a surgical implant are discussed. It is shown how lifetime of the ceramic material BIOLOX®*delta* can be described and evaluated. The unique microstructure and reinforcing mechanisms of the material not only support the short-term performance like fracture toughness and strength but also improve substantially the long-term reliability.

2.2   Description of BIOLOX®*delta*

BIOLOX®*delta* is an alumina-based composite ceramic. Eighty vol % of the matrix consists of fine-grained high-purity alumina which is very similar to the well-known material BIOLOX®*forte*. As it is the case in any other composite material, the basic physical properties like stiffness, hardness and thermal conductivity are mainly predetermined from the dominating phase. It was the basic idea for the development of the new material to preserve all the desirable properties of BIOLOX®*forte* which has millions of components in service but to increase its strength and toughness.

These properties are rigorously improved by implementation of reinforcing elements. Figure 2.1 shows the microstructure of BIOLOX®*delta*.

Two reinforcing components are integrated in BIOLOX®*delta*. Seventeen vol % of the matrix consists of tetragonal zirconia particles. The average grain size of the zirconia is around 0.2 µm. As a further reinforcing element, approx. Three vol % of the matrix is built by platelet-shaped crystals of the ceramic composition strontium aluminate. The platelets stretch to a maximum length of approx. Three micrometer with an aspect ratio of 5:10. The reinforcing ability of these ingredients is explained below.

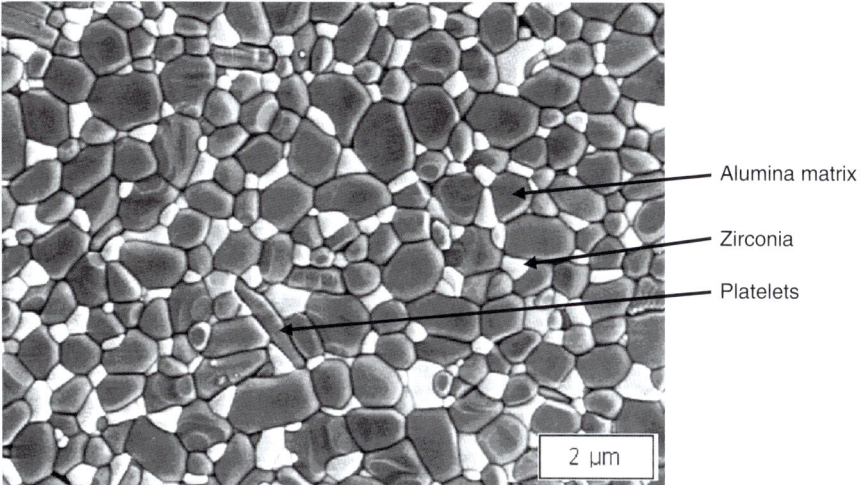

Alumina matrix

Zirconia

Platelets

2 μm

Fig. 2.1 Microstructure of BIOLOX®*delta*

Additionally to the reinforcing components, there are also stabilising elements doped to the material. Chromium is added, which is soluble in the alumina matrix and which increases the hardness of the composite. The minor amount of chromium is the reason for the mauve colour of the material. Furthermore, some yttrium is added to the composite which is solved in the zirconia and which supports the stabilisation of the tetragonal phase (Ohmichi et al. 1999).

The reinforcing elements, in particular the zirconia, substantially increase fracture toughness and strength of the material (Hannink et al. 2000; De Aza et al. 2002). Fracture toughness (K_{IC}) is a measure for the ability of the material to withstand crack extension. Strength (s_c) is defined as the maximum stress within a structure that causes failure of the component. Consequently, when the fracture toughness of the alumina is increased, the strength also is directly improved. This basic principle is the concept of the development of BIOLOX®*delta*. The microstructure is designed in order to provide a maximum of resistance against crack extension.

The benefit in crack resistance which is obtained from incorporating zirconia into an alumina matrix is well known in the science of high-performance ceramics, as it is shown in Fig. 2.2.

The figure represents a realistic part of the microstructure. In the case of severe overloading, crack initiation and crack extension will occur. High tensile stresses in the vicinity of the crack tip trigger the tetragonal–monoclinic phase transformation of the zirconia particles. The accompanied volume expansion leads to the formation of compressive stresses which are very efficient for blocking the crack extension.

As it is shown this reinforcing mechanism is fully activated within a region of a few micrometers. For the macroscopic performance of the material, it is extremely important that immediately at the beginning of crack initiation the reinforcing mechanisms also are activated. Regarding Fig. 2.2, one should keep in mind that the average distance between the reinforcing zirconia particles is approx. 0.2 μm, i.e.

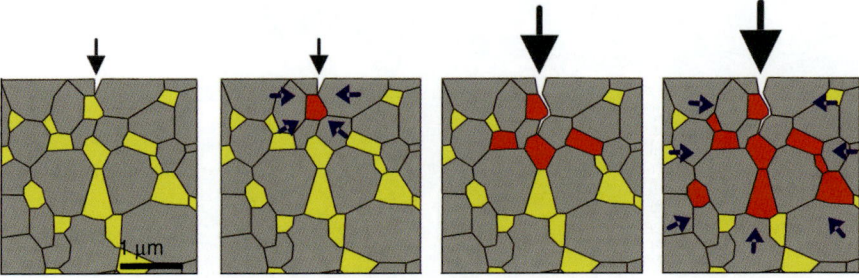

Fig. 2.2 Reinforcing mechanism in BIOLOX®*delta* at crack initiation and propagation

similar to the grain size. Thus, the reinforcement is activated immediately when any microcrack is initiated.

The reinforcing ability of zirconia particles is a consequence of the phase transformation, i.e. the spontaneous change from the tetragonal to the monoclinic phase. The phase transformation is accompanied by a volume change of 4 % of the zirconia particle, i.e. a linear expansion of 1.3 %. Spontaneous phase transformation is a well-known principle in material science. For example, the properties of high-performance steels also rely on spontaneous phase transformation from austenite to martensite.

It should be emphasised that the ability of phase transformation is the precondition for any benefit of the zirconia within the material. The composite is designed such that phase transformation occurs when it is needed, i.e. in the case of microcrack initiation. In contrast to pure zirconia (which draws its high strength from the same principle), the main source of the stability of the tetragonal phase is the embedding of the zirconia particles in the alumina matrix. In contrast, the stability of pure zirconia only relies on the chemical stabilisation (i.e. doping with yttria) and the grain size, which should not exceed a certain range. This is the most important distinction of the composite material BIOLOX®*delta* to pure zirconia. In particular, the mechanical stabilisation of the stiff alumina matrix is not sensitive to any aging effect.

2.3   Comparison of Component and Material Testing

As described above, it is the objective of this chapter to show the intrinsic stability of the material BIOLOX®*delta* against any lifetime-limiting effects. This is mainly accomplished by using well-defined specimens according to the requirements of international standards for surgical materials (e.g. ISO 6474 or ASTM F 603).

However, it may be useful to compare the data obtained from test specimens like bending bars to the properties of hip components. For this purpose, in Fig. 2.3 the results of ball head fracture tests and of 4-point bending tests of several powder batches are presented.

The burst tests on BIOLOX®*delta* ball heads (Fig. 2.3 left) refer to a standard design diameter of 28 mm, taper 12/14. Each individual data point in the figure

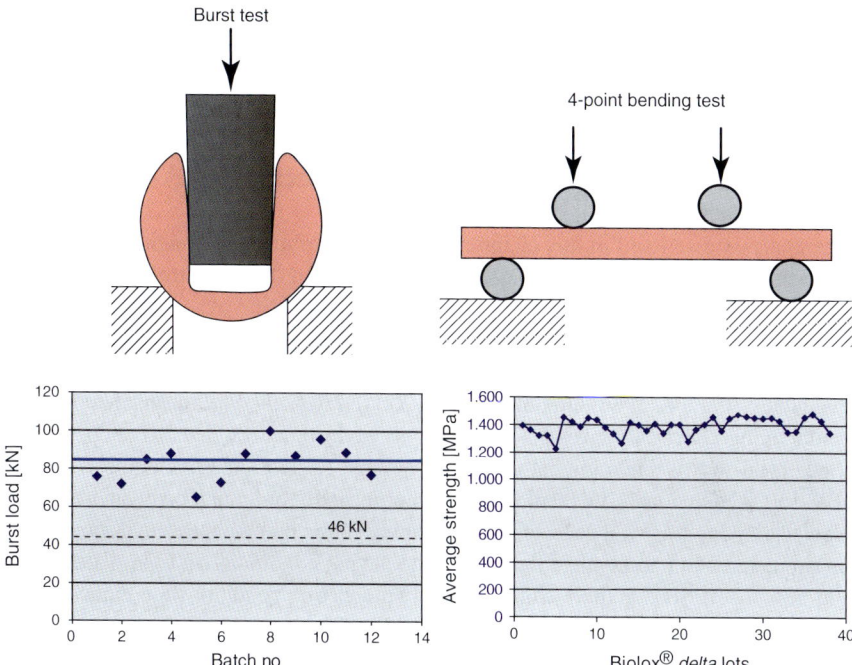

Fig. 2.3 Burst load of BIOLOX®*delta* ball heads (28 +3.5) and strength of bending tests

represents the average value of a test series of at least seven ball heads. The strength (Fig. 2.3 right) refers to 4-point bending tests according to ASTM F 603. The strength as it is derived from bending tests represents the maximum stress in the specimen at the moment of fracture. Each individual data point represents the average of 30 specimens. As it is shown, plenty of data is available for either ball head burst tests and strength. The larger scatter in the burst tests is a consequence of the smaller number of specimens used in this test.

From these data, one is able to compare the strength of the material to the performance of the components. The average burst load is 83 kN and the average strength 1,400 MPa. Usually the load acting on an artificial hip joint is expressed as multiples of the body weight (BW). A reasonable value for 1 BW is 1 kN (approx. 100 kg). From various experiments and calculations, it is derived that the maximum load which can occur in vivo in an extreme situation (e.g. one-leg balancing of a stumble) is approx. $9 \times BW$. This result gives an impressive indication of the large safety margin that is provided from the use of the material BIOLOX®*delta* as a surgical material.

On this basis, the lifetime experiments were designed. The long-term stress on the specimens was chosen such that a reasonable margin in comparison to maximum in vivo loading is provided. Thus, for the cyclic loading tests, two stress levels of 300 and 600 MPa were chosen. From the comparison discussed under Fig. 2.3, the stress level of 300 MPa is equivalent to a component loading of $18 \times BW$, i.e. double the maximum in vivo load (300 MPa/1,400 MPa $\approx$ 18 BW/83 BW). Analogous,

600 MPa corresponds to fourfold maximum in vivo load. Using these stress levels, it is analysed whether the material is able to resist extreme conditions over a lifetime relevant period.

2.4   Discussion of Lifetime-Limiting Effects

The analysis discussed in this chapter refers to a combination of aging and fatigue experiments. Any degradation of the material after long-term treatment is evaluated by comparison of residual strength to the as-received state.

Aging is a relevant issue for all zirconia-containing materials. The transformation from the tetragonal to the monoclinic phase can be triggered by the so-called hydrothermal attack (Pezzotti 2006; Gremillard et al. 2004). *Hydrothermal* means that this particular aging effect only takes place in aqueous environment at elevated temperatures. It has been shown that a critical temperature range for hydrothermal aging is around 134–150 °C. Obviously, this temperature is not realistic for human body environment. However, today it is well accepted that the aging in the human body environment can be simulated in an accelerated test using autoclaving conditions of 2-bar water steam and 134 °C. Various authors claim that 1-h autoclaving conditions are equivalent to 2–4 years in the human body (Hannink et al. 2000; De Aza et al. 2002). Consequently, accelerated aging is also required as a standard test for pure zirconia as a material for surgical implants. Usually, it is investigated whether the residual strength of the material deteriorates after aging. The concept which is presented here does not only rely on the residual strength but also to the performance of the material at cyclic loading.

Fatigue is defined as the material sensitivity against cyclic loading. Limited fatigue resistance is usually observed when the material's ability of crack resistance is continuously deteriorating during the cycling. Even materials, which offer plastic deformation and high crack resistance like metals, can substantially lose their strength during cyclic loading and exhibit brittle fracture. In general, ceramics show higher fatigue resistance in comparison to metals. However, the fatigue effects of ceramics also depend on their specific crack resistance mechanisms. As it was shown under Fig. 2.2, the crack resistance of BIOLOX®*delta* is rather complex. Thus, it is necessary to demonstrate whether this material may show any degradation at cyclic loading.

As a special feature of this investigation, hydrothermal aging and fatigue are combined. According to the theoretical background, one should consider if any aging effect may also impair the fatigue resistance or vice versa.

2.5   Result of Lifetime Experiments

The experiments were designed to simulate a combination of worst-case conditions on BIOLOX®*delta*. The specimens were prepared according to the four-point bending configuration as it is shown in Fig. 2.3 (right). As discussed above, the lifetime-limiting effects of aging and cyclic fatigue were combined in these tests.

Table 2.1 Test matrix with number of tested samples

Autoclaving (h)	No cyclic load	300 MPa, 20*10⁶ cycles	600 MPa, 5*10⁶ cycles
0	30	6	6
5	30	6	6
100	30	6	6

Table 2.2 Residual strength and monoclinic phase content after diverse treatments

Autoclaving		No cyclic load	300 MPa, 20*10⁶ cycles	600 MPa, 5*10⁶ cycles
0	Strength [MPa]	1,346	1,433	1,284
	Monoclinic phase content	18 %	33 %	43 %
5	Strength [MPa]	1,332	1,248	1,361
	Monoclinic phase content	22 %	35 %	42 %
100	Strength [MPa]	1,234	1,308	1,300
	Monoclinic phase content	30 %	33 %	47 %

Two stress levels (300 and 600 MPa) are chosen for the cyclic loading tests. The lower stress level was applied for 20 Mio cycles, the higher stress level for 5 Mio cycles. All tests were performed in Ringer's solution. The accelerated aging was simulated by 5-h and 100-h treatment in autoclaving conditions, which is equivalent to 10 years and 200 years in vivo. All specimens used for cyclic loading were proof tested prior to the cycling. Table 2.1 shows the test matrix including the number of specimens used.

Using 30 specimens is usually required for determination of strength. However, due to the time-consuming experiments applying the cyclic loading, it was decided to use only six specimens for each cyclic loading test. After the treatment, the residual strength of the specimens was determined and compared to the initial strength. Furthermore, the monoclinic phase content was measured for each treatment.

As the most amazing result, the yield of specimens surviving all the tests was 100 % in all cases. Even most severe conditions (i.e. 100-h autoclaving, 600-MPa cyclic load) did not reveal any premature failure. It should be recalled that this stress level represents four times the highest load level at worst-case conditions in vivo. We can thus conclude that the reliability of BIOLOX®*delta* exceeds by far the necessary requirements for reliable surgical components.

Table 2.2 shows the results of the posttest analysis including residual strength and monoclinic phase content. There is a marginal natural scatter in residual strength that is always expected for ceramic materials. However, statistical analysis using student's *t*-test did not reveal any significant deviation of all strength results.

In contrast, there is a clear tendency of an increase in monoclinic phase content both after autoclaving and after cyclic loading, which is illustrated in Fig. 2.4. For example, the test series without autoclaving shows an increase of monoclinic phase content from 18 % in the initial state to 43 % after 5 Mio cycles at 600 MPa. It must

Fig. 2.4 Increase of monoclinic phase content at cyclic loading

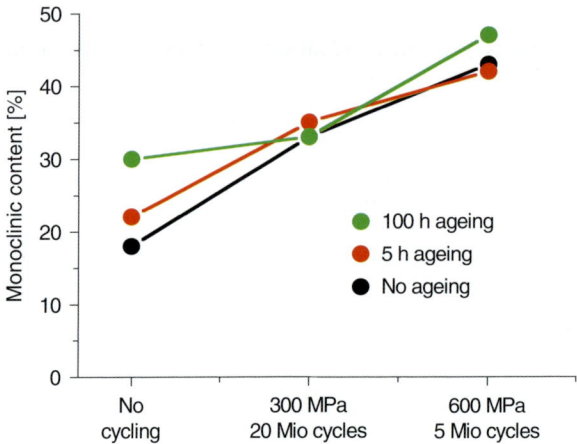

be concluded that the cyclic mechanical loading at a high stress level (600 MPa) of almost half the strength (1,400 MPa) activated the reinforcing ability of the material. As discussed under Fig. 2.2, a high mechanical stress triggers localised phase transformation that prevents any further crack propagation. Obviously the increased amount of monoclinic phase content does not deteriorate the strength of the material. This important conclusion is independent from the source of the phase transformation. In other words, when the phase transformation is activated either by accelerated aging, cyclic fatigue or a combination of both, the residual strength remains on the initial level.

The reported monoclinic phase content should be discussed with respect to the composition of the material. The monoclinic phase content shown in Fig. 2.4 is related to the total zirconia. As described above, the total volume content of zirconia in the alumina matrix is 17 %. In order to assess the effect of the zirconia content, one should refer the amount of monoclinic phase relative to the total volume of the material. For example, the highest amount of monoclinic phase in a region close to the surface measured in this study is 47 %. This equals a total monoclinic content of only 8 % (= 47 % × 17 %). Obviously, even under extreme conditions, the amount of monoclinic phase in this material is well under control. In this context it is elucidative to remind that in pure zirconia an amount of 20 % monoclinic phase is allowed according to the standard ISO 13356 already in the initial state before accelerated aging. It is thus concluded that the specific composition of BIOLOX®*delta* provides inherent protection against improper phase transformation.

Conclusions

The material BIOLOX®*delta* has been exposed to extreme conditions (accelerated aging and cyclic loading in Ringer's solution). It has been shown that even a combination of worst-case conditions does not reveal any premature failure. Furthermore, it was shown that the residual strength remains on the initial level. A certain amount of phase transformation was observed during the tests. The highest amount of monoclinic phase relative to the total volume of the specimen was 47 %. The residual strength was not affected by the phase transformation.

In other studies it was shown that BIOLOX®*delta* performs extremely well in severe wear tests (Clarke et al. 2005). These results are also attributed to the reinforcing mechanism in the material. These exciting results promote the confidence that BIOLOX®*delta* offers the highest probability of long-term durability in well-designed artificial joint systems.

References

Clarke IC, Pezzotti G, Green DD, Shirasu H, Donaldson T (2005) Severe simulation test for run-in ear of all-alumina compared to alumina composite THR. Proceedings 10th BIOLOX symposium, Steinkopff Verlag, Darmstadt Springer 11–20

De Aza AH, Chevalier J, Fantozzi G, Schehl M, Torrecillas R (2002) Crack growth resistance of alumina, zirconia and zirconia toughened alumina ceramics for joint prostheses. Biomaterials 23:937–945

Gremillard L, Chevalier J, Epicier T, Deville S, Fantozzi G (2004) Modeling the ageing kinetics of zirconia ceramics. J Eur Cerm Soc 24:3483–3489

Hannink RHJ, Kelly PM, Muddle BC (2000) Transformation toughening in zirconia-containing ceramics. J Am Ceram Soc 83(3):461–487

Ohmichi N, Kamioka K, Ueda K, Matsui K, Ohgai M (1999) Phase transformation of zirconia ceramics by annealing in hot water. J Ceram Soc Japan 107(2):128–133

Pezzotti G (2006) Environmental phase stability of next generation ceramic composite for hip prostheses. Key Eng Mater 309–311:1223–1226

Ceramic-Ceramic Bearing in Difficult Hips (Primary and Revision)

3

Francesco Benazzo, Loris Perticarini, Claudia Russo, and Alberto Combi

3.1   Introduction

The primary goal of total hip arthroplasty (THA) is to provide the patient with end-stage arthritis of the hip with a long-lasting, pain-free, functional hip joint.

The average age of a primary THA patient is decreasing, and younger, more active patients require hip implants that will last for decades (Manley and Sutton 2008).

Furthermore, patients with severe osteoarthritis secondary to developmental dysplasia of the hip (DDH), initial diagnosis of avascular necrosis of femoral head, posttraumatic arthritis, and rheumatoid arthritis are known to adversely influence the long-term outcome of THA.

Total hip arthroplasty in these patients is technically difficult because of the disturbed anatomy of the proximal femur and the modified shape of the acetabulum; the soft tissues are contracted and usually there is an abductor insufficiency and adductor retraction and shortening.

Various designs, coating, tridimensional structure, and superficial finish of threaded uncemented cups have been introduced, achieving initial stability by interference of the threads with acetabular bone as well as different bearings applied to improve the implants' tribological properties.

This patient expects a long durability implying low wear and minimization of the risk of bone reabsorption, an optimization of function (increased range of motion, low risk of dislocation), and a long-term resistance to high loading.

The use of large-diameter heads (>28 mm) provides increased range of motion and their higher stability and reduced tendency for dislocation (Pandorf 2007).

F. Benazzo (✉) • L. Perticarini • C. Russo • A. Combi
Clinica Ortopedica e Traumatologica, Fondazione IRCCS Policlinico S. Matteo,
Viale Golgi 19, Pavia 27100, Italy
e-mail: fbenazzo@unipv.it; loris.perticarini@gmail.com;
claudia_russo82@hotmail.it; albertocombi.84@gmail.com

K. Knahr (ed.), *Total Hip Arthroplasty*,
DOI 10.1007/978-3-642-35653-7_3, © EFORT 2013

For many years, metal-on-polyethylene bearings have been one of the mainstays of THA. This type of implant has improved the quality of life for hundreds of thousands of patients but is not without problems. Several studies have demonstrated osteolysis due to wear debris generated within the articulating bearing surface using polyethylene (D'Antonio et al. 2005; Anissian et al. 2001; Bierbaum et al. 2002).

Nowadays, the ceramic-on-ceramic bearing represents an important option in total hip replacement. Clinical results reported for alumina-on-alumina bearings indicate that they are an excellent choice for young and active patients because they exhibit significantly greater survivorship and significantly less osteolysis than metal-on-conventional polyethylene controls at more than 10 years' clinical follow-up (Murphy et al. 2006).

Clinical retrievals of alumina-alumina bearings have indicated steady-state wear rates of alumina bearings to be a few microns per year (Mittelmeier and Heisel 1992; Boutin et al. 1988) and sphericity, surface roughness, and wear volume to be directly related to alumina grain size. In some instances, wear was as low as a few microns for a 15-year period in use, which is 2,000 times less than a regular metal-on-polyethylene sliding couple and 100 times less than a metal-on-metal prosthesis (Clarke et al. 2000). Advantages of ceramic-ceramic include its extreme hardness and scratch resistance, improved lubrication that creates a low coefficient of friction resulting in excellent wear resistance, and decreased and less bioactive particulate debris than polyethylene or metal (Bierbaum et al. 2002; Clarke 1992; Saikko et al. 1993).

However, a number of authors have raised concerns regarding the use of titanium acetabular components coupled with ceramic press-fit liners including malseating of the ceramic liner, fracture of the liner (HA et al. 2007), and the occurrence of noise (Ranawat and Ranawat 2007; Walter et al. 2008; Jarrett et al. 2009).

A major concern about ceramic-bearing couples is fracture. Early ceramics had insufficient purity, low density, and a coarsely grained microstructure, which resulted in less mechanical strength of the ceramic material (Willmann 2000).

Today, the number of ceramic fractures is very low, especially thanks to the introduction of new ceramics. Alumina showed head fracture in 0.021 % (21 per 100,000 implants), but now with Biolox® delta the rate dropped to 0.003 % (3 per 100,000 implants). The complication rate for Biolox® delta inserts fractured in vivo was 0.02 % (20 in every 100,000) (Pandorf 2009). Biolox® delta is a zirconia-toughened, platelet-reinforced alumina ceramic (ZPTA) designed to incorporate the wear properties and stability of alumina with vastly improved material strength and toughness. It contains approximately 74 % alumina and 25 % zirconia. Additives of chromium dioxide and strontium oxide enhance the performance of the material.

Numerous mechanisms have been proposed to explain the etiology of noisy ceramic-on-ceramic bearings. Mismatch of the bearing surface (Morlock et al. 2001) was once thought to be the main etiology. Other investigators have suggested that impingement between the femoral neck and the metal acetabular rim leads to generation of metal debris that gains access to the bearing surface acting as third body and results in generation of noise (Walter et al. 2004). Lack of appropriate lubrication or so-called slip stick was offered as another potential etiological factor in generation of noise with hard-on-hard bearing surfaces (Rieker et al. 1998).

Over the last few years, attention of orthopedic surgeons had turned to studies by Walter et al. (Walter et al. 2004) that proposed component malpositioning as

Fig. 3.1 Distribution of patients according to the diagnosis

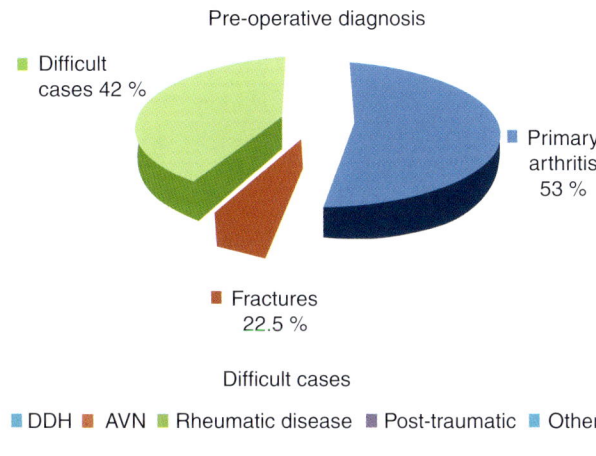

Pre-operative diagnosis

Difficult cases 42 %

Primary arthritis 53 %

Fractures 22.5 %

Fig. 3.2 Diagnosis distribution of difficult cases. The DDH is the most frequent

Difficult cases

■ DDH ■ AVN ■ Rheumatic disease ■ Post-traumatic ■ Other

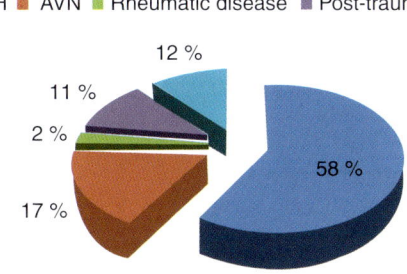

12 %

11 %

2 %

58 %

17 %

the major etiological problem in generating squeaking in ceramic-on-ceramic hips.

The aim of this chapter is to provide the reader with basic concepts, tricks, and tips of ceramic-on-ceramic bearing in difficult hips, reviewing the results of our experience at midterm follow-up in total hip arthroplasty.

3.2   Patients and Methods

3.2.1   Study Population

Between January 2002 and December 2009, 442 THAs were performed using ceramic-on-ceramic coupling. The average age was 54 years (range, 16–94 years). There were 214 females and 191 males (23 women and 14 men had bilateral procedures). The mean body mass index was 26.8 (range, 22.1–32.0). The implant was on the right side in 231 cases and on the left in 211 cases. The average follow-up was 6 years (range, 3–10 years). The main etiology was primary osteoarthritis in 235 hips and secondary arthritis in 180 hips; of these 180, 30 were caused by avascular necrosis, 20 by a trauma, 4 by rheumatic disease, and 105 owing to developmental dysplasia of the hip (Fig. 3.1). The remaining cases were 22 subcapital hip fractures and 5 cases of ceramic-on-polyethylene implant substitution. These last categories were classified as difficult cases (Fig. 3.2). Implantation distribution throughout the period in question is shown in Fig. 3.3.

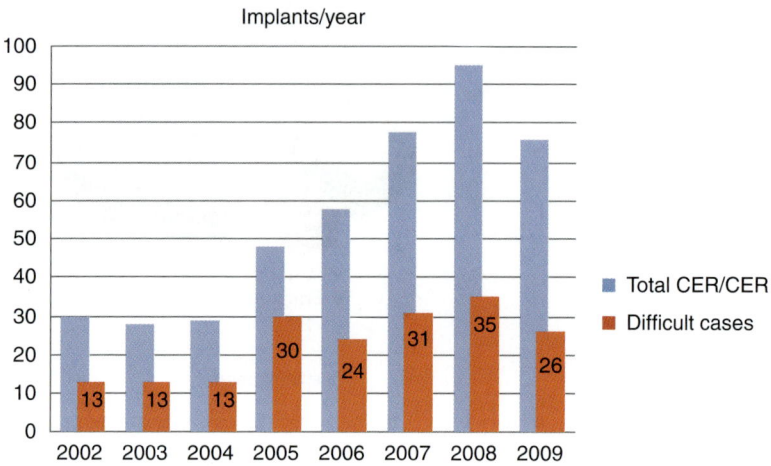

Fig. 3.3 The *blue columns* represent the implant division for years; the red ones represent the number of difficult cases

3.2.2 Surgical Procedure

Four senior surgeons carried out all the prostheses using a posterolateral approach, with the patient in lateral decubitus position, both in primary and in revision surgery.

Anteversion was guided by the bone contours and care was taken to avoid cup edge protrusion which can easily occur at the anterior wall of the acetabulum. Additional screw fixation was provided when there was insufficient hold after impaction or in case of dysplastic acetabulum. Hip stability was tested using trial implants in extension, in external rotation, and in flexion and internal rotation. The final setting was then the implantation of the definitive components. We also checked for leg length equality and evaluated the tensor fasciae latae.

3.2.3 Acetabular and Femoral Components

Uncemented Primary Delta Acetabular Cups (Lima Corporate, San Daniele del Friuli, ITA) were used in 335 patients, Primary Blind Acetabular Cups in 61 patients, and other type in the remaining 46 cases. Implanted cup diameter ranged from 44 to 68 mm. The size of the femoral head ranged from 28 to 40 mm (Fig. 3.4) and was made of alumina until 2004 and of Biolox® delta thereafter. Cups were associated with straight stems (C2, Lima Corporate) in 203 cases, with modular conical stems in 201 cases (Modulus, Lima Corporate), and with various other types in the remaining 38 cases.

3.2.4 Follow-Up

All patients were contacted to be evaluated by a surgeon who had not operated them. Patients were clinically evaluated both preoperatively and postoperatively at

Fig. 3.4 Diameters of femoral heads used in total ceramic-ceramic implants and in difficult cases implant. The head most used is 36 mm, but in difficult cases we implanted small cups with 32-mm head in 41 % of cases

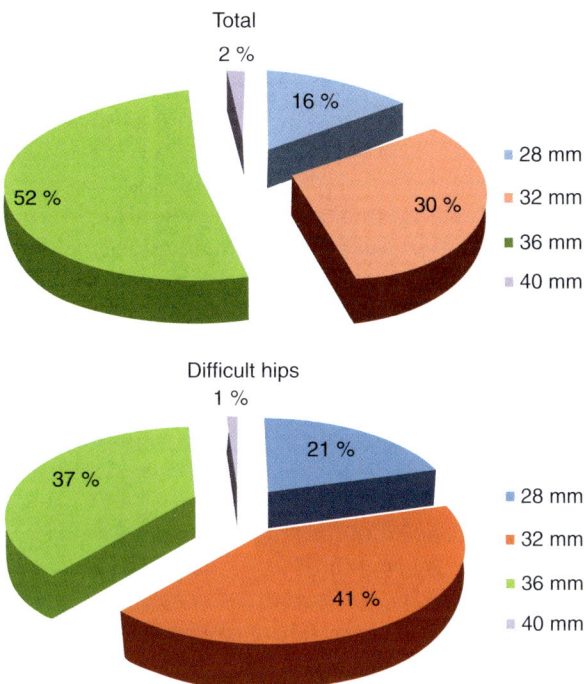

regular follow-up intervals (at 1, 3, 6, 12 months; every year for 3 years; and then every 2 years) using the Harris Hip Score. Standard anterior-posterior and lateral radiographs were taken at regular follow-up intervals and evaluated for cup inclination angle, the presence of radiolucent lines, the osteolysis, and the sclerosis around the implant. A single observer made all measurements. Patients were monitored in order to check intra- and postoperative complications, including infections, nerve injuries, dislocations, deep vein thrombosis, pulmonary embolisms, and fractures. All the patients seen were questioned as if other people could hear any noise coming from their hips.

3.3   Results

The acetabulum was reamed and the cup impacted at a mean abduction angle of $41.7° + -6.2$ SD (range, 34–54) with anteversion adapted to the patient's anatomy, or corrected according to need, in dysplastic cases (Fig. 3.5).

Cup abduction angles in the squeaking hips did not differ from the average abduction angles of the non-squeaking hips. The average preoperative Harris Hip Score was 49.5 (range, 35–52), which improved to 93.2 (range, 85–100; $P < 0.05$) at the last follow-up.

Except for two patients who had died from unrelated causes and six patients who did not show for follow-up, the 397 remaining patients (434 hips) had a complete clinical and radiological file. All the patients with implants still in

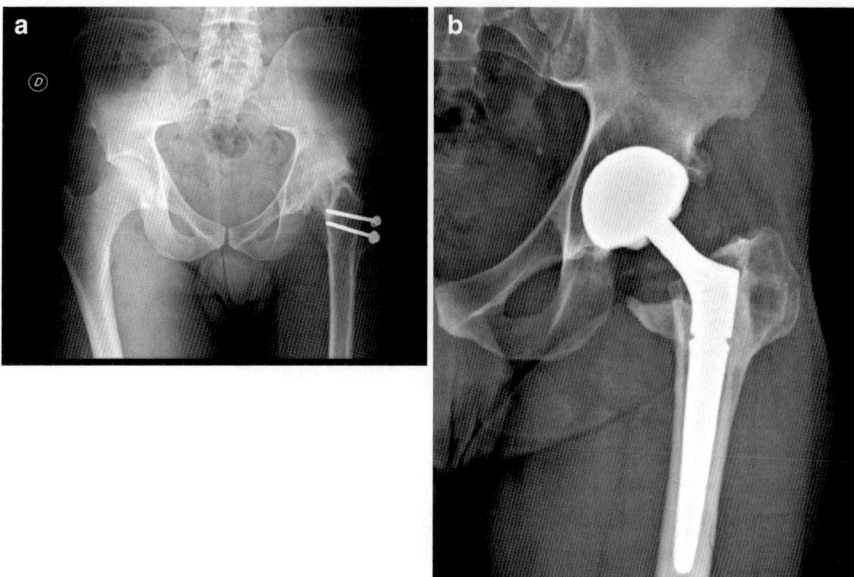

Fig. 3.5 Preoperative X-ray (**a**) and at 4 years (**b**) of DDH case already treated with femoral osteotomy

place had a documented follow-up ranging from 3 to 10 years (mean follow-up 6 years).

Hip dislocation occurred postoperatively in five cases and they were treated conservatively except for one case in which the acetabular insert and the femoral head were replaced. There were no cases of sciatic nerve injury, deep vein thrombosis, pulmonary embolism, prosthetic infection, or fracture. One case of pericarditis was reported 1 month after surgery and treated with antibiotics for 6 months. No postoperative wound healing disorders or infections occurred.

One patient underwent a stem revision 42 months after surgery for modular neck rupture, with implantation of a Revision stem. Another patient complained of thigh and hip pain 11 months after the first implant and was subjected to a reimplant with Revision stem also.

During follow-up, four of the patients reported bothersome hip noise ("squeaking"), two were solved with three local injections administered under image intensification by low molecular weight hyaluronic acid, and the other two spontaneously resolved.

In two cases the implant was replaced due to alumina ceramic insert rupture. There was one case of impingement without dislocation and trochanteritis which was treated with lateral and posterior release, removal of anterior osteophyte, and femoral head substitution.

There were two cases of aseptic loosening, one in a Crowe 4 DDH patient 9 months after surgery, caused by the high dislodging forces of the lengthened abductor muscles (no femoral shortening was performed); the patient underwent revision

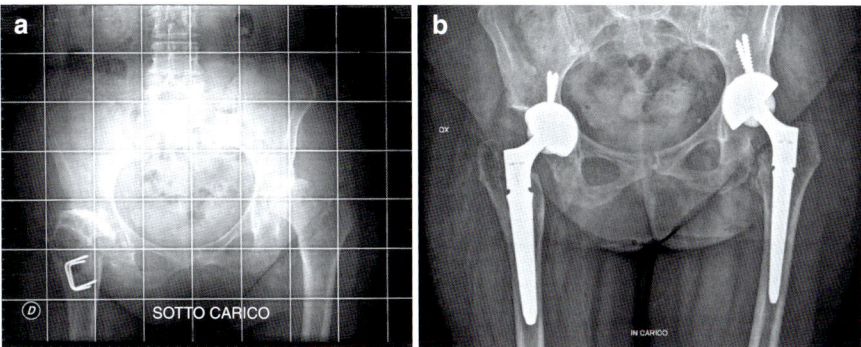

Fig. 3.6 Preoperative X-ray (**a**) and at 5 years (**b**) of bilateral DDH case operated in the same session. Left hip was already treated with femoral osteotomy

with a second Delta TT cup showing excellent results at 4 years of follow-up. The other case of aseptic loosening occurred 18 months after surgery and was revised with a second Delta TT cup with good results at 19 months of follow-up.

In conclusion implants failed in nine unilateral cases (2 %), and failure did not subsequently reoccur.

None of the remaining 388 patients (417 hips) showed osteolysis upon plain imaging. All implants were radiographically stable at latest checkup; radiographic analysis demonstrated bone integration in all patients with no radiolucent zones (Fig. 3.6). No clinically relevant leg length and offset discrepancy were recorded in our patients.

3.4   Guidelines and Tip and Tricks in Ceramic-on-Ceramic Application

As previously described, in order to enable the proper functioning of the implant, it is necessary to implant the cup at approximately 45° of inclination, with a suitable anteversion for the correct biomechanic reconstruction, while avoiding any possible cause of impingement. It is also important that the cup has a high grip, in order to allow high primary stability that enables us to forgive a partial uncovering of the cup edge, especially in case of DDH in which it is necessary to implant small cups in an elusive roof acetabulum. Anyway the ceramic allows us to implant large-diameter heads in cups of small dimension.

In order to minimize the risk of complication, it is also useful to adopt some tricks.

For example, during liner implantation, we must use a trial insert to check the cup position, rinse and clean the metal shell, remove all tissues and particles from the taper, implant the insert, and check for tilting.

Any remaining osteophytes, protruding from the metal shell, must be removed with an osteotome after the implantation of the final liner. If the liner is not seated properly, the vibration produced by the hits of the hammer will make the liner to pop out. The sequence described above can be repeated to assure the proper final seating of the liner.

In head implantation instead we must rinse and dry the metal taper, remove all tissues and particles from the stem taper, and put on ball head with slight turn. Final reduction must be performed without scratching the head, also using an introducer to avoid strip wear.

To overcome any femur deformity, modular stem has to be taken into consideration.

3.5   Discussion

In our experience the results of ceramic-ceramic bearing are comparable to those reported in the literature, having a follow-up of 30 years.

Given the progress achieved in total hip arthroplasty design and the introduction of the Biolox® delta, we anticipate extremely positive results in the future of ceramic-on-ceramic prosthesis.

In our series, the number of "difficult" cases is high; for difficult cases, we intend the DDH patients, the posttraumatic hips, and all cases where the reconstruction can only be achieved with releases, modular stems, and cup downplacing. The association of a modular stems, and a large-diameter bearing in small cups (minimum 32 mm), can bring a huge benefit in difficult hip reconstruction providing in the same time a high-quality bearing.

The low incidence of squeaking in our series can be explained as follows:
– The cups utilized have been conceived to accept a ceramic liner, whose stability inside the metal shell guarantees a substantial lack of reciprocal micromotion and vibrations; the liner remains in all sizes at the level of the metal edge.
– The accuracy in cleaning the ceramic surfaces before implantation.
– The accuracy in avoiding scratches during reduction.

In case of squeaking, the lubrication provided by LMW hyaluronic acid has been sufficient to decrease or eliminate the unwanted sounds.

The introduction of ZPTA (Biolox® delta) has dramatically decreased the incidence of rupture of the components; still, the liner is always thinner if compared to the heads; therefore, edge loading for misplaced cups (vertical position) can cause chipping of the material and start the avalanche progression typical of the ceramic failure.

Finally, we can also consider the high cost of implants; therefore, we recommend the use in young patients with high functional demands, such as patients with DDH (where a long-lasting overload, due to the young age of the patient and difficult joint reconstruction, can be expected), posttraumatic osteoarthritis, and avascular necrosis (same reasons) of femoral head.

References

Anissian HL, Stark A, Good V et al (2001) The wear pattern in medical-on-medical hip prostheses. J Biomed Mater Res 58:673

Bierbaum BE, Nairus J, Kuesis D, Morrison JC, Ward D (2002) Ceramic-on-ceramic bearings in total hip arthroplasty. Clin Orthop 405:158

Boutin P, Christel P, Dorlot JM, Meunier A, de Roquancourt A, Blanquaert D, Herman S, Sedel L, Witvoet J (1988) The use of dense alumina-alumina ceramic combination in total hip replacement. J Biomed Mater Res 22:1203–1232

Clarke IC (1992) Role of ceramic implants: design and clinical success with total hip prosthetic ceramic-to-ceramic bearings. Clin Orthop 282:19

Clarke IC, Good V, Williams P, Schroeder D, Anissian L, Stark A, Oonishi H, Schuldies J, Gustafson G (2000) Ultra-low wear rates for rigid-on-rigid bearings in total hip replacements. Proc Inst Mech Eng H 214:331–347

D'Antonio JA, Capello WN, Manley MT (2005) Alumina ceramic bearings for total hip arthroplasty: five-year results of a randomized study. Clin Orthop 436:164

Ha YC, Kim SY, Kim HJ, Yoo JJ, Koo KH (2007) Ceramic liner fracture after cementless alumina-on-alumina total hip arthroplasty. Clin Orthop Relat Res 458:106–110

Jarrett CA, Ranawat AS, Bruzzone M, Blum YC, Rodriguez JA, Ranawat CS (2009) The squeaking hip: a phenomenon of ceramic-on-ceramic total hip arthroplasty. J Bone Joint Surg Am 91:1344–1349

Manley MT, Sutton K (2008) Bearings of the future for total hip arthroplasty. J Arthroplasty 23(Suppl 1):47–50

Mittelmeier H, Heisel J (1992) Sixteen-years' experience with ceramic hip prostheses. Clin Orthop 282:64–72

Morlock M, Nassutt R, Janssen R et al (2001) Mismatched wear couple zirconium oxide and aluminum oxide in total hip arthroplasty. J Arthroplasty 16:1071

Murphy SB, Ecker TM, Tannast M (2006) Two- to 9-year clinical results of alumina ceramic-on-ceramic THA. Clin Orthop Relat Res 453:97

Pandorf T (2007) Bioceramics and alternative bearings in joint arthroplasty: wear of large ceramic bearings. In: Chang J-D, Billau K (eds) Ceramics in Orthopaedics, Session 3, 12th BIOLOX® Symposium Seoul, Republic of Korea, Springer, pp 91–97 http://www.springer.com/medicine/orthopedics/book/978-3-7985-1782-0

Pandorf T (2009) CeramTec satellite symposium, EFORT Vien 2009

Ranawat AS, Ranawat CS (2007) The squeaking hip: a cause for concern-agrees. Orthopedics 30(738):743

Rieker CB, Kottig P, Schon R et al (1998) Clinical wear performance of metal on metal hip arthroplasties. In: Jacobs JJ, Craig TL (eds) Alternative bearing surfaces in total joint replacement. ASTM International, West Conshohocken, p 144

Saikko VO, Paavolaenen PO, Slatis PS (1993) Wear of the polyethylene acetabular cup: metallic and ceramic heads compared in a hip simulator. Acta Orthop Scand 64:391

Walter WL, Insley GM, Walter WK et al (2004) Edge loading in third generation alumina ceramic-on-ceramic bearings: stripe wear. J Arthroplasty 19:402

Walter WL, Waters TS, Gillies M, Donohoo S, Kurtz SM, Ranawat AS, Hozack WJ, Tuke MA (2008) Squeaking hips. J Bone Joint Surg Am 90(Suppl 4):102–111

Willmann G (2000) Ceramic femoral head retrieval data. Clin Orthop 379:22

Alumina-on-Alumina Bearings in Hip Arthroplasty: What Every Surgeon Should Know

4

P. Hernigou, Y. Homma, J. Hernigou, I. Guissou, and D. Julian

The history of alumina-alumina (Al-Al) bearing surfaces for total hip arthroplasty started in France with Boutin et al. (1988) who implanted the first alumina hip in 1970. Alumina heads are used because of their wear characteristics (Jazrawi et al. 1999) and because of their superior smoothness. In the earliest designs, a bulk alumina acetabular component was implanted either with cement by Boutin et al. (1988) or as a press fit by Mittelmeier and Heisel (1992). Fixation proved to be insufficient (Hamadouche et al. 1999, 2002), and at the beginning the predominant cause of failure was aseptic loosening. Another complication was alumina fracture (Fritsch and Gleitz 1996), and for many surgeons, revision procedure was noted difficult when fracture of alumina ceramic head occurs. The success of contemporary Al-Al bearings (Capello et al. 2008; Chevillotte et al. 2011; Garino 2000; Kim et al. 2010; Mesko et al. 2011) is due both to the absence of osteolysis (Bascarevic et al. 2010; Hernigou and Bahramy 2003; Hernigou et al. 2009) demonstrated in studies with long-term follow-up and to the failures of metal-on-metal friction (Medicines and Healthcare products Regulatory Agency (MHRA) 2012). The aim of this chapter is to explain some clinical and engineering characteristics of Al-Al hips that are specific to this arthroplasty.

P. Hernigou (✉) • J. Hernigou • I. Guissou • D. Julian
Orthopedic Department, Hospital Henri Mondor,
University Paris-East, Creteil 94000, France
e-mail: philippe.hernigou@wanadoo.fr

Y. Homma
Orthopedic Department, Juntendo University,
Tokyo, Japan

K. Knahr (ed.), *Total Hip Arthroplasty*,
DOI 10.1007/978-3-642-35653-7_4, © EFORT 2013

4.1   Fixation of the Cup with a Titanium Shell

High rates of aseptic loosening were reported for Al-Al bearings in the 1970s and 1980s, because of the method of fixation of the components (loosening between the cement and alumina). Since the early 1990s, it is recognized that alumina liner should never be fixed with cement (Nizard et al. 1992; Petsatodis et al. 2010; Sedel et al. 1990, 1994); the dominant design is a porous-coated titanium shell (Bizot et al. 2000; Chang et al. 2009; Garcia-Cimbrelo et al. 2008) with an alumina liner. This design has generated excellent rates of survival and patient satisfaction results. However, assembling the acetabular component intraoperatively into the shell is not so easy, and some rules need to be respected. A sufficient force across the interface between the titanium shell and bone is required to maintain the friction force that keeps the titanium component shell fixed in bone. Impacting the shell into the acetabulum should slightly expand the bone and generate circumferential tensile stress in the bone. The bone then acts like an elastic band on the shell and generates circumferential compressive stress in the interface between the titanium metal back and the bone. Appropriate surgical technique is essential in order to properly fix the shell in the bone but this is not always achieved due to surgical difficulties sometimes. Intraoperatively using the reamer in an asymmetric method can deform (Squire et al. 2006) the cavity performed in the bone by 2 mm diametrically which will give a larger diameter than the shell and a poor fixation. If the hole in the bone is not perfectly circular but elliptic, this may be sufficient to limit the contact of the shell with the bone to two diametrically opposing areas which decreases the fixation. Increased bone stiffness and soft tissue entrapments are other possible mechanisms that may prevent uniform seating of the shell and generate nonuniform loading of the shell on the bone, and this may compromise the bone fixation. Increasing the diameter of the shell to improve fixation will report the problem on the bone with a risk of fracture of the acetabulum at the time of impaction.

4.2   Alumina Liner and Morse Taper

Appropriate surgical technique is essential in order to properly assemble the acetabular component, but this is not always achieved, and a number of factors may contribute to this. Intraoperatively, the titanium shell can deform diametrically because the titanium shell has a thinner wall than the alumina, and the material stiffness of titanium is lower than that of alumina. The risk is to obtain a limited contact of the shell with the liner to two diametrically opposing areas, which increased the risk of poor fixation of the liner, micro-mobility, and fracture. Reduced shell thickness and increased bone stiffness may increase deformation of the shell. Soft tissue entrapment and bone or hydroxyapatite (HA) fragments are other possible mechanisms that may generate nonuniform loading of the liner. The design (Langdown et al. 2007) may also be relevant in poor liner canting, and particularly the mating taper angle. A small angle generates a smaller window of insertion for which the taper will engage. Increasing the taper angle may allow easier insertion of the liner, but the required force at the interface for static friction to keep the assembly together will be higher.

4.3   Alumina Head Morse Taper

The alumina ceramic for femoral head arthroplasty is a polycrystalline form of industrial sapphire. It is obtained from aluminum oxide powder pressed under hot isostatic pressure at a temperature between 1,600 and 1,800 °C and then sintered and polished to obtain a smooth surface. The ceramic head has an excellent compression strength, and currently a 32-mm head tested in compression sustains a 102-kN load. This exceeds the mechanical resistance of the femoral diaphysis to static load of only 20 kN. So probably the risk of fracture with alumina has nothing to do with the activity or the weight of the patients. According to the high level of this excellent compression strength, jumping and sports may be allowed if the compression load is not reached during these activities. However, improper selection, placement, positioning, alignment, and fixation of the femoral head on the Morse taper (Willmann 2000) may result in unusual stress conditions which may lead to a fracture. Inadequate cleaning of the Morse taper (removal of surgical debris) can lead to abnormal impaction of and position of the head on the trunnion. It is necessary to use clean gloves when handling or touching the Morse taper (Pandorf 2009). It is also important to avoid the contact of a metallic hammer when seating an alumina head. A nylon or a polyethylene-seating instrument most be used. It is necessary to avoid an excessive force but it is also necessary to impact the head on the Morse taper with enough force to seat the head on the taper. The impact has to be exactly in the direction of the axis of the taper. Twisting the head allows only a position but is not enough because the weight of the patient will impact later the head on the taper in a direction that is not exactly the direction of the axis of the cone.

4.4   Alumina Fracture

Contemporary alumina materials (Chang et al. 2009; Yoo et al. 2005) are very different to those associated with the high rates of fracture (Mittelmeier and Heisel 1992) reported in the 1970s. The introduction of improved materials and hot isostatic pressing during manufacture served to reduce the grain size and increase the density of the alumina with improvement in its mechanical properties. Ceramic fractures can be explained by the propagation of a crack initiated in the material by the imperfection of the material or by a specific event that initiates the crack. Because of the grain structure of the material, the initial crack will grow and lead to a fracture fatigue. Aluminas are vulnerable to point loading that can occur if there is debris at the taper mating surfaces. This is applicable at the femoral head/stem interface and the acetabular shell/liner interface and can lead to fractures in both scenarios. Clean assembly (Pandorf 2009) of the components is therefore important but sometimes difficult to achieve during surgery. Failure to engage the tapers of the titanium shell and alumina liner properly may also be responsible for fracture of the liner or for liner chipping on insertion.

4.5   How to Perform Revision of a Ceramic Hip in Absence of Fracture

Due to the cone technology, a cone that had already received a ceramic head is theoretically damaged and the engineers and manufacturers will advise to replace the cone for a new ceramic head. When another ceramic head is seated on the same taper, there is an increased risk of alumina fracture if the cone is damaged. If during a revision you need to remove a ceramic head, the alumina should not be directly stroked to avoid a fracture of the head or to avoid damaging the taper. A hammer stroke should be done on the shoulder of the stem in the same direction of the stroke that had fixed previously the femoral head. With the reaction force, the femoral head moves proximally on the taper and is gently removed with the hand without taper damage. When the ceramic femoral head is removed, the taper has caused an imprint (Willmann 2000) in the bore of the head. The imprint is normally a homogenous ring. When the direction of the stroke that has fixed the head is out of the taper axis, the imprint is asymmetric. If the imprint is asymmetric, this means that the femoral head was not correctly fixed on the taper and that probably the taper may be damaged; a new alumina head should not be used on such a taper. If the imprint is a perfectly symmetric ring, this means that the taper has no damage and that a new alumina head could probably be used.

4.6   How to Perform a Revision for a Fracture of a Component

It is important to recognize a fracture of a ceramic (Fritsch and Gleitz 1996) component early, because the abrasive effect of alumina particles can cause catastrophic destruction of bone or metallosis because of metallic debris originated from the metallic stem, neck taper, or socket metal back. When the fracture arrives on the alumina head with an alumina liner without fracture, the cup can be conserved, but of course it is necessary to use a new alumina femoral head. But according to the fact that the breakage of the ceramic head may have altered the surface of the Morse taper, this may lead to a mismatch between the bore of the head and the metal taper and this can cause an area of high point pressure; this may be responsible for the initiation and propagation of a crack that predispose the new ceramic femoral head to re-fracture! Therefore, a ceramic femoral head probably should not be used on an existing Morse taper at the time of revision for a fracture of the femoral head. This concept necessitates removal of the femoral stem to get a new taper (this may be difficult if the stem is stable). When the fracture arrives on the alumina head with a PE cup, it is necessary to remove the cup at the time of revision for a fracture of an alumina head, even when it appears normal macroscopically. If the polyethylene cup is not removed, these particles will be at the origin of a three-body abrasive wear. After the cup has been removed, a new bearing couple has to be chosen. Because of the risk of alumina particles in the joint or in the neosynovial even after debridement and extensive synovectomy, the best bearing surfaces are alumina on alumina. But as previously mentioned (with a ceramic cup), this may necessitate to remove the stem to implant a new alumina head on a new taper. A metal-on-metal bearing surface should be avoided because the alumina is harder than metal and a quick three-body abrasive wear can occur. If the surgeon does not want to remove the stem (old patient, stable stem difficult to remove), the femoral head should be made with reinforced special forged cobalt chromium, or metal with the surface reinforced with diamond, or made of oxinium which has the advantage of the metal for the fracture and the advantage of ceramic for the bearing surface, and the new PE cup should be highly cross-linked since wear is less even in presence of a rough head. A revision arthroplasty after a fracture of the femoral head should be followed every 6 months because there is a high risk of repeated revision in this situation particularly if a metal femoral had been implanted (risk of three-body abrasive wear) or if a new alumina head has been implanted on the original old taper without changing the stem (risk of fracture). For a fracture of a liner, the problem is exactly the same: the new liner should be an alumina liner; for the same reasons, it will be necessary to remove the shell to obtain a new Morse taper.

References

Bascarevic Z, Vukasinovic Z, Slavkovic N et al (2010) Alumina-on-alumina ceramic versus metal-on-highly cross-linked polyethylene bearings in total hip arthroplasty: a comparative study. Int Orthop 34:1129–1135

Bizot P, Banallec L, Sedel L, Nizard R (2000) Alumina-on-alumina total hip protheses in patients 40 years of age or younger. Clin Orthop 379:68–76

Boutin P, Christel P, Dorlot JM et al (1988) The use of dense alumina-alumina ceramic combination in total hip replacement. J Biomed Mater Res 22:1203–1232

Capello WN, D'Antonio JA, Feinberg JR, Manley MT, Naughton M (2008) Ceramic-on- ceramic total hip arthroplasty: update. J Arthroplasty 23:39–43

Chang JD, Kamdar R, Yoo JH, Hur M, Lee SS (2009) Third-generation ceramic-on-ceramic bearing surfaces in revision total hip arthroplasty. J Arthroplasty 24:1231–1235

Chevillotte C, Pibarot V, Carret JP, Bejui-Hugues J, Guyen O (2011) Nine years follow up of 100 ceramic on ceramic total hip arthroplasty. Int Orthop 35:1599–1604

Fritsch EW, Gleitz M (1996) Ceramic femoral head fractures in total hip arthroplasty. Clin Orthop Relat Res 328:129–136

Garcia-Cimbrelo E, Garcia-Rey E, Murcia-Mazon A, Blanco-Pozo A, Marti E (2008) Alumina-on-alumina in THA: a multicenter prospective study. Clin Orthop Relat Res 466: 309–316

Garino JP (2000) Modern ceramic-on-ceramic total hip systems in the United States: early results. Clin Orthop Relat Res 379:41–47

Hamadouche M, Nizard RS, Meunier A, Bizot P, Sedel L (1999) Cementless bulk alumina socket: preliminary results at 6 years. J Arthroplasty 14:701–707

Hamadouche M, Boutin P, Daussange J, Bolander ME, Sedel L (2002) Alumina-on-alumina total hip arthroplasty: a minimum 18.5-year follow-up study. J Bone Joint Surg Am 84-A:69–77

Hernigou P, Bahramy T (2003) Zirconia and alumina ceramics in comparison with metal heads: polyethylene wear after a minimum ten year follow-up. J Bone Joint Surg Br 85:504–509

Hernigou P, Zilber S, Filippini P, Poignard A (2009) Ceramic-ceramic bearing decreases osteolysis: a 20-year study versus ceramic-polyethylene on the contralateral hip. Clin Orthop Relat Res 467:2274–2280

Jazrawi LM, Bogner E, Della Valle CJ et al (1999) Wear rates of ceramic-on-ceramic bearing surfaces in total hip implants: a 12-year follow-up study. J Arthroplasty 14:781–787

Kim YH, Choi Y, Kim JS (2010) Cementless total hip arthroplasty with ceramic-on-ceramic bearing in patients younger than 45 years with femoral-head osteonecrosis. Int Orthop 34: 1123–1127

Langdown AJ, Pickard RJ, Hobbs CM et al (2007) Incomplete seating of the liner with the Trident acetabular system: a cause for concern? J Bone Joint Surg Br 89-B:291–295

Mesko JW, D'Antonio JA, Capello WN, Bierbaum BE, Naughton M (2011) Ceramic-on-ceramic hip outcome at a 5- to 10-year interval: has it lived up to its expectations? J Arthroplasty 26: 172–177

Mittelmeier H, Heisel J (1992) Sixteen-years' experience with ceramic hip prostheses. Clin Orthop Relat Res 282:64–72

Nizard RS, Sedel L, Christel P et al (1992) Ten-year survivorship of cemented ceramic-ceramic total hip prosthesis. Clin Orthop Relat Res 282:53–63

No authors listed. Medicines and Healthcare products Regulatory Agency (MHRA) (2012) Medical device alert: all metal-on-metal (MoM) hip replacements, (MDA/2012/ 008). http://www.mhra. gov.uk/Publications/Safetywarnings/MedicalDeviceAlerts/CON079157. (Date last accessed 28 Feb 2012)

Pandorf T (2009) How important it is to use clean taper fixations? Procs 13th international BIOLOX symposium: ioceramics and alternative bearings in joint arthroplasty. Edinburgh

Petsatodis GE, Papadopoulos PP, Papavasiliou KA et al (2010) Primary cementless total hip arthroplasty with an alumina ceramic-on-ceramic bearing: results after a minimum of twenty years of follow-up. J Bone Joint Surg Am 92-A:639–644

Sedel L, Kerboull L, Christel P (1990) Alumina-on-alumina hip replacement. Results and survivorship in young patients. J Bone Joint Surg Br 72:658–663

Sedel L, Nizard R, Kerboull L, Witwoet J (1994) Alumina-alumina hip replacement in patients younger than 50 years old. Clin Orthop Relat Res 298:175–183

Squire M, Griffin WL, Mason JB, Peindl RD, Odum S (2006) Acetabular component deformation with press-fit fixation. J Arthroplasty 21:72–77

Willmann G (2000) Ceramic femoral head retrieval data. Clin Orthop Relat Res 379:22–28

Yoo JJ, Kim YM, Yoon KS et al (2005) Alumina-on-alumina total hip arthroplasty: a five year minimum follow-up study. J Bone Joint Surg Am 87-A:530–535

Part II

Metal-on-Metal Articulations

Metal-on-Metal Resurfacing and the Cost to the Nation: A Conservative Estimate of the Unexpected Costs Required to Implement the New Metal-on-Metal Follow-Up Programme in the UK

5

John Lloyd, Ian Starks, Tom Wainwright, and Robert Middleton

5.1   Introduction

The past 15 years has seen resurgence in the interest in metal-on-metal hip replacements following the introduction of the hip resurfacing (HR) in the mid-1990s. Marketing of these implants has placed strong emphasis on the advantages of HRs over more conventional total hip replacements (THRs), especially for younger active individuals. Frequently cited advantages include, preservation of femoral bone stock (Schmalzried et al. 1996), less bearing surface wear (Chan et al. 1999; McMinn et al. 1996) and lower dislocation rates (Hing et al. 2007). Superior function and activity scores have also been observed (Mont et al. 2009; Vendittoli et al. 2006). However, there are a number of complications that are specific to HR. These include femoral neck fracture (Schimmin and Back 2005; Treacy et al. 2005) and avascular necrosis (Amstutz et al. 2004; Daniel et al. 2004). More recently, concerns have been raised about the effects of increased serum metal ion levels

J. Lloyd, FRCS (T&O) (✉)
Department of Orthopaedics, The Royal Bournemouth Hospital,
Castle Lane East, Bournemouth, UK
e-mail: jelloyd1@btinternet.com

I. Starks, BA FRCSEd (T&O)
Department of Orthopaedics, The Royal Bournemouth Hospital, Bournemouth, UK

T. Wainwright, PgDip PgCert BSc (Hons) MCSP AIC MIHM • R. Middleton, MA FRCS
Department of Orthopaedics, The Royal Bournemouth Hospital,
Bournemouth, UK

Centre of Postgraduate Medicine, Research and Education,
The School of Health and Social Care, Bournemouth University,
Bournemouth, UK

K. Knahr (ed.), *Total Hip Arthroplasty*,
DOI 10.1007/978-3-642-35653-7_5, © EFORT 2013

(de Souza et al. 2010), metal hypersensitivity and pseudotumour formation (Beaule et al. 2011; Glyn-Jones et al. 2009; Pandit et al. 2008).

A number of different designs of HR have been marketed over the last decade with differing success rates (Amstutz and Le Duff 2010; Daniel et al. 2010; McMinn et al. 2010). The National Joint Registry (NJR) has collected data on HR since 2003. The 7th Annual Report (2010) confirmed concerns that some implants were failing prematurely, in particular, the ASR (DePuy Orthopaedics Inc., Warsaw, Indiana) and Cormet 2000 (Corin Group PLC, Cirencester, UK) with revision rates of 12 and 10 %, respectively, at 5 years (National Joint Registry for England and Wales 2010). DePuy issued a Field Safety Notice in March 2010 for the ASR hip, and by May 2010 the Medicines and Healthcare products Regulatory Agency (MHRA) had published a medical device alert. In September 2010, DePuy withdrew the ASR device (Medicines and Healthcare products Regulatory Agency 2010).

In response to the withdrawal of the ASR and growing concerns over metal ion disease, the British Orthopaedic Association (BOA) and the British Hip Society (BHS) published guidance on the use of metal-on-metal implants and, in particular, on how to responsibly manage and follow up these patients (Large diameter metal on metal bearing total hip replacements 2011; Withdrawal of Depuy ASR resurfacing and XL metal on metal bearings – information for and advice to surgeons 2010). It is advised that all patients with a metal-on-metal prosthesis undergo a minimum of annual clinical and radiological follow-up. The use of cross-sectional imaging (magnetic resonance imaging (MRI) or ultrasound) and serum metal ion levels should be used as adjuncts in patients with symptomatic replacements. These guidelines are more rigorous than the 2006 BOA "Guide to Good Practice" on long-term follow-up for primary hip replacement patients (Primary total hip replacement: a guide to good practice 2006). For patients who have received the recalled ASR implant, DePuy have agreed to fund all additional follow-up costs for up to 7 years postoperatively. However, the new BOA/BHS guidelines apply to all metal-on-metal bearings, and so hospitals are now required to follow up all HR patients according to the new protocol. In a National Health Service facing intense financial pressures over the coming years, this has huge financial implications (Appleby et al. 2010).

The aim of this study was to estimate the additional financial burden on the National Health Service for implementing the 2011 BHS/BOA recommendations for postoperative follow-up of HR patients.

5.2   Methods

The total number of HRs performed nationally between 2003 and 2010 was obtained from the NJR annual reports (Van der Weegen et al. 2011) (Table 5.1).

A 10-year cost analysis for the increased postoperative surveillance now required for this cohort of patients was completed. All indicative costs were taken from the NHS Payment by Results Tariff, except for metal ion levels which were obtained from the Biochemistry Department at our institute (Table 5.2). In order to simplify

Table 5.1 Number of HR by year

	2003	2004	2005	2006	2007	2008	2009	2010
Number of resurfacings	2,637	4,981	6,198	6,484	6,662	5,750	4,327	2,577
Cumulative total	2,637	7,618	13,816	20,300	26,962	32,712	37,039	39,616

Table 5.2 Cost details

Department of Health national framework costing (2011–2012) was used to calculate the individual NHS tariffs. They are as follows:

Outpatient follow-up appointment	£84
X-ray AP pelvis and lateral hip	£164
MRI	£216
Ultrasound	£49
Serum cobalt and chromium ion blood test	£30

Table 5.3 Protocol details

Protocol name	Details of protocol
Standard	Clinic review at 6 weeks postoperation and then clinical and x-ray review at 1, 5, 10 years postoperation
MOM 1	Clinic review at 6 weeks postoperation and then clinical and x-ray review at 1, 2, 3, 4, 5, 6, 7, 8, 9, 10 years postoperation
MOM 2	Clinic review at 6 weeks postoperation and then clinical and x-ray review at 1, 2, 3, 4, 5, 6, 7, 8, 9, 10 years postoperation, with the addition of one single MRI and metal ion review in 2012
MOM 3	Clinic review at 6 weeks postoperation and then clinical and x-ray review at 1, 2, 3, 4, 5, 6, 7, 8, 9, 10 years postoperation, with the addition of one single ultrasound and metal ion review in 2012
MOM 4	Clinic review at 6 weeks postoperation and then clinical, x-ray, MRI and metal ion review at 1, 2, 3, 4, 5, 6, 7, 8, 9, 10 years postoperation
MOM 5	Clinic review at 6 weeks postoperation and then clinical, x-ray, ultrasound and metal ion review at 1, 2, 3, 4, 5, 6, 7, 8, 9, 10 years postoperation

the analysis, the outpatient attendance and associated investigations were the only costs compared. For the purpose of this study, these costs have been assumed to remain constant throughout the analysis. It was also assumed that current practice in all hospitals was currently in accordance with the 2006 BOA Guide to Good Practice guidelines.

The MHRA, BOA and BHS guidance on investigation and follow-up for HR was applied to the data. For the purposes of this cost analysis, a standard protocol (2006 BOA Guide to Good Practice guidelines) was compared with five example follow-up templates based on the new guidelines (Table 5.3). These ranged from the minimum of yearly follow-up and x-ray (protocol 1) to yearly follow-up with metal ion levels and cross-sectional imaging at each visit (protocols 4 and 5).

Table 5.4 Ten-year costing table in pounds

Year	Standard	MOM 1	MOM 2	MOM 3	MOM 4	MOM 5
2012	1,652,176	9,824,768	19,570,304	12,954,432	19,570,304	12,954,432
2013	2,079,976	9,824,768	9,824,768	9,824,768	19,570,304	12,954,432
2014	2,308,384	9,824,768	9,824,768	9,824,768	19,570,304	12,954,432
2015	2,176,200	9,824,768	9,824,768	9,824,768	19,570,304	12,954,432
2016	1,608,032	9,824,768	9,824,768	9,824,768	19,570,304	12,954,432
2017	1,652,176	9,824,768	9,824,768	9,824,768	19,570,304	12,954,432
2018	2,079,976	9,824,768	9,824,768	9,824,768	19,570,304	12,954,432
2019	2,308,384	9,824,768	9,824,768	9,824,768	19,570,304	12,954,432
2020	2,176,200	9,824,768	9,824,768	9,824,768	19,570,304	12,954,432
2021	1,608,032	9,824,768	9,824,768	9,824,768	19,570,304	12,954,432
Total	19,649,536	98,247,680	107,993,216	101,377,344	195,703,040	129,544,320

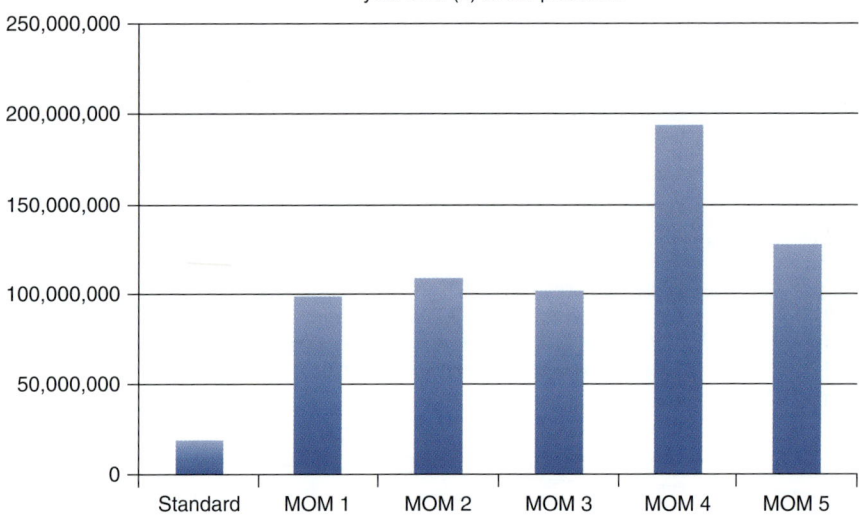

Graph to show comparative 10 year cost (£) of the protocols

Graph 5.1 The comparative costs of the various HR follow-up protocols are compared with the standard cost of conventional THR follow-up

5.3   Results

Between 2003 and 2010, a total of 39,616 HRs were recorded in the NJR (Table 5.1). The cost of 10-year follow-up for these patients ranges from £98,247,680 to £195,703,040 dependent upon the follow-up protocol used (Table 5.4). This compares with a 10-year follow-up cost of £19,649,536 for a conventional hip replacement using the "Guide to Good Practice" guidelines.

The comparative costs of the various HR follow-up protocols are compared with the standard cost of conventional THR follow-up in Graph 5.1.

5.4   Discussion

This is the first study to estimate the financial implications of the recent BOA/BHS guidelines on following up metal-on-metal hip resurfacings to the NHS. At a conservative estimate, over the next 10 years, the new follow-up regimen for HR will cost somewhere between an extra £78,598,144 and £176,053,504 nationally. This will be 5–10 times more expensive than that budgeted and expected for following up a similar cohort of patients undergoing a non-metal-on-metal THR. In a time when we are facing £21 billion cuts in funding, this is a huge financial blow to the NHS (Appleby et al. 2010).

While the NJR performs a vital service, their figures are incomplete. The NJR has 82 % compliance rate (sales figures vs. returned NJR forms) between 2003 and 2009, which may indicate our calculations are underpowered by up to 20 % (National Joint Registry for England and Wales 2010). Also, our calculations do not take into consideration inflation and thus only provide a conservative guide as to the real problem. They also do not include costs associated with any hip resurfacings inserted between 2010 and the present date. For the purpose of this study, we have excluded the metal-on-metal large bearing THRs; however, it should be noted that these implants are subject to the same follow-up guidelines. It is estimated from NJR figures that a minimum of 22,051 large metal-on-metal THRs were implanted over the same time frame 2003–2010 (National Joint Registry for England and Wales 2011).

Since National Institute of Clinical Excellence's (NICE) approval for HR in 2002, there has been no obligation for the surgeon or hospital trust to provide regular clinical or radiographic follow-up of their HR (NICE recommends the selective use of metal on metal hip resurfacing 2002). Until recently BOA's good practice guidance for primary THR follow-up could be reasonably applied to HR (Primary total hip replacement: a guide to good practice 2006). They recommend radiographic and clinical reviews at one, five and each subsequent 5 years after surgery. However, many surgeons have chosen to follow up their patients closely, publishing their experiences and results, which have been summarised by Van der Weegen et al. in a systematic review (Van der Weegen et al. 2011).

As we enter the next phase of HR, it is imperative that all patients be followed up on an annual basis with a clinical and radiological review as advised by the BOA, BHS and MHRA (Large diameter metal on metal bearing total hip replacements 2011; Medicines and Healthcare products Regulatory Agency 2010; Withdrawal of Depuy ASR resurfacing and XL metal on metal bearings – information for and advice to surgeons 2010). Since our true understanding of the correlation of serum metal ion levels, pseudotumour and implant failure remains in its infancy, it is conceivable that we could see a move towards the addition of annual metal ion levels and Ultra-sound scan (USS) or MRI for the duration of the implant's life, further increasing costs.

In addition to the increased cost of adhering to the new guidelines is the impending financial burden of revision surgery. The mean 5-year revision rate for hip resurfacings are 6.3 % but range from 4.3 to 12 % (National Joint Registry for England and Wales 2010). The mean 5-year revision rate for large metal-on-metal THRs fares slightly worse at 7.8 %. It is predicted that revision rates will increase above current levels because of a greater understanding of the natural history of metal-on-metal implants, a lower threshold to investigate unexplained pains and a lower threshold to offer a revision operation.

An important consideration, in addition to the financial burden, is the impact on workload and capacity required to create additional follow-up clinics, additional x-ray and MRI or additional USS appointments. MRI is probably the most reliable investigation but also the most time consuming and expensive. In our hospital trust an unreported MRI pelvis takes 30 min to perform which equates to an additional 19,808 h of unplanned and unbudgeted MRI scans nationally if each resurfacing patient has only one MRI over the duration of their implant's life. All of these unplanned and unbudgeted investigations will have a huge impact on local resources including staffing levels in order to coordinate the appointments, run the clinics and provide the expertise to report the additional investigations.

What is clear from this chapter is that every orthopaedic department is going to have to review the number of metal-on-metal hip arthroplasties they have implanted and plan and budget for appropriate follow-up arrangements. Whilst DePuy have agreed funding for those patients with ASR hip components, this only accounts for about 10 % of all implanted HR. The vast majority of HRs implanted over the last 10 years were from other manufacturers (National Joint Registry for England and Wales 2011). Thus, orthopaedic departments are going to have to find more funding, or redirect existing funds, to address this problem. The additional cost to the patients in terms of potential distress and anxiety, as well as the potential increasing revision load, is immeasurable.

Conclusion

In summary, it is important for the department of health, local hospital trusts and individual surgeons to be aware of the huge financial and logistical implications for implementing close follow-up of HR in accordance with national guidelines. Surgeons should carefully weigh these new costs when considering a patient for HR. We predict a huge swing away from Metal on metal (MOM) bearings for both cost and longevity reasons.

References

Amstutz HC, Le Duff MJ (2010) Hip resurfacing results for osteonecrosis as good as for other etiologies at 2 to 12 years. Clin Orthop 468:375–381

Amstutz HC, Beaule PE, Dorey FJ et al (2004) Metal-on-metal hybrid surface arthroplasty: two to six year follow-up study. J Bone Joint Surg Am 86:28–39

Appleby J, Ham C, Imison C et al (2010) Improving NHS productivity: more with the same not more of the same. The Kings Fund. www.kingsfund.org.uk/.../improving-nhs-productivity

Beaule PE, Kim PR, Powell J et al (2011) A survey on the prevalence of pseudotumours with metal-on-metal hip resurfacing in Canadian academic centers. J Bone Joint Surg Am 93(Suppl 2): 118–121

Chan F, Bobyn D, Medley J et al (1999) Wear and lubrication of metal-on-metal hip implants. Clin Orthop 369:10–24

Daniel J, Pynsent PB, McMinn DJ (2004) Metal-on-metal resurfacing of the hip in patients under the age of 55 years with osteoarthritis. J Bone Joint Surg Br 86:177–184

Daniel J, Ziaee H, Kamali A et al (2010) Ten-year results of a double-heat-treated metal-on-metal hip resurfacing. J Bone Joint Surg Br 92:20–27

de Souza RM, Parsons NR, Oni T et al (2010) Metal ion levels following resurfacing arthroplasty of the hip. J Bone Joint Surg Br 92:1642–1647

Glyn-Jones S, Pandit HP, Kwon YM et al (2009) Risk factors for inflammatory pseudotumour formation following hip resurfacing. J Bone Joint Surg Br 91:1566–1574

Hing C, Back D, Schimmin A (2007) Hip resurfacing: indications, results, and conclusions. Instr Course Lect 56:171–178

Large diameter metal on metal bearing total hip replacements (2011) www.britishhipsociety.com/pdfs/BHS_MOM_THR.pdf Published by BOA and BHS www.boa.ac.uk/PP/Pages/clin-issues.aspx

McMinn D, Treacy R, Lin K et al (1996) Metal on metal surface replacement of the hip: experience of the McMinn prosthesis. Clin Orthop 329(Suppl):89–98

McMinn D, Daniel J, Ziaee H et al (2010) Hip resurfacing. In: Bentley G (ed) European instructional lectures: 11 EFFORT Congress, Madrid, Spain. Springer, New York, pp 133–142

Mont MA, Marker DR, Smith JM et al (2009) Resurfacing is comparable to total hip arthroplasty at short-term follow-up. Clin Orthop 467:66–71

National Joint Registry for England and Wales (2010) 7th annual report. www.njrcentre.org

National Joint Registry for England and Wales (2011) 8th annual report. www.njrcentre.org

NICE recommends the selective use of metal on metal hip resurfacing (2002) National Institute Clinical Excellence 2002/34. Issued: 19 June 2002

Pandit H, Glyn-Jones S, McLardy-Smith P et al (2008) Pseudotumours associated with metal-on-metal hip resurfacings. J Bone Joint Surg Br 90:847–851

Primary total hip replacement: a guide to good practice (2006) Published by BOA 1998

Medicines and Healthcare products Regulatory Agency (2010) Medical device alert. ref: MDA/2010/069 www.mhra.gov.uk

Schimmin AJ, Back D (2005) Femoral neck fractures following Birmingham hip resurfacing: a national review of 50 cases. J Bone Joint Surg Br 87:463–464

Schmalzried TP, Peters PC, Maurer BT et al (1996) Long duration metal-on-metal total hip arthroplasties with low wear of the articulating surfaces. J Arthroplasty 11:322–331

Treacy RB, McBryde CW, Pynsent PB (2005) Birmingham hip resurfacing arthroplasty: a minimum follow-up of 5 years. J Bone Joint Surg Br 87:167–170

Van der Weegen W, Hoekstra HJ, Sijbesma T et al (2011) Survival of metal-on-metal hip resurfacing arthroplasty. A systematic review of the literature. J Bone Joint Surg Br 93:298–306

Venddittoli PA, Lavingne M, Roy AG et al (2006) A prospective randomized clinical trial comparing metal-on-metal total hip arthroplasty and metal-on-metal total hip resurfacing in patients less than 65 years old. Hip Int 16(Suppl 4):73–81

Withdrawal of Depuy ASR resurfacing and XL metal on metal bearings – information for and advice to surgeons (2010) Published by BOA and BHS

A Clinicopathological Study of Metal-on-Metal Hips Revised for Suspected Adverse Reactions to Metal Debris

6

Gulraj S. Matharu, Matthew P. Revell, Vaiyapuri Sumathi, Paul B. Pynsent, and Peter A. Revell

Abbreviations

ALVAL	aseptic lymphocytic vasculitis and associated lesions
ARMD	adverse reaction to metal debris
MHRA	Medicines and Healthcare products Regulatory Agency
MoM	metal-on-metal
THR	total hip replacement

6.1 Introduction

Total hip replacement (THR) is well established as the most successful surgical procedure for the long-term alleviation of pain and disability in patients with arthritis of the hip joint (Learmonth et al. 2007). A total of 68,907 primary hip replacements were performed in England and Wales during 2010 (National Joint Registry 2011). In recent times metal-on-metal (MoM) bearings for THR have gradually been reintroduced, mainly because of the substantially lower wear rates compared to that of metal-on-polyethylene articulations and the decreased wear rates with increasing head diameters (Fisher et al. 2006). This has subsequently led to a resurgence of MoM hip resurfacing in young and active patients with hip arthritis (Amstutz et al. 2004; Treacy et al. 2011). Hip resurfacing has the added advantages of femoral bone preservation and the potential ease of future revision (Ball et al. 2007; Matharu et al. 2013). In carefully selected patients excellent medium- to long-term survival has been reported for MoM hip resurfacing by the designer surgeons (McMinn et al. 2011; Treacy et al. 2011) and independent centres (Coulter et al. 2012; Holland et al. 2012; Murray et al. 2012).

G.S. Matharu • M.P. Revell (✉) • V. Sumathi • P.B. Pynsent • P.A. Revell
Department of Arthroplasty, Royal Orthopaedic Hospital,
Northfield, Birmingham B31 2AP, UK
e-mail: matthew.revell@nhs.net

K. Knahr (ed.), *Total Hip Arthroplasty*,
DOI 10.1007/978-3-642-35653-7_6, © EFORT 2013

Over recent years concerns have mounted regarding abnormal periprosthetic tissue reactions associated with MoM bearings. A number of reports have observed these abnormal reactions with both MoM THRs (Bolland et al. 2011; Langton et al. 2011a) and MoM hip resurfacings (Pandit et al. 2008; Langton et al. 2010, 2011b) ultimately leading to implant failure and the need for revision arthroplasty, which itself can be an extensive procedure (Grammatopoulos et al. 2009). Failure rates due to these reactions for MoM THRs and hip resurfacings have been reported to be as high as 48.8 % and 25 % at 6 years, respectively, for some devices (Langton et al. 2011a), whilst with other MoM hip resurfacing designs, the prevalence of these reactions may be considerably lower at 0.3 % at a mean 7.1 year follow-up (Carrothers et al. 2010). This has led to the Medicines and Healthcare products Regulatory Agency (MHRA) issuing guidance with regard to the investigation and management of these periprosthetic reactions and the market withdrawal of certain MoM THRs and hip resurfacings with unacceptably high failure rates (MHRA 2010, 2012).

Although the pathogenesis of these abnormal periprosthetic tissue reactions is not fully understood, they are likely to represent the local tissue response caused as a result of metal wear debris generated from the bearing surfaces (Hart et al. 2009; Haddad et al. 2011). A variety of terms have been used in the literature to describe these reactions; however, presently there is no clear consensus defining the boundaries of each of these terms (Haddad et al. 2011; Murray et al. 2011). Adverse reaction to metal debris (ARMD) is one of the most commonly used and accepted terms in the literature. It was originally coined as an umbrella term (Langton et al. 2010, 2011b) and includes the following clinical and histopathological features:

- Metallosis: Macroscopic staining of the soft tissues which is associated with abnormal wear (Haddad et al. 2011).
- Pseudotumour: Non-neoplastic, non-infective, solid or semi-liquid soft-tissue periprosthetic masses (Pandit et al. 2008; Murray et al. 2011). These masses may progress and cause significant soft-tissue destruction (Grammatopoulos et al. 2009).
- Aseptic lymphocytic vasculitis and associated lesions (ALVAL): Specific histological reaction observed in association with both MoM (Willert et al. 2005) and non-MoM bearings (Fujishiro et al. 2011), characterised by perivascular lymphocytes, lymphoid aggregates containing follicles with B and T cells, plasma cells, tissue necrosis, fibrin exudation, high endothelial venules and the accumulation of macrophages (Willert et al. 2005).
- Macroscopic tissue necrosis: Observed at the time of revision surgery and initial histopathological specimen analysis.

Despite ARMD being a useful term to group together reactions reported in association with MoM bearings, it is becoming increasingly apparent that ARMD encompasses a spectrum of clinical and histopathological findings (Campbell et al. 2010; Matharu et al. 2012b). Such a broad classification does little to clarify the aetiology and pathogenesis of what appears to represent a complex condition.

6.2   Study Aims

The study aims were to characterise the clinical features in patients with MoM hip bearings revised for suspected ARMD and to determine the nature of the local histopathological responses observed in these individuals.

6.3   Patients and Methods

This was a retrospective study performed at a single-specialist arthroplasty centre. The study was approved and registered with the institutional review board.

6.3.1   Inclusion and Exclusion Criteria

Patients were included if they had undergone revision arthroplasty at this centre between 1998 and 2010 for a MoM hip resurfacing or MoM THR revised for a suspected adverse reaction to metal debris. For the purposes of this study, a diagnosis of suspected ARMD was made if, on review of both the clinical and histopathological information, there were features compatible with those consistently reported in the literature, namely, clinical evidence of periprosthetic joint effusions or solid masses, metallosis, macroscopic tissue necrosis or foreign body granulomas and histopathological evidence of aseptic foreign body or phagocytic reactions, significant metal wear debris, lymphocytic reactions and tissue necrosis (Willert et al. 2005; Pandit et al. 2008; Campbell et al. 2010; Langton et al. 2010, 2011b; Matharu et al. 2012b).

Patients with evidence of infection from the samples sent at the time of revision surgery for microbiological and histopathological analysis were excluded. All patients with fractures sustained as a clear result of trauma and in the absence of prior neck thinning were also excluded from the final cohort. Cases referred to this centre from other institutions for specialist management were also included providing they met the necessary criteria.

6.3.2   Case Selection and Clinical Data Collection

Cases were identified by retrospectively searching the hospital's clinical and histopathological databases. Each case identified was screened using the aforementioned criteria to determine whether it was suitable for inclusion in the final cohort. In addition, cases were contributed from the arthroplasty surgeons, radiologists and histopathologists in instances where patients had been identified as having features compatible with a reaction to metal debris requiring revision hip arthroplasty.

Data collection was performed using the prospectively maintained hospital databases, the electronic imaging system and patient case notes. Data were collected on patient demographics, all previous surgery on the ipsilateral hip, the presence of a contralateral MoM hip bearing, date of presentation with ipsilateral hip symptoms and all investigations performed prior to revision hip arthroplasty. The latter included the results of blood tests (white cell count, C-reactive protein and erythrocyte sedimentation rate) and imaging (hip radiographs, ultrasound, computerised tomography, magnetic resonance imaging and bone scans). The presence of femoral neck thinning on radiographs following hip resurfacing was defined as thinning of greater than 10 % between the initial postoperative radiograph following the index procedure and the most recent radiograph prior to revision arthroplasty (Heilpern et al. 2008). Data were extracted from the operation notes at revision surgery using a standardised pro-forma. This was used to record features regarding the explanted prosthesis, the prospective clinical indication for performing revision surgery and the presence or absence of intraoperative metallosis, periprosthetic effusions or masses, component loosening, femoral neck thinning, osteolysis, soft-tissue damage, foreign body granuloma, tissue necrosis, femoral neck fracture or infection.

6.3.3   Histopathological Analysis

In all cases the histopathological specimens from the revision procedure had been analysed and reported as part of the patient's routine clinical care. These reports were used initially to identify suitable cases of suspected ARMD for inclusion in the final cohort as already described. The archival formalin-fixed paraffin-embedded haematoxylin and eosin stained sections of periprosthetic tissue removed at revision arthroplasty were subsequently anonymised by the allocation of a study number. All sections were reviewed by two senior histopathologists (PAR and VS) blinded to any clinical details and the original cellular pathology diagnostic report.

Each case was examined for the presence of individual histopathological features which may be found in relation to failed prosthetic joints in the literature (Willert et al. 2005; Pandit et al. 2008; Revell 2008; Campbell et al. 2010; Langton et al. 2010). Features of interest were lymphocytes, macrophages, metal wear debris, necrosis, plasma cells and neutrophils (to exclude infection). Particular attention was paid to the nature of the lymphocytic and macrophage infiltrate, with the former scored for the presence or absence of a distribution which was diffuse, perivascular or in focal aggregates, which were with or without a follicular appearance. Each feature was scored as nought (not seen), one (present but only in small numbers) and two (plentiful and abundant). Twenty cases were examined by two histopathologists together in order to agree about the features present in each case and allocate scores for the specific features. Both histopathologists then examined all of the sections for the individual cases independently, scoring each of the features present as previously agreed. After completing examination of the sections, a diagnostic category was assigned for each case. Cases were only diagnosed as ALVAL if they showed all the features described when this condition was originally reported, namely, the presence of perivascular lymphocytes, lymphoid aggregates containing follicles with B and T cells, plasma cells, tissue necrosis, fibrin exudation, high endothelial venules and the accumulation of macrophages (Willert et al. 2005). Those showing lymphoid aggregates were stained with CD3 (T cell) and CD20 (B cell) markers using immunohistochemistry to confirm the presence of these cells.

6.4   Results

6.4.1   Patient Demographics

During the study period, a total of 3,994 primary MoM hip bearings were implanted at this centre (3,457 hip resurfacings and 537 THRs). A total of 60 MoM hip revisions were performed for suspected ARMD and eligible for study inclusion. Mean age of these patients at index surgery was 50.4 years (range 24.5–77.0 years), and 73 % ($n=44$) were female.

Of the revisions, 80 % ($n=48$) were hip resurfacings (35 Birmingham Hip Resurfacings, Smith & Nephew, Warwick, United Kingdom; 11 Corin McMinn, Corin, Cirencester, United Kingdom; 2 Conserve Plus, Wright Medical Technology, Memphis, Tennessee), and 20 % ($n=12$) were THRs (6 Corail Pinnacle, DePuy, Leeds, United Kingdom; 6 other different MoM THR implants). There were 43 % ($n=26$) of patients with a contralateral MoM bearing in situ at the time of the revision surgery (13 hip resurfacings and 13 THRs). Of the 60 revisions performed for suspected ARMD, 32 % ($n=19$) had the index hip surgery at another institution and were subsequently referred to this centre for treatment.

6.4.2   Clinical Features

The mean time from the index MoM procedure to becoming symptomatic was 4.2 years (range 0–19.5 years) and mean time from index MoM procedure to revision hip arthroplasty was 6.0 years (range 0.27–19.6 years). Prior to revision surgery, the mean blood results were as follows: white cell count 7.5×10^9/L, C-reactive protein 16.2 mg/L and erythrocyte sedimentation rate 22.9 mm/h.

The prospective clinical indications for revision hip arthroplasty are detailed in Table 6.1, with the majority of revisions performed for aseptic loosening (32 %), component malposition (27 %) and unexplained pain (27 %). Features observed on preoperative hip radiographs were acetabular component loosening (23 %; $n=14$), femoral component loosening (23 %; $n=14$) and femoral neck thinning (20 %; $n=12$). Periprosthetic effusions of variable sizes (largest measuring 9 cm × 5 cm × 9 cm) were

Table 6.1 Prospective clinical indications for revision hip arthroplasty of metal bearings

Clinical indication for revision	Number of cases (%)
Aseptic component loosening	19 (32)
Component malposition	16 (27)
Unexplained pain	16 (27)
Femoral neck fracture	2 (3.3)
Presumed infection	2 (3.3)
Dislocation/subluxation	2 (3.3)
Avascular necrosis (femoral head)	1 (1.7)
Bone impingement	1 (1.7)
Femoral component failure	1 (1.7)

Table 6.2 Clinical findings at revision hip arthroplasty

Intraoperative findings	Number of cases (%)
Metallosis	24 (40)
Loosening (acetabular component)	21 (35)
Periprosthetic effusion[a]	19 (32)
Femoral neck thinning	16 (27)
Osteolysis	16 (27)
Soft-tissue damage	12 (20)
Foreign body granuloma	11 (18)
Loosening (femoral component)	6 (10)
Femoral neck fracture	5 (8)
Infection	5 (8)
Tissue necrosis	0 (0)

[a]Effusions of variable sizes were present ($n=19$); however, there were no cases of solid periprosthetic masses described at the time of revision hip arthroplasty

demonstrated on ultrasound (17 %; $n=10$), computerised tomography (8 %; $n=5$) and magnetic resonance imaging (5 %; $n=3$). Clinical findings observed at revision hip arthroplasty are recorded in Table 6.2.

6.4.3 Histopathological Features

Histopathological analysis demonstrated lymphocytic populations were present in 32 % ($n=19$) of cases. These cases were subsequently categorised as follows: ALVAL in 8 % ($n=5$; Fig. 6.1), marked lymphocytic infiltration without lymphoid follicles or plasma cells in 12 % ($n=7$; Fig. 6.2) and low-grade chronic inflammation in 12 % ($n=7$; Fig. 6.3). A further 5 % ($n=3$) of cases demonstrated histopathological evidence of infection. The remaining 63 % ($n=38$) showed no convincing evidence of an immunological or infectious process. Of this latter group, 61 % (23 of 38; Fig. 6.4) demonstrated a phagocytic macrophage response to metal wear debris, whilst in the other 39 % (15 of 38) a variety of other changes were observed, such as the presence of detritic bone fragments.

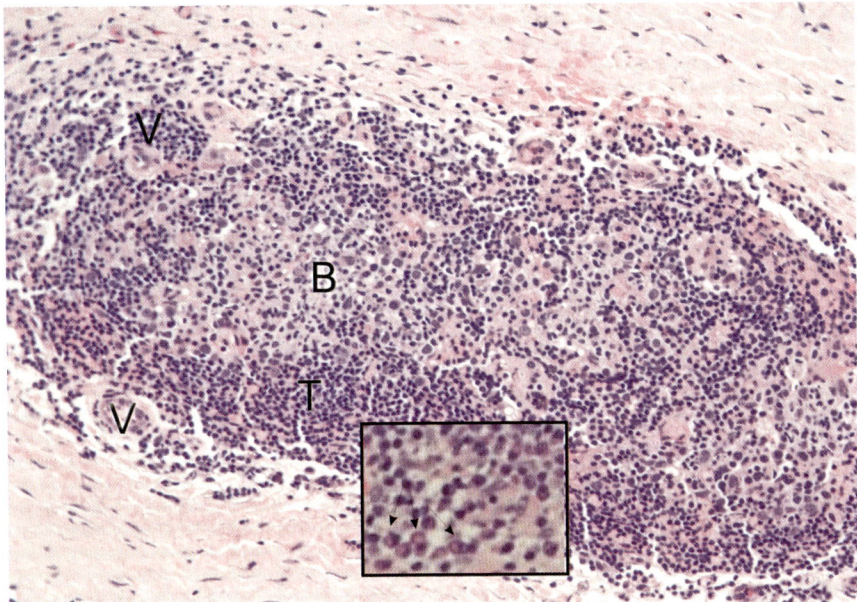

Fig. 6.1 Aseptic lymphocytic vasculitis and associated lesions (ALVAL). Lymphocyte aggregate with a central B cell area (B) which also contains macrophages, with surrounding smaller T lymphocytes (T). High endothelial cell vessels are present (V). Plasma cells are found at the periphery of the lymphoid aggregate as shown by arrows in the magnified inset. The identity of B and T cells was confirmed by immunohistochemistry (not shown)

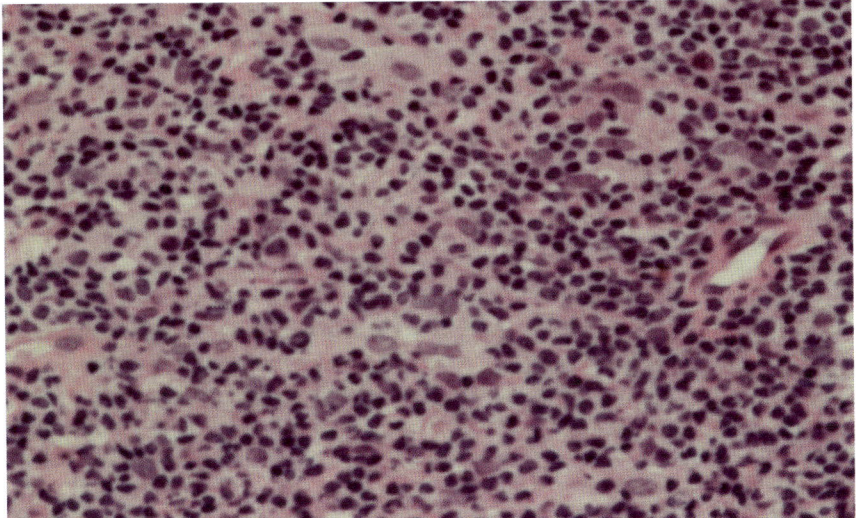

Fig. 6.2 Marked lymphocytic infiltration. There is a heavy and diffuse lymphocytic infiltrate present. However, important features, including lymphoid follicles and plasma cells, are absent and therefore this histopathological appearance cannot be described as ALVAL

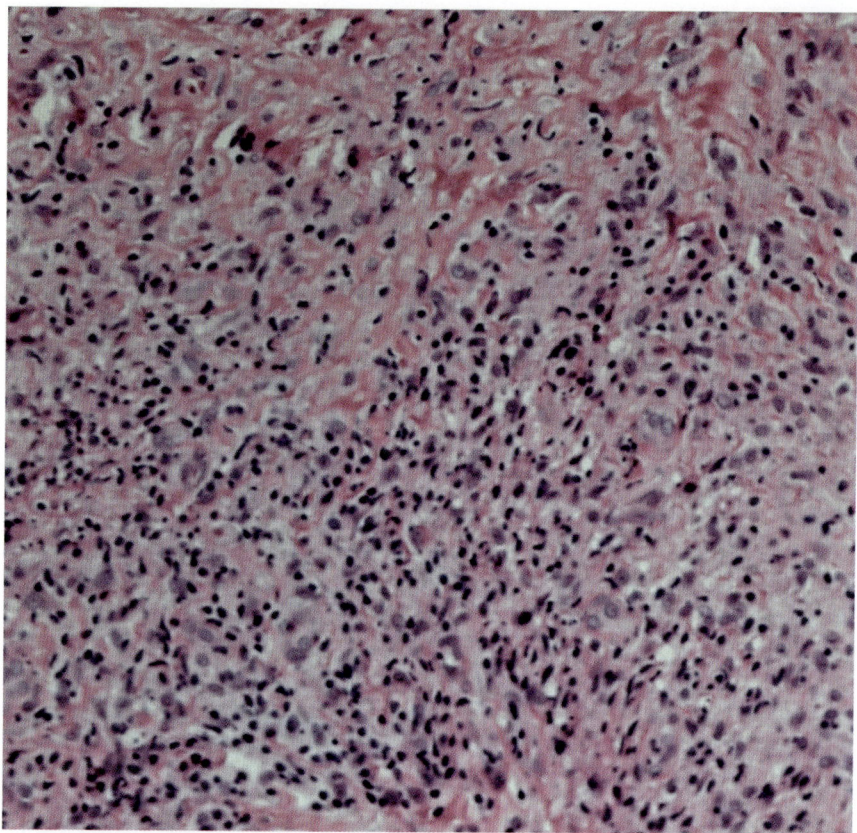

Fig. 6.3 Low-grade chronic inflammation. There is evidence of a low-grade chronic inflammatory reaction with lymphocytes mixed in with the macrophage infiltrate. Fibrin is also present (*top*)

6.5   Discussion

The present study represents a comprehensive review of a large series of MoM hip bearings revised for suspected ARMD. The findings demonstrate that whilst the clinical features of patients revised for suspected ARMD were similar to those reported in the literature, the histopathological findings were diverse with lack of a convincing immunologically driven process in the majority of cases.

6.5.1   Clinical Features

A number of studies have reported on the clinical features observed in MoM hips revised for ARMD (Pandit et al. 2008; Glyn-Jones et al. 2009; Browne et al. 2010; Langton et al. 2010, 2011b; Rajpura et al. 2011; Matharu et al. 2012b). Typically a

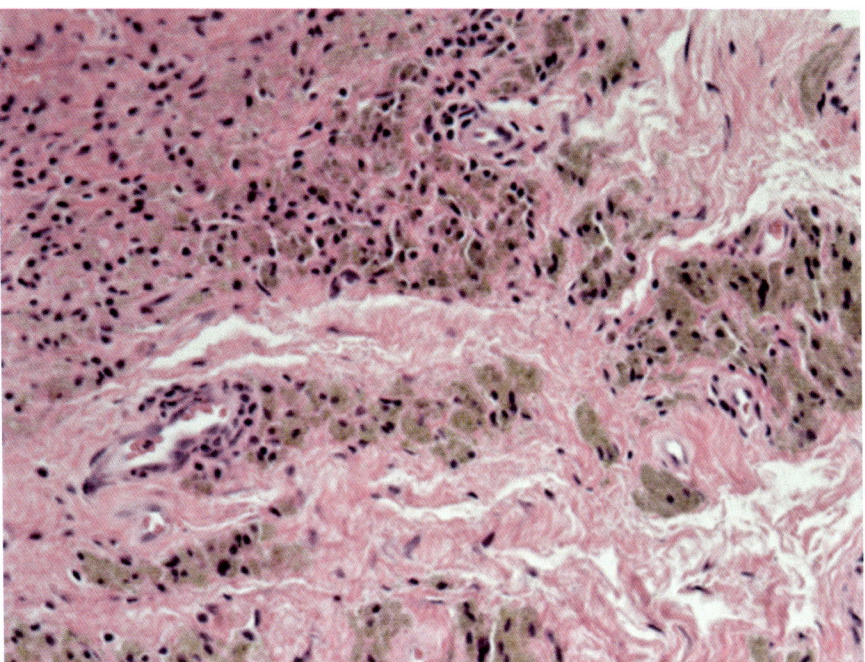

Fig. 6.4 Phagocytic response to metal wear debris. This demonstrates a pure phagocytic response with macrophages containing metal wear debris. There is no associated lymphocytic response

patient (usually female) presents with groin pain, with or without mechanical symptoms, a number of months after implantation of a MoM hip bearing, with normal or mildly raised blood inflammatory markers and imaging findings which can include femoral neck thinning, periprosthetic effusions and evidence of component loosening or malposition. At the time of revision surgery, these imaging findings can be appreciated in more detail, in addition to assessing for other common features suggestive of the diagnosis such as metallosis, soft-tissue damage and foreign body reactions. The clinical features observed in the present study (Table 6.2) broadly support those previously reported in ARMD patients. However, it is important to remember that whilst patients with ARMD can present with component loosening or malposition, individuals may present in more unusual manners such as with a femoral neck fracture subsequent to neck thinning or dislocation, as observed in a few cases in this study (Table 6.1). A high index of suspicion should therefore be exercised by the surgeon when dealing with patients with hip pain following MoM arthroplasty to ensure the correct diagnosis is made and that an alternate bearing surface is considered at revision.

In the present study periprosthetic effusions of variable sizes ($n = 19$) and soft-tissue damage ($n = 12$) were recorded at the time of revision surgery. Similar findings were observed when a subgroup of patients with ARMD undergoing revision at this centre were previously reviewed (Matharu et al. 2012b). However, in the present series, there were no cases of solid periprosthetic masses (termed 'pseudotumour' in the literature) or macroscopic tissue necrosis, findings which have been described previously in association with MoM bearings revised for ARMD (Pandit et al. 2008; Grammatopoulos et al. 2009; Langton et al. 2011b; Natu et al. 2012). One explanation for these observed differences may be because a spectrum of clinical findings exists in ARMD, and solid 'pseudotumour' masses along with tissue necrosis represent more advanced stages of these abnormal reactions. If this is indeed the case, it further highlights the need for early diagnosis of ARMD and revision arthroplasty as poor outcomes have been reported following revision of these destructive soft-tissue lesions (Grammatopoulos et al. 2009). An alternate explanation for the variation in clinical findings is that they may each represent different pathological processes yet to be defined. A recent report suggested that these 'pseudotumour' lesions are not always associated with increased wear and that they occur in well-positioned MoM hips (Matthies et al. 2012), further highlighting the complexity of these reactions associated with metal bearings.

6.5.2   Histopathological Features

The histopathological features observed in patients revised for suspected ARMD were diverse in the present cohort with the majority of cases lacking evidence of a convincing immunologically driven process. Approximately one-third (32 %) of cases demonstrated evidence of a lymphocytic reaction, and only 8 % of cases fulfilled all the criteria originally described for ALVAL (Willert et al. 2005). Most of the remaining cases demonstrated a pure phagocytic response with macrophages containing metal wear debris. A similar diversity of histopathological findings in hips revised for ARMD has been described previously (Mahendra et al. 2009; Campbell et al. 2010; Hart et al. 2010; Natu et al. 2012).

There are a number of possible explanations for the diversity of histopathological features observed in ARMD patients. The most important is that different pathological processes may be responsible for adverse MoM reactions. Both high implant wear (Langton et al. 2010, 2011b; Kwon et al. 2010a) and a host susceptibility to metal resulting in a local delayed type IV hypersensitivity reaction (Willert et al. 2005; Mahendra et al. 2009; Campbell et al. 2010; Natu et al. 2012) have been suggested. Analysis of pseudotumour-like tissues from revised MoM hips suggested specific histological features relate to the likely pathogenesis, with hips revised for suspected high implant wear containing more macrophages and metal particles whilst those revised for suspected metal hypersensitivity being characterised by a predominant and dense lymphocytic infiltrate with varying degrees of tissue necrosis (Campbell et al. 2010). The lymphocytic patterns seen in ALVAL (perivascular lymphocytic infiltrates with lymphoid aggregates) bear a remarkable resemblance to that seen in a number of chronic inflammatory conditions, such as in patients with rheumatoid arthritis (Takemura et al. 2001; Weyand and Goronzy 2003; Aloisi and Pujol-Borrell 2006). It is therefore plausible that the small subgroup of patients with ALVAL in this study have a true immune reaction to metal. At the histopathological level this subgroup may be quite different from the majority of other MoM hips revised for ARMD which were characterised by a phagocytic reaction to metal debris with or without diffuse and perivascular lymphocytes. These latter appearances are similar to those associated with failed metal-on-polyethylene bearings (Revell 2008).

Another explanation for the variability of histopathological features reported in hips revised for ARMD relates to the definitions used for ALVAL. In this study a strict definition was used for ALVAL which required all the features to be present when the condition was originally described (Willert et al. 2005). However, in previous studies the term has been used more loosely with cases lacking lymphoid aggregates or plasma cells defined as ALVAL (Browne et al. 2010; Natu et al. 2012). A recent histopathological review of 120 ARMD revisions reported ALVAL in as many as 86 % of cases with the remaining 14 % demonstrating pure metallosis and no lymphocytic component (Natu et al. 2012). These findings are contradictory to the present study. The majority of cases classed as ALVAL in this recent report had a diffuse chronic lymphocytic infiltrate not organised into follicles or aggregates, with plasma cells present in only 38 % of ALVAL cases (Natu et al. 2012). Such cases would have been classified as marked lymphocytic infiltration without lymphoid follicles or plasma cells in the present study (12 % of cases; Fig. 6.2) and not ALVAL. In addition, it is important to remember that sampling errors may account for some of the reported variability between studies of the histopathological appearances in hips revised for ARMD, as well as disparities observed within the same cohort (Hart et al. 2010).

6.5.3   Limitations

This study has some recognised limitations. First, this was a retrospective study with data collection from the operative notes dependent on the accuracy of the individual making the recording. Secondly, the definition used for suspected ARMD may have been considered fairly inclusive. Although there is currently no universally accepted method for classifying reactions associated with metal bearings, it is felt the definition used in the present study was comprehensive and took into account both the clinical and histopathological features consistently reported in the literature. Thirdly, despite utilising all available sources to identify cases of MoM bearings revised for suspected ARMD, it is possible some may have been overlooked. Therefore, this study does not represent a consecutive series. Finally, during the study period it was not routine practice at this centre to measure blood metal ion levels or perform forensic analysis of explanted MoM bearings which would have allowed an assessment of component wear to have been made.

6.5.4   Future Work

Further studies are needed to characterise the likely complex pathogenesis of these abnormal periprosthetic reactions to metal. Knowledge of the pathogenetic mechanisms involved would allow these reactions to be better classified, improve universal reporting and avoid the somewhat confusing nomenclature presently in the literature. These studies will require detailed histopathological and immunohistochemical analysis of the periprosthetic tissues as well as mechanical analysis of the explanted hip components. Although similar studies have already been performed, contradictory findings have been reported with some suggesting a type IV metal hypersensitivity reaction is likely to be responsible (Willert et al. 2005; Mahendra et al. 2009; Campbell et al. 2010; Natu et al. 2012) whilst others concluding this may not be the dominant biological reaction (Kwon et al. 2010b). With these issues in mind, detailed immunohistochemical analysis of the present study cohort is currently being undertaken.

Conclusions

The present study has demonstrated that periprosthetic tissue responses in MoM hips revised for suspected ARMD were diverse with most lacking evidence of a convincing immunologically driven process. Where there is clinical suspicion of ARMD, only a small proportion showed all the true features of ALVAL. Given the diversity of histopathological responses observed, it is suspected different pathogenetic processes are responsible for periprosthetic tissue reactions to metal debris. Future studies should aim to define the pathogenesis of what appears to be a complex condition and subsequently devise a more robust classification system for the reporting of adverse reactions to metal debris.

Acknowledgement The authors received funding from Smith & Nephew PLC which was used to undertake the work presented in this manuscript.

References

Aloisi F, Pujol-Borrell R (2006) Lymphoid neogenesis in chronic inflammatory diseases. Nat Rev Immunol 6:205–217

Amstutz HC, Beaulé PE, Dorey FJ et al (2004) Metal-on-metal hybrid surface arthroplasty: two to six-year follow-up study. J Bone Joint Surg Am 86-A:28–39

Ball ST, Le Duff MJ, Amstutz HC (2007) Early results of conversion of a failed femoral component in hip resurfacing arthroplasty. J Bone Joint Surg Am 89-A:735–741

Bolland BJ, Culliford DJ, Langton DJ et al (2011) High failure rates with a large-diameter hybrid metal-on-metal total hip replacement: clinical, radiological and retrieval analysis. J Bone Joint Surg Br 93-B:608–615

Browne JA, Bechtold CD, Berry DJ et al (2010) Failed metal-on-metal hip arthroplasties: a spectrum of clinical presentations and operative findings. Clin Orthop Relat Res 468:2313–2320

Campbell P, Ebramzadeh E, Nelson S et al (2010) Histological features of pseudotumor-like tissues from metal-on-metal hips. Clin Orthop Relat Res 468:2321–2327

Carrothers AD, Gilbert RE, Jaiswal A et al (2010) Birmingham hip resurfacing: the prevalence of failure. J Bone Joint Surg Br 92-B:1344–1350

Coulter G, Young DA, Dalziel RE et al (2012) Birmingham hip resurfacing at a mean of ten years: results from an independent centre. J Bone Joint Surg Br 94-B:315–321

Fisher J, Jin Z, Tipper J et al (2006) Tribology of alternative bearings. Clin Orthop Relat Res 453:25–34

Fujishiro T, Moojen DJ, Kobayashi N et al (2011) Perivascular and diffuse lymphocytic inflammation are not specific for failed metal-on-metal hip implants. Clin Orthop Relat Res 469:1127–1133

Glyn-Jones S, Pandit H, Kwon YM et al (2009) Risk factors for inflammatory pseudotumour formation following hip resurfacing. J Bone Joint Surg Br 91-B:1566–1574

Grammatopoulos G, Pandit H, Kwon YM et al (2009) Hip resurfacings revised for inflammatory pseudotumour have a poor outcome. J Bone Joint Surg Br 91-B:1019–1024

Haddad FS, Thakrar RR, Hart AJ et al (2011) Metal-on-metal bearings: the evidence so far. J Bone Joint Surg Br 93-B:572–579

Hart AJ, Sabah S, Henckel J et al (2009) The painful metal-on-metal hip resurfacing. J Bone Joint Surg Br 91-B:738–744

Hart AJ, Masters JP, Sandison A et al (2010) Histological and immunohistochemical response in tissue around metal on metal hips – the UK experience. Podium presentation number 010 at the American Academy of Orthopaedic Surgeons Annual Meeting, New Orleans, USA

Heilpern GN, Shah NN, Fordyce MJ (2008) Birmingham hip resurfacing arthroplasty: a series of 110 consecutive hips with a minimum five-year clinical and radiological follow-up. J Bone Joint Surg Br 90-B:1137–1142

Holland JP, Langton DJ, Hashmi M (2012) Ten-year clinical, radiological and metal ion analysis of the Birmingham Hip Resurfacing: from a single, non-designer surgeon. J Bone Joint Surg Br 94-B:471–476

Kwon YM, Glyn-Jones S, Simpson DJ et al (2010a) Analysis of wear of retrieved metal-on-metal hip resurfacing implants revised due to pseudotumours. J Bone Joint Surg Br 92-B:356–361

Kwon YM, Thomas P, Summer B et al (2010b) Lymphocyte proliferation responses in patients with pseudotumors following metal-on-metal hip resurfacing arthroplasty. J Orthop Res 28:444–450

Langton DJ, Jameson SS, Joyce TJ et al (2010) Early failure of metal-on-metal bearings in hip resurfacing and larger diameter total hip replacement. A consequence of excess wear. J Bone Joint Surg [Br] 92-B:38–46

Langton DJ, Jameson SS, Joyce TJ et al (2011a) Accelerating failure rate of the ASR total hip replacement. J Bone Joint Surg Br 93-B:1011–1016

Langton DJ, Joyce TJ, Jameson SS et al (2011b) Adverse reaction to metal debris following hip resurfacing: the influence of component type, orientation and volumetric wear. J Bone Joint Surg Br 93-B:164–171

Learmonth ID, Young C, Rorabeck C (2007) The operation of the century: total hip replacement. Lancet 370:1508–1519

Mahendra G, Pandit H, Kliskey K et al (2009) Necrotic and inflammatory changes in metal-on-metal resurfacing hip arthroplasties. Acta Orthop 80:653–659

Matharu GS, McBryde CW, Revell MP et al (2013) Femoral neck fracture after Birmingham Hip Resurfacing arthroplasty: prevalence, time to fracture, and outcome after revision. J Arthroplasty 28:147–153

Matharu GS, Revell MP, Pynsent PB et al (2012) A review of hip resurfacings revised for unexplained pain. Hip Int 22:633–640

Matthies AK, Skinner JA, Osmani H et al (2012) Pseudotumors are common in well-positioned low-wearing metal-on-metal hips. Clin Orthop Relat Res 470:1895–1906

McMinn DJ, Daniel J, Ziaee H et al (2011) Indications and results of hip resurfacing. Int Orthop 35:231–237

Medicines and Healthcare products Regulatory Agency (MHRA) (2010) Medical Device Alert: ASR™ hip replacement implant manufactured by DePuy International Ltd. MDA/2010/069. http://www.mhra.gov.uk/. Accessed 29 Sept 2012

Medicines and Healthcare products Regulatory Agency (MHRA) (2012). Medical Device Alert: all metal-on-metal (MoM) hip replacements. MDA/2012/036. http://www.mhra.gov.uk/. Accessed 29 Sept 2012

Murray DW, Grammatopoulos G, Gundle R et al (2011) Hip resurfacing and pseudotumour. Hip Int 21:279–283

Murray DW, Grammatopoulos G, Pandit H et al (2012) The ten-year survival of the Birmingham hip resurfacing: an independent series. J Bone Joint Surg Br 94:1180–1186

Natu S, Sidaginamale RP, Gandhi J et al (2012) Adverse reactions to metal debris: histopathological features of periprosthetic soft tissue reactions seen in association with failed metal on metal hip arthroplasties. J Clin Pathol 65:409–418

Pandit H, Glyn-Jones S, McLardy-Smith P et al (2008) Pseudotumours associated with metal-on-metal hip resurfacings. J Bone Joint Surg Br 90:847–851

Rajpura A, Porter ML, Gambhir AK et al (2011) Clinical experience of revision of metal on metal hip arthroplasty for aseptic lymphocyte dominated vasculitis associated lesions (ALVAL). Hip Int 21:43–51

Revell PA (2008) The combined role of wear particles, macrophages and lymphocytes in the loosening of total joint prostheses. J R Soc Interface 5:1263–1278

Takemura S, Braun A, Crowson C et al (2001) Lymphoid neogenesis in rheumatoid synovitis. J Immunol 167:1072–1080

The National Joint Registry Centre (2011) National Joint Registry for England and Wales 8th annual report. http://www.njrcentre.org.uk/. Accessed 9 Sept 2012

Treacy RB, McBryde CW, Shears E et al (2011) Birmingham hip resurfacing: a minimum follow-up of ten years. J Bone Joint Surg Br 93-B:27–33

Weyand CM, Goronzy JJ (2003) Ectopic germinal center formation in rheumatoid synovitis. Ann N Y Acad Sci 987:140–149

Willert HG, Buchhorn GH, Fayyazi A et al (2005) Metal-on-metal bearings and hypersensitivity in patients with artificial hip joints. A clinical and histomorphological study. J Bone Joint Surg [Am] 87-A:28–36

Metal-on-Metal Hip Resurfacing and Surgical Techniques in Active Patients with Severe Hip Deformity

7

Antonio Moroni, A. Hoang-Kim, R. Orsini, and G. Micera

Hip resurfacing is now becoming an established alternative to total hip replacement in the young, high-demand patient with end-stage hip arthritis. Many of the complications and early failures of the previous generations of hip resurfacing appear to have been eliminated with the most recent hip resurfacing systems. The literature now contains excellent short- and medium-term results of the new generation of hip resurfacing (Amstutz et al. 2004a; Amstutz and Le Duff 2008; Daniel et al. 2004; McMinn and Daniel 2006; Treacy 2006). The advantages of preservation of proximal bone stock, low dislocation risk and excellent bearing wear characteristics make hip resurfacing an attractive alternative to total hip replacement. However, concerns over the risk of implant failure persist.

An increased risk of implant failure has been attributed to two major failure modes in hip resurfacing. In up to 70 % of the failures, aseptic implant loosening can occur as the result of bone degradation and loss surrounding the implant (Harris 1995). This loss of supportive bone construct is particularly prominent on the femoral side and may be the result of vascular insult to the femoral head during reaming preparation or stress shielding by the stiff femoral component. The second and more catastrophic failure mode is femoral neck fracture. Neck fracture occurs in approximately 1–2 % of patients (Amstutz et al. 2004a, b; McMinn and Daniel 2006; Beaulé et al. 2004; De Smet 2005; Marker 2007; Shimmin et al. 2005; Siebel et al. 2006) within the first 3–4 months postoperatively (Amstutz et al. 2004a, b; Siebel et al. 2006;

A. Moroni, MD (✉)
Department of Quality of Life Science, University of Bologna,
237, Corso d'Augusto, Rimini, Italy
e-mail: antoniomoroni@usa.net

A. Hoang-Kim
St. Michael's Hospital,
30 Bond Street, M5B 1W8, Toronto, Ontario, Canada

R. Orsini • G. Micera
University of Bologna, Rizzoli Institute,
1, G.C. Pupilli, Bologna, Italy

K. Knahr (ed.), *Total Hip Arthroplasty*,
DOI 10.1007/978-3-642-35653-7_7, © EFORT 2013

Shimmin et al. 2005). Failure within this short time frame has lead to the suggestion that iatrogenic mechanical error during preparation of the femoral head, including femoral neck notching, varus implant alignment and failure to fully seat the femoral component, may be the root cause of early resurfacing failure (Amstutz et al. 2004a; McMinn and Daniel 2006; Treacy et al. 2005; Beaulé et al. 2004; De Smet 2005; Marker et al. 2007; Shimmin et al. 2005; Siebel et al. 2006; Freeman 1978a, b).

Femoral head malpreparation may be the result of a number of different surgical factors including inappropriate implant selection due to an inaccurate or poorly executed pre-operative plan, inaccurate femoral guidewire insertion with the use of conventional guidewire alignment instrumentation, reliance on inaccurate computer-generated data during navigation and careless reaming preparation of the femoral head.

7.1   Bearings

Over decades of development, polyethylenes, metallica alloys and ceramics have become the primary materials for bearing surfaces in total hip arthroplasty. Polyethylene has been used since the origins of total joint arthroplasty in the hip. With metal-on-polyethylene and ceramic-on-ceramic bearings, the prosthetic head is significantly smaller than the femoral head. In these traditional bearings, the small head is a potential cause of instability. Ceramic-on-ceramic bearings have the advantage of chemical inertness, but cup fixation and head or insert fracture risk are major concerns (Allain et al. 2003; Hamadouche et al. 2002). In contrast, metal-on-metal (MM) bearings have no concerns regarding breakage and do not adversely influence component fixation (Baad-Hansen et al. 2011; Pabinger et al. 2003). Unlike other bearing options, with MM bearings it is possible to replicate the patient's original femoral head size (Moroni et al. 2012).

Metal-on-metal hip resurfacing is an alternative surgical procedure to standard total hip replacement for young active patients, with the advantage of preserving the femoral head. Younger and more active people have higher expectations with respect to the use of their joints and it is perceived that MM hip resurfacing results in a greater range of motion and would better suit the active lifestyle of younger people who place additional stress on their prostheses and for a longer period of time (Murphy et al. 2009). While some surgeons recommend that patients refrain from running and participating in high-impact activities after total hip arthroplasty, patients undergoing MM hip resurfacing are allowed to perform high-impact activities such as jogging (Klein et al. 2007). Encouraging medium- to long-term results have been reported in the literature (Amstutz 2007; McMinn et al. 2011; Shimmin 2008; Treacy et al. 2011). Recently high failure rates have been reported with certain MM bearings (Australian Orthopaedic Association 2010; Langton et al. 2011; Naal et al. 2011). However, well-designed and properly positioned hip resurfacing implants continue to show 96–98 % survival rate at 10–13 years (McMinn et al. 2011; Treacy et al. 2011).

A recent literature review identified studies published from January 1, 2009 to February 13, 2012 evaluating the revision rate of different MM hip resurfacing systems in comparison to the benchmark set by the National Institute for Health and Clinical Excellence (NICE), was recently published (Sehatzadeh et al. 2012).

The authors found long-term studies for MM hip resurfacing with three implants [Birmingham Hip Resurfacing (BHR) (Smith & Nephew Orthopaedics Ltd, Memphis, Tennessee), ConservePlus (Wright Medical technology Inc, Arlington, Tennessee) and Cormet (Corin Ltd, Cirencester, Gloucestershire)]. The revision rates for MM hip resurfacing with these implants appear to meet the NICE criteria for a revision rate of 10 % or less at 10 years. Metal-on-metal hip resurfacing with the ReCap (Biomet Orthopaedics, Warsaw, Indiana) implant had excellent outcomes at a mean follow-up of 2.9 years. One RCT with a mean follow-up of 4.7 years compared the revision rate of MM Hip resurfacing using the Durom implant (Zimmer Inc, Warsaw, Indiana) with that for THA and reported a higher revision rate for MM hip resurfacing with the Durom implant than for THA, but the observed difference was not statistically significant. One implant (Articular Surface Replacement (ASR), DePuy International Ltd, Leeds, Yorkshire) failed to meet the NICE criteria.

7.2   Surgical Technique

End-stage degenerative disease of the hip in younger patients is frequently the result of conditions such as congenital hip dysplasia (CDH), Perthes disease or osteonecrosis (ON). In these patients, the affected hip is characterised by a loss of bone which has historically been a contraindication to MM hip resurfacing due to the risks of impingement and insufficient off-set. In this instance of CDH, we may conduct surgeries using head lengthening with bone chip augmentation. If there is a short head or short femoral neck, the standard hip resurfacing cannot be used.

In one study, we wanted to analyse the midterm functional and radiographic outcomes in patients with osteonecrosis of the femoral head treated with MM hip resurfacing. Pre-operative planning was aimed at relocating the hip centre of rotation in an anatomical position at the level of the true acetabulum, with a cup inclination of 40° and slight medialisation. When templating, care was taken not to excessively medialise the socket, as this was considered to constitute a risk for future dislocation. We aimed at a valgus inclination of 2–5° more than the patient's femoral neck-shaft angle, as this is considered to be a factor safeguarding against postoperative femoral neck fractures (Freeman 1978a, b). We perform all surgeries using a posterolateral approach. The acetabulum was reamed vertically to expose the medial wall. Reaming begins with a reamer of the same diameter as the selected femoral head component. After exposure of the medial wall, reamers of increasing diameter were oriented with the correct inclination, aiming at a positioning of 40° on the frontal plane. Socket anteversion is chosen based on the degree of anteversion of the patient's femoral neck. In patients with excessive femoral neck anteversion, the acetabular component is implanted in a less anteverted position, as the total anteversion of the neck and cup should equal 45° (McMinn et al. 2008). Acetabular components with supplementary screw fixation are used if the amount of superolateral uncoverage was greater than 1 cm with the trial component in place. After seating the acetabular component, the protruding osteophytes are removed with an osteotome.

After chamfering, the head is examined and all the necrotic bone with no visible blood supply is removed using a curette. There are two stages of treatment decision-making in whether we proceeded with MM hip resurfacing. First, at least 50 % of the femoral head must be viable; second, the integrity of the head-neck junction must be preserved (i.e. there should not be a major loss of bone at the junction). If these conditions are met, MM hip resurfacing is performed; otherwise THA is chosen.

In cases where a large amount of necrotic bone was removed, resulting in gaps larger than 3 mm between the chamfered bone and the seated head/neck template, a bone grafting technique was employed. This technique is also used to fill cysts in the femoral head which were larger than 3 mm.

A special set of surgical instruments is manufactured to carry out the surgical procedure (Finsbury Orthopaedics, Leatherhead, UK; Smith & Nephew, TN, USA). It comprises containing rings of various diameters and cannulated impactors which replicate the shape and size of both the chamfers and the interior superior part of the femoral components. The deficient femoral head is reamed with standard sleeve cutters, the guide rod is inserted and the head or neck template is seated until the feet overlap the head-neck junction. All the cartilage is removed from the bone chips, which are less than 2 mm in size. With the guide rod still in place, the chips are placed in a containing ring on the patient's femoral head. As the containing ring is filled, the appropriate cannulated impactor is used to impact the grafted area. The inner part of the cannulated impactor used for the Adept femoral component and the BHR femoral component differ slightly due to the differing implant designs. With the foot of the containing ring placed at the femoral head/neck junction, a pin is inserted in a hole located within the ring in order to secure it to the head. The desired femoral head reconstruction is obtained when the top of the end of the cannulated impactor overlaps the top of the containing ring. This is checked by reapplying the measuring device and comparing the length prior to augmentation. Finally, the containing ring, the cannulated impactor and the guide rod are removed and the femoral component is cemented according to the standard implantation technique.

We recommend no weight bearing in the first month and only partial weight bearing in the second month. Full weight bearing was allowed at 8 weeks following surgery. The peri-operative antibiotic and thromboprophylaxis treatment was the same for all patients and consisted of 2 g of cefalexin at induction, then 1 g every 8 h for 5 days, and 100 mg of tobramycin at induction, then 100 mg every 8 h for 3 days. For prophylaxis, a dose of 4,000 U of enoxaparin per day was administered for 60 days.

This was a retrospective study on 48 patients treated by a single surgeon with MM hip resurfacing for end-stage OB of the femoral head. Thirty-three hips were treated with the BHR and 16 hips were treated with the Adept hip resurfacing implant. The mean pre-operative oxford hip score was 29 ± 7 (range, 16–40). At the time of the final postoperative follow-up, the mean score was 47 ± 1.

We believe that an accurate surgical technique with the augmentation of the femoral head with bone chips contributed to the success rate observed in these patients with AVN.

7.3   Soft Tissue Reactions

A massive soft tissue reaction has been identified in some patients with metal-on-metal articulations. Termed a pseudotumour, this lesion has been associated with pain, a mass, nerve palsy, dislocation and a rash (Pandit et al. 2008). Pseudotumours appear to be more common than metal hypersensitivity reactions. The risk of developing a pseudotumour is roughly estimated to be 0.1–3 % in patients who undergo MM resurfacing within 5 years after implantation (Beaulé et al. 2011; Pandit et al. 2008). Literature indicates that the most important surgical risk factor for development of a pseudotumour is acetabular component orientation (Shimmin et al. 2010).

7.4   Metal Ion Release

Modern metal-on-metal hip resurfacing was introduced as a bone-preserving method of joint reconstruction for young and active patients; however, the large diameter of the bearing surfaces is of concern for potential increased metal ion release (Clarke et al. 2003). It is certain that metal ions are released because of the combined effect of corrosion of the implant surface and wear particles (Moroni et al. 2008). Metal wear particles are in the nanometer size range and therefore have a high surface area to volume ratio and are capable of releasing metal ions (Doorn et al. 1998). Because the amount of wear and corrosion is considered related to the area of the bearing surfaces, the introduction of large-diameter MM bearings, as used in hip resurfacing, has prompted even more concern. However, we support that the classic elastohydrodynamic theory, which suggests fluid film lubrication, believed responsible for reduced wear, is more likely to occur with large-diameter MM bearings (Smith 2001). Considering that the potentially negative effect of metal ion release resulting from corrosion associated with large-diameter bearings could be balanced by the potentially positive effect of increased fluid film lubrication, we expected no differences in metal ion release between large- and small-diameter metal bearings. In one of our studies, we tested the hypothesis that there were no differences in serum concentrations of Cr, Co and Mo between two groups of patients who had either hip resurfacing with a mean head diameter of 48 mm or 28-mm MM THA (Moroni et al. 2008). Serum concentrations of Cr, Co, Mo and Ni in the patients who had resurfacing also were compared with those observed in control subjects. The relationship between levels of metal ions, age, length of follow-up, implant size and the Harris hip scoring system also was investigated in patients who had resurfacing (Moroni et al. 2008).

Clinical interpretation of increased ion levels is difficult because the in vivo threshold limit is still unknown. International and national working groups are discussing only the reference values to be set for hazardous occupational toxicants in body fluids, i.e. "exposure equivalents for carcinogenic substances" (EKA values) and "biological tolerance values for occupational exposure" (BAT values) of the Deutsche Forschungsgemeinschaft Commission (Greim and Lehnet 1995) and "Biological Exposure Indices" (BEI) of the American Conference of Governmental Industrial Hygienists (Morgan 1997).

In another study, we asked whether (1) serum chromium (Cr), cobalt (Co) and molybdenum (Mo) concentrations would differ between patients with either MM-BHR or MM-THA at 5 years; (2) confounding factors such as gender would influence ion levels; and (3) ion levels would differ at 2 and 5 years for each implant type (Moroni et al. 2011). At follow-up of 5 years, we found ion concentrations in patients with MM-BHR were similar to those in patients who had MM-THA. In addition, we found time of follow-up and age had no influence on serum ion levels, whereas gender in association with implant type influenced Cr levels, with females who had MM-BHR showing an increase in Cr levels compared with males who had MM-BHR. Our results confirm those reported by Vendittoli et al. (2007), who evaluated blood ion concentrations in patients with MM Durom hip resurfacing. Vendittoli suggested that the female gender contributed to higher metal ion levels with resurfacing implants. They proposed that the difference in ion levels between genders may be secondary to differences in metal ion metabolism, such as different lean body mass, cellular or extracellular storage or renal excretion. Another possible explanation for the gender difference could be the different hip anatomy and biomechanics between genders. However, there is no evidence to substantiate these hypotheses.

Conclusions

Metal-on-metal hip resurfacing can be beneficial for appropriately selected patients, provided the surgeon has the surgical skills required for performing this procedure. We believe that if the surgeon does not completely remove the necrotic bone from the femoral head, its presence at the bone-cement interface could jeopardise the longevity of the procedure. When necessary, grafting the deficient head with bone chips collected when reaming the socket and trimming the femoral head could be viable, and future studies are warranted. Future studies should involve the long-term biological effects of high levels of metal ions in the blood and urine of patients who have received metal implants.

References

Allain J, Roudot-Thoraval F, Delecrin J et al (2003) Revision total hip arthroplasty performed after fracture of a ceramic femoral head. A multicenter survivorship study. J Bone Joint Surg Am 85:825–830

Amstutz HC, Ball ST, Le Duff MJ, Dorey FJ (2007) Resurfacing THA for patients younger than 50 years: results of 2- to 9-year follow up. Clin Orthop Relate Res 460:159–164

Amstutz HC, Le Duff MJ (2008) Eleven years of Experience with metal-on-metal hybrid hip resurfacing: a review of 1000 conserve plus. J Arthroplasty 23:36–43

Amstutz HC, Beaulé P, Dorey F et al (2004a) A metal-on-metal hybrid surface arthroplasty: two to six year follow-up study. J Bone Joint Surg Am 86-A:28–39

Amstutz HC, Campbell P, Le Duff MJ (2004b) Fracture of the Neck of the Femur after surface arthroplasty of the hip. J Bone Joint Surg Am 86-A(9):1874–1877

Australian Orthopaedic Association (2010) National Joint Replacement Registry. Annual report 2010. Available at http://www.scribd.com/doc/61660967/National-Joint-Replacement-Registry-Aoanjrrreport-2010. Accessed on Feb 5, 2013

Baad-Hansen T, Storgaard Jakobsen S, Soballe K (2011) Two-year migration results of the ReCap hip resurfacing system—a radiostereometric follow-up study of 23 hips. Int Orthop 35: 497–502

Beaulé PE, Lee J, Le Duff MJ et al (2004) Orientation of the femoral component in surface arthroplasty of the hip. A biomechanical and clinical analysis. J Bone Joint Surg Am 86:2015–2021

Beaulé PE, Kim PR, Powell J, Canadian Hip Resurfacing Study Group (2011) A survey on the prevalence of pseudotumors with metal-on-metal hip resurfacing in Canadian academic centers. J Bone Joint Surg Am 93:118–121

Clarke MT, Lee PT, Arora A et al (2003) Levels of metal ions after small- and large-diameter metal-on-metal hip arthroplasty. J Bone Joint Surgc Br 85:913–917

Daniel J, Pynsent P, McMinn D (2004) Metal-on-metal resurfacing of the hip in patients under the age of 55 years with osteoarthritis. J Bone Joint Surg Br 86(2):177–184

De Smet K (2005) Belgium experience with metal-on-metal surface arthroplasty. Orthop Clin North Am 36:203–213

Doorn PF, Campbell PA, Worrall J et al (1998) Metal wear particle characterization from metal on metal total hip replacements: transmission electron microscopy study of periprosthetic tissues and isolated particles. J Biomed Mater Res 42:103–111

Freeman MA (1978a) Some anatomical and mechanical considerations relevant to the surface replacement of the femoral head. Clin Orthop Relat Res 134:19–24

Freeman MA (1978b) Total surface replacement hip arthroplasty. Clin Orthop Relat Res 134:2–4

Greim H, Lehnet G (1995) Critical data evaluation for BAT and EKA values, vol 2, Biological exposure values for occupational toxicants and carcinogens H. Wiley, Weinheim

Hamadouche M, Doutin P, Daussange J et al (2002) Alumina-on-alumina total hip arthroplasty: a minimum 18.5 year follow-up study. J Bone Joint Surg Am 84:69–77

Harris WH (1995) The problem is osteolysis. Clin Orthop Relat Res 311:46–53

Klein GR, Levine BR, Hozaxk WJ et al (2007) Return to athletic activity after total hip arthroplasty. Consensus guidelines based on a survey of the Hip Society and American Association of Hip and Knee Surgeons. J Arthroplasty 22:171–175

Langton DJ, Jameson SS, Joyce TJ et al (2011) Accelerating failure rate of the ASR total hip replacement. J Bone Joint Surg Br 93:1011–1016

Marker D, Seyler T, Jinnah R et al (2007) Femoral neck fractures after metal-on-metal total hip resurfacing: a prospective cohort study. J Arthroplasty 22:66–71

McMinn D, Daniel J (2006) History and Modern concepts in surface replacement. Proc Inst Mech Eng 220(2):239–251

McMinn DJ, Daniel J, Ziaee H et al (2008) Results of the Birmingham Hip Resurfacing dysplasia component in severe acetabular insufficiency: a six- to 9.6-year follow-up. J Bone Joint Surg Br 90:715–723

McMinn DJ, Daniel J, Ziaee H et al (2011) Indications and results of hip resurfacing. Int Orthop 35:231–237

Morgan MS (1997) The biological exposure indices: a key component in protecting workers from toxic chemicals. Environ Health Perspect 105(suppl 1):105–115

Moroni A, Savarino L, Cadossi M et al (2008) Does ion release differ between hip resurfacing and metal-on-metal THA? Clin Orthop Relat 466:700–707

Moroni A, Savarino L, Hoque M et al (2011) Do ion levels in hip resurfacing differ from metal-on-metal THA at midterm? Clin Orthop Relat Res 469:180–187

Moroni A, Nocco E, Hoque M et al (2012) Cushion bearings versus large diameter head metal-on-metal bearings in total hip arthroplasty: a short-term metal ion study. Arch Orthop Trauma Surg 132:123–129

Murphy TP, Trousdale RT, Pagnano MW et al (2009) Patients' perceptions of hip resurfacing arthroplasty. Orthopaedics 32(10):730

Naal FD, Pilz R, Munzinger U et al (2011) High revision rate at 5 years after hip resurfacing with the Durom implant. Clin Orthop Relat Res 469:2598–2604

Pabinger C, Biedermann R, Stockl B et al (2003) Migration of metal-on-metal versus ceramic-on-polyethylene hip prostheses. Clin Orthop Relat Res 412:103–110

Pandit H, Glynn-Jones S, McLardy-Smith P et al (2008) Pseudotumours associated with metal-on-metal hip resurfacings. J Bone Joint Surg Br 90:847–851

Sehatzadeh S, Kaulback K, Levin L (2012) Metal-on-metal hip resurfacing arthroplasty: an analysis of safety and revision rates. Ont Health Technol Assess Ser 12(19):1–63

Shimmin AJ, Bare J, Back D (2005) Complications associated with hip resurfacing arthroplasty. Orthop Clin North Am 36:187–193

Shimmin A, Beaulé PE, Campbell P (2008) Metal-on-metal hip resurfacing arthroplasty. J Bone Joint Surg Am 90(3):637–54. doi:10.2106/JBJS.G.01012. Review

Shimmin AJ, Walter WL, Esposito C (2010) The influence of the size of the component on the outcome of resurfacing arthroplasty of the hip: a review of the literature. J Bone Joint Surg Br 92(4):469–476

Siebel T, Maubach S, Morlock M (2006) Lessons learned from early clinical experience and results of 300 ASR hip resurfacing implantations. Proc Inst Mech Eng 220:345–353

Smith SL, Dowson D, Goldsmith AA (2001) The effect of femorale head diameter upon lubrication and wear of metal-on-metal total hip replacements. Proc Inst mech Eng H. 215(2): 161–170

Treacy RB, McBryde C, Pynsent P (2005) Birmingham hip resurfacing arthroplasty. A minimum follow up of five years. J Bone Joint Surg Br 87(2):167–170

Treacy RB (2006) To resurface or replace the hip in the under 65-years old: the case of resurfacing. Ann R Coll Surg Engl 88(4):349–353

Treacy RB, Mcbryde CW, Shears E et al (2011) Birmingham hip resurfacing: a minimum follow-up of ten years. J Bone Joint Surg Br 93:27–33

Vendittoli P, Mottard S, Roy A et al (2007) Chromium and cobalt ion release following the Durom high carbon content, forged metal-on-metal surface replacement of the hip. J Bone Joint Surg Br 89:441–448

The Incidence of Pseudotumour in Metal-on-Metal Hip Resurfacing and the Results of a Screening Tool for Patient Recall

8

G. Erturan, A. Taylor, K. Barker, S. Masterson, R. Marsh, D. Beard, P. McLardy-Smith, M. Gibbons, A. Carr, and S. Glyn-Jones

8.1 Introduction

Metal-on-metal hip resurfacing arthroplasty (MoMHRA) was introduced in 1997 and has become an established surgical option, especially for younger patients with end-stage osteoarticular disease (Daniel et al. 2011). Designer and non-designer data continue to support the use of MoMHRA for this cohort of patients despite pseudotumour becoming an acknowledged complication (Murray et al. 2012; Treacy et al. 2011). The rates of pseudotumour are variable, and concern amongst the general public, healthcare providers and government is increasing together with the potential revision burden on hip services particularly compounded by poor reported outcomes post-revision (Glyn-Jones et al. 2009; Pandit et al. 2008; Hart et al. 2009; Kwon et al. 2011; Grammatopolous et al. 2009; Carrothers et al. 2010).

We wanted to determine whether a simple screening tool would be effective in picking up pseudotumours in our MoMHRA population. In addition, we aimed to assess our department's ability to predict incidence and prevalence of pseudotumours in MoMHRA by comparing our recall data to our department's previously published theoretical predictions based on survivorship studies that expected a 4 % revision rate at 8 years (Glyn-Jones et al. 2009).

G. Erturan (✉) • A. Taylor • K. Barker • S. Masterson • R. Marsh • D. Beard • P. McLardy-Smith
M. Gibbons • A. Carr • S. Glyn-Jones
Nuffield Department of Orthopaedics,
Rheumatology and Musculoskeletal Sciences,
University of Oxford, Nuffield Orthopaedic Centre,
Oxford, UK
e-mail: erturan@doctors.org.uk

K. Knahr (ed.), *Total Hip Arthroplasty*,
DOI 10.1007/978-3-642-35653-7_8, © EFORT 2013

The study was started in 2011; however, due to increasing concerns in the UK, British Government Legislation drove the Department of Health to issue a management and recall protocol through its Medicines and Healthcare products Regulatory Agency (MHRA) (Medical Device Alert 2012). A summary of the MHRA protocol is featured in Table 8.1.

Although the recent MHRA guidelines have surpassed the original indication for this work in the UK, it may still prove valuable for healthcare providers outside of the National Health Service who need a foundation for pseudotumour recall and surveillance.

8.2   Method

Over a 9-year period, 1,102 patients have undergone a MoMHRA at our institute. They were all sent a postal screening questionnaire that included the Oxford Hip Score (OHS) and a set of four discriminatory questions. We aimed to recall all patients who gave one positive answer to the discriminatory questions and/or had an OHS of under 30.

The four questions were:
- Q1: "Are you experiencing pain from your hip?"
- Q2: "Have you any swelling around your hip?"
- Q3: "Are you experiencing any squeaking sound from hip?"
- Q4: "Have you been seen in a clinic in the last year?"

Question 4 was designed to trigger a search into recent clinical consultations that may include a problematic hip prosthesis and ensure that we were not replicating recall and investigations performed elsewhere.

Upon recall, a range of movement and blood parameters, in particular, cobalt and chromium levels, were measured together with ultrasound scanning (USS), magnetic resonance imaging (MRI) or both. Specifically, MRI was triggered for those with blood ion levels above 5 parts per billion (ppb). Although current MRHA guidelines now use 7 ppb as a trigger, Hart et al. demonstrated that although blood metal ions had good discriminant ability to separate failed from well-functioning hip replacements, a cut-off level of 7 ppb provided a specific test but had poor sensitivity (Hart et al. 2011). Their research suggested that the optimal cut-off level for the maximum of cobalt or chromium was 4.97 ppb and had sensitivity 63 % and specificity 86 % (Hart et al. 2011).

8.3   Results

Of 1,102 patients who were sent the postal screen, 719 (65 %) replied, and 82 of 719 (11 %) fitted the criteria for recall to clinic. From these 82 patients, 11 failed to attend clinic and 1 patient declined to do so, leaving 70 (85 %) patients in our investigation pool.

Table 8.1 Medicines and Healthcare products Regulatory Agency (MHRA) protocol for the screening of pseudotumour

MoM hip resurfacing (no stem)	Follow-up	Imaging: MARS* MRI or USS	1st blood metal ion level	Results of 1st blood metal ion	2nd blood metal ion level	Results of 2nd blood metal ion	Consider need for revision
Symptomatic patients	Annually (>5 years)	All cases	Yes	>7 ppb indicates potential for soft tissue reaction	Yes – 3 months after 1st blood test if >7 ppb	>7 ppb indicates potential especially if greater than previous	Abnormal imaging and/or blood metal ion levels rising
Asymptomatic patients	According to local protocol	No – unless concern for cohort or patient becomes symptomatic	No – unless concern for cohort or patient becomes symptomatic				

*MARS = Metal artefact reduction sequence

Table 8.2 Oxford Hip Score (OHS) and relation to diagnosis of pseudotumour. No significant difference was found between tumour-positive and tumour-negative groups

	Pseudotumour positive	Pseudotumour negative
Median OHS	30	29
OHS range	6–48	2–48

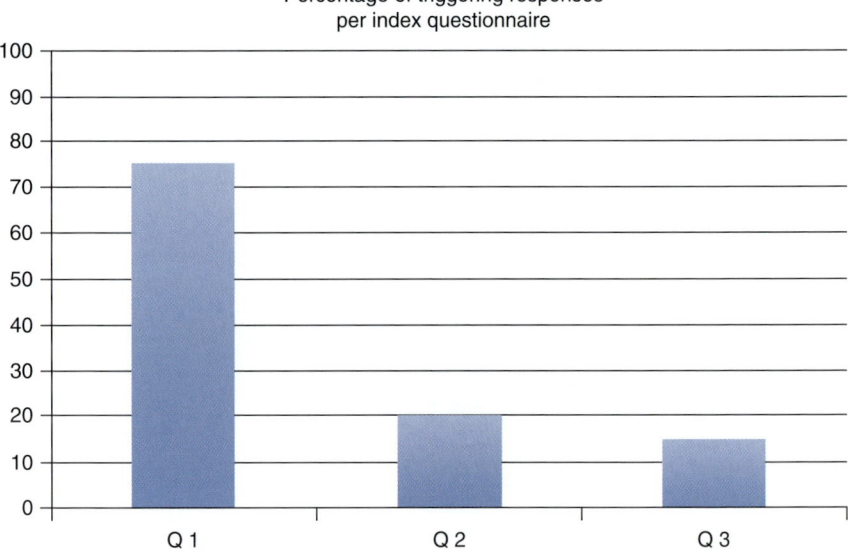

Fig. 8.1 Table demonstrating the percentage of recall triggering answers per index questionnaire

The ages at surgery and time to follow-up for those diagnosed with a pseudotumour were similar for both sexes, median age: 44 years (range 32–54) and median follow-up time post-surgery of just over 5 years (63 months, range 22–110).

Of those recalled, there was no significant difference in the hip scores between those who were then diagnosed with a pseudotumour and those who were not, see Table 8.2.

Results from the screening questionnaire revealed Question 1: "Are you experiencing pain from your hip?" as being the most commonly given positive trigger for recall to clinic at 75 %; see Fig. 8.1.

8.3.1 Ultrasound Scanning Results

Ultrasound scanning demonstrated the appearance of pseudotumour in 27 of 70 (39 %) of patients. Subsequent MRI confirmed USS diagnosis in 22 of these patients; see Fig. 8.2.

A completely unremarkable USS was seen in 26 of 70 (37 %), with MRI revealing pseudotumour in 2 from this group; see Fig. 8.3.

There were 17 (24 %) patients whose USS revealed a small effusion. Pseudotumour was later confirmed in one patient; see Fig. 8.4.

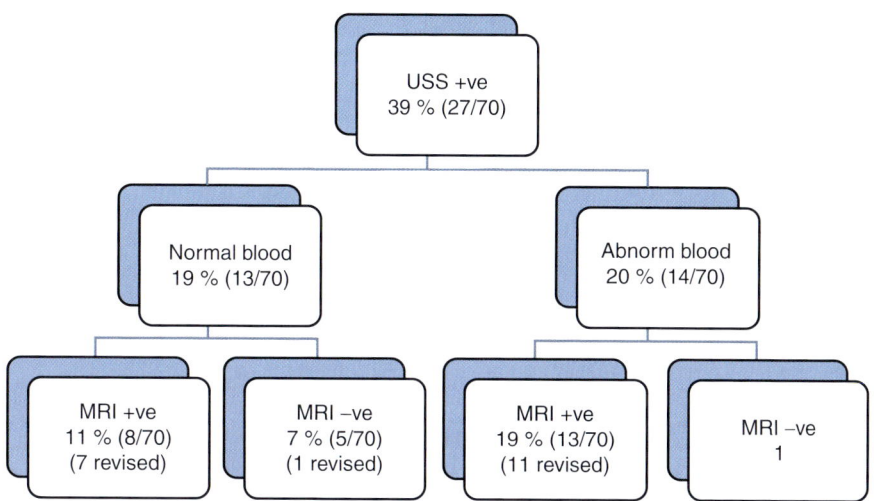

Fig. 8.2 Outcome following a positive ultrasound scan for pseudotumour

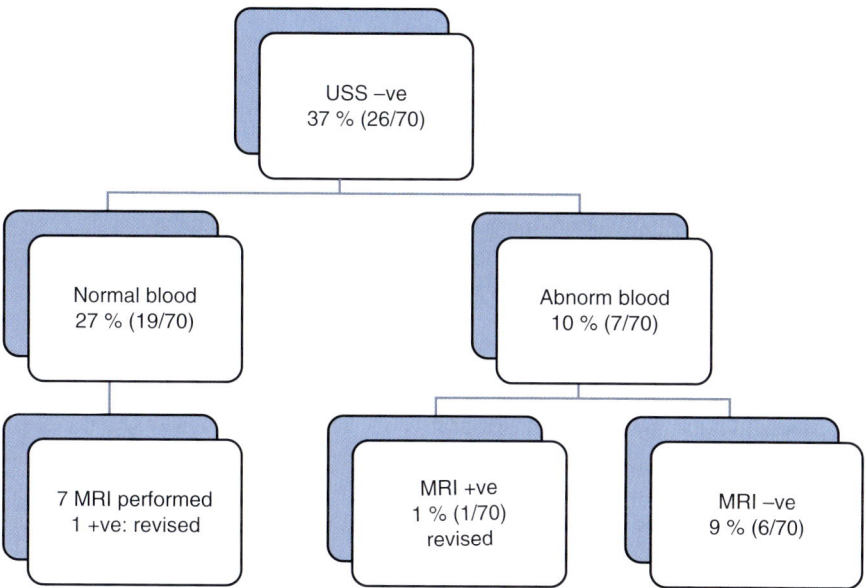

Fig. 8.3 Outcome following a negative ultrasound scan for pseudotumour

8.3.2   Blood Ion Results

Abnormal blood results (>5 ppb) were seen in 27 (39 %) of patients. Of these, 11 (16 %) had a normal MRI.

Normal blood results were found in 43 (61 %) of patients; however, 9 (13 %) had a positive MRI scan for pseudotumour.

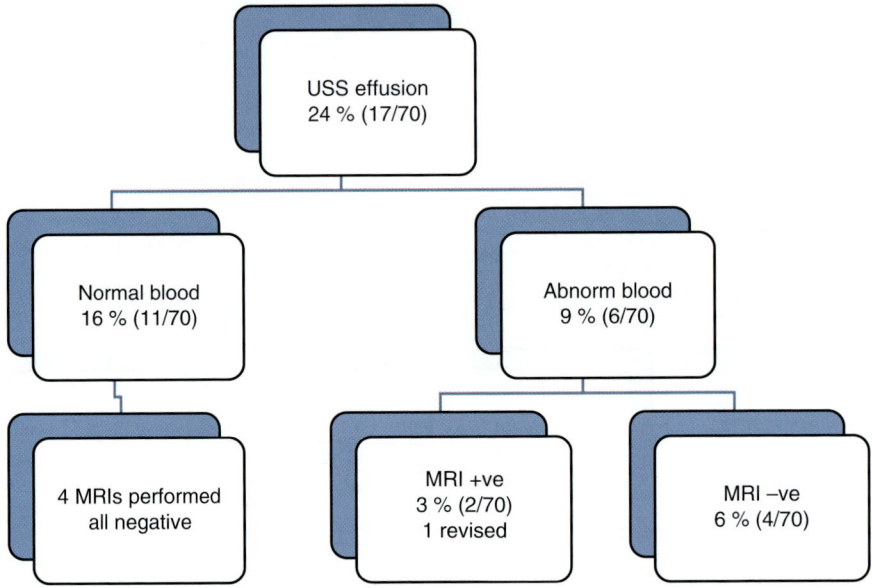

Fig. 8.4 Outcome following the demonstration of a small effusion when ultrasound scanning for a pseudotumour

Table 8.3 The sensitivity and specificity of blood ions and ultrasound scanning in the diagnosis of pseudotumour after hip resurfacing

	Blood tests	Ultrasound
Sensitivity	64 % (16/25)	91 % (21/23)
Specificity	67 % (22/33)	80 % (24/30)

Blood ion levels of chromium and cobalt were not sensitive or specific markers for pseudotumour (64 and 67 %, respectively). The sensitivity and specificity of ultrasound scanning in comparison was significantly better than blood test; see Table 8.3.

We did not observe a significant correlation between radiographically measured tumour volume and blood ion level. Nor was there a significant correlation between hip score and blood ion level in either the positive tumour group or those with either normal radiological appearances or an effusion.

8.3.3 Revision Results

Of the 719 responders to the questionnaire, 38 (5 %) had had their resurfacing revised to a total hip replacement. As a proportion of our recall to clinic group, this was 22 of the 70 (31 %) with a median Oxford Hip Score of 23; see Table 8.4.

Table 8.4 Revision rate and Oxford Hip Score related to the results of a recall patient ultrasound scan (USS) positive (+ve), small effusion (?), negative (−ve) and in general over the whole recall group (Total)

	Revision rate	Oxford hip score
USS +ve	70 % (19/27)	30
USS ?	1 % (1/17)	38
USS −ve	8 % (2/26)	28
Total	31 % (22/70)	23

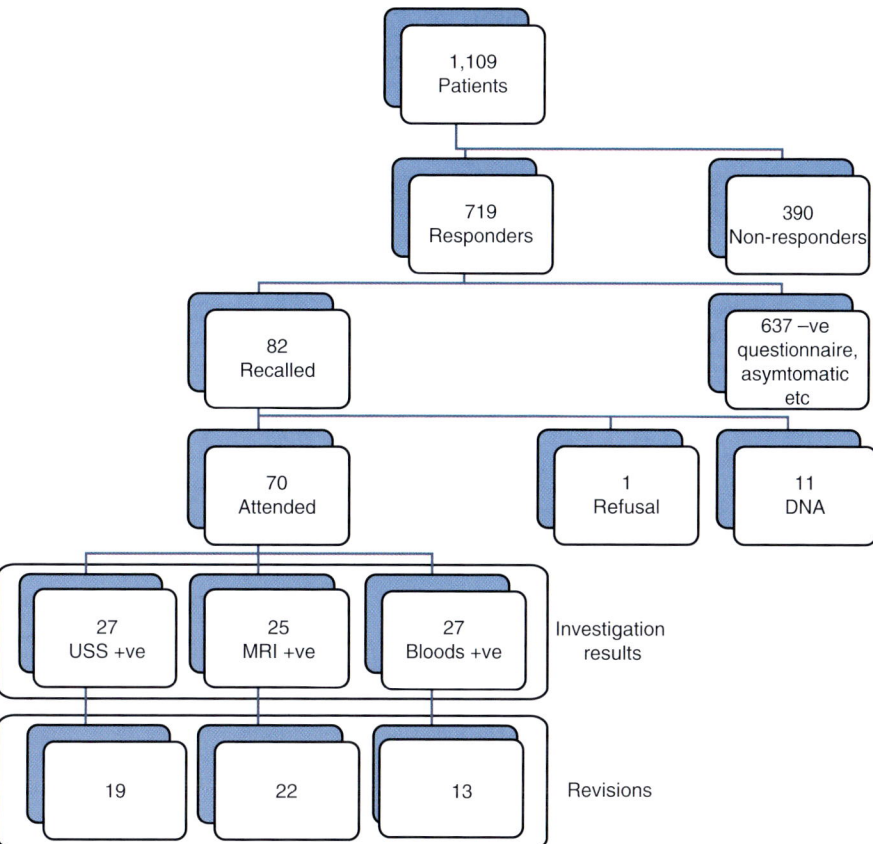

Fig. 8.5 Flow diagram summarising the results of the screening questionnaire to detect pseudotumour after hip resurfacing

8.3.4 Results Summary

Figure 8.5 demonstrates a flow diagram summary of the study results from the screening questionnaire. We have seen that 31 % of those recalled are positive for pseudotumour as compared with approximately 5 % of the MoMHRA population.

Conclusion

The problem of pseudotumour development and its sequelae are proving to be significant with a revision rate of 5 % at present in the general population. Our basic screening test demonstrated that a third of those patients recalled had already developed a pseudotumour and almost a quarter of the group may be at high risk of doing so based on radiographic and blood markers.

We understand that the limitation of this study is the unknown pseudotumour status in the non-recall cohort. However, due to government legislation, all patients are now being followed up, and as such we hope to strengthen the sensitivity and specificity of our results.

The potential pseudotumour burden and hence need for recall and investigation is apparent. Individual parameters fail to act as a threshold for recall, but a questionnaire is a seemingly effective and pragmatic initial approach.

Although there is growing awareness of the serious complication profile of pseudotumours secondary to metal-on-metal hip resurfacing, the extent of the global problem amongst the resurfaced population is not fully understood. To date, there have been no published attempts of screening this population for investigation and treatment; however, health regulatory bodies need to prepare for the clinical impact both directly and indirectly as a result of the health economic burden and potential to stress other clinical services.

References

Daniel J, Ziaee H, Pradhan C (2011) Indications and results of hip resurfacing. Int Orthop 35(2):231–237 (Epub 2010/11/17)

Murray DW, Grammatopoulos G, Pandit H, Gundle R, Gill HS, McLardy-Smith P (2012) The ten-year survival of the Birmingham hip resurfacing: an independent series. J Bone Joint Surg Br 94(9):1180–1186 (Epub 2012/08/31)

Treacy RB, McBryde CW, Shears E, Pynsent PB (2011) Birmingham hip resurfacing: a minimum follow-up of ten years. J Bone Joint Surg Br 93(1):27–33 (Epub 2011/01/05)

Glyn-Jones S, Pandit H, Kwon YM, Doll H, Gill HS, Murray DW (2009) Risk factors for inflammatory pseudotumour formation following hip resurfacing. J Bone Joint Surg Br 91(12):1566–1574 (Epub 2009/12/02)

Pandit H, Glyn-Jones S, McLardy-Smith P, Gundle R, Whitwell D, Gibbons CL et al (2008) Pseudotumours associated with metal-on-metal hip resurfacings. J Bone Joint Surg Br 90(7):847–851 (Epub 2008/07/02)

Hart AJ, Sabah S, Henckel J, Lewis A, Cobb J, Sampson B et al (2009) The painful metal-on-metal hip resurfacing. J Bone Joint Surg Br 91(6):738–744 (Epub 2009/06/02)

Kwon YM, Ostlere SJ, McLardy-Smith P, Athanasou NA, Gill HS, Murray DW (2011) "Asymptomatic" pseudotumors after metal-on-metal hip resurfacing arthroplasty: prevalence and metal ion study. J Arthroplasty 26(4):511–518 (Epub 2010/07/02)

Grammatopolous G, Pandit H, Kwon YM, Gundle R, McLardy-Smith P, Beard DJ et al (2009) Hip resurfacings revised for inflammatory pseudotumour have a poor outcome. J Bone Joint Surg Br 91(8):1019–1024 (Epub 2009/08/05)

Carrothers AD, Gilbert RE, Jaiswal A, Richardson JB (2010) Birmingham hip resurfacing: the prevalence of failure. J Bone Joint Surg Br 92(10):1344–1350 (Epub 2010/10/05)

Medical Device Alert: all metal-on-metal (MoM) hip replacements (MDA/2012/036). 2012 [cited 31 October 2012]. Available from: http://www.mhra.gov.uk/Publications/Safetywarnings/MedicalDeviceAlerts/CON155761

Hart AJ, Sabah SA, Bandi AS, Maggiore P, Tarassoli P, Sampson B et al (2011) Sensitivity and specificity of blood cobalt and chromium metal ions for predicting failure of metal-on-metal hip replacement. J Bone Joint Surg Br 93(10):1308–1313 (Epub 2011/10/05)

Part III

Polyethylene – Standard and New Improvements

New Polys and Large Heads: Clinical Aspects

9

Eduardo García-Rey

Total hip replacement (THR) has become one of the most successful procedures in the last decades (Learmonth et al. 2007). Sir John Charnley developed low-friction arthroplasty using cemented fixation, a 22.225 mm stainless-steel femoral head and an all-polyethylene (PE) cup during the early 1960s of the last century, an operation with excellent long-term results worldwide (Charnley 1961) (Fig. 9.1). Cemented THRs usually show higher survivorship rates than uncemented designs; nevertheless some contemporary implants are providing very low rates of loosening with their improved primary and secondary bone fixation. In a study from the Swedish Hip Arthroplasty Register, Hailer et al. observed increased use of uncemented THR despite a lower revision rate at 10 and 15 years (Hailer et al. 2010). In their analysis they found better results for cemented arthroplasties regardless of the age or the diagnosis of the patient; when they assessed the cup and the stem, they concluded that the worse outcomes of uncemented THR were due to a higher revision rate of the cup produced by wear-related problems. So the most important problem in a long term is PE wear in both cemented and uncemented THRs as this is the main source of osteolysis and loosening (Harris 1995).

9.1 Polyethylene Wear

Conventional PE is gamma sterilised in air, a method that favours cross-linking but produces free radicals that can oxidise in vivo and decrease the mechanical properties of the plastic. This process would start the process of wear debris that is the principal

This manuscript was read in part at the EFORT Congress Berlin Tribology Day 25 May 2012, Large diameter heads: Risk/Benefits?

E. García-Rey, MD, PhD, EBOT
Orthopaedics Department, Hospital La Paz-Idi Paz, P° Castellana 261,
28046 Madrid, Spain
e-mail: edugrey@yahoo.es

K. Knahr (ed.), *Total Hip Arthroplasty*,
DOI 10.1007/978-3-642-35653-7_9, © EFORT 2013

Fig. 9.1 Radiograph of a female patient who underwent surgery at our hospital with a low-friction arthroplasty at 32 years of age secondary to congenital hip disease at 30 year of follow-up. Left hip was operated 15 years later

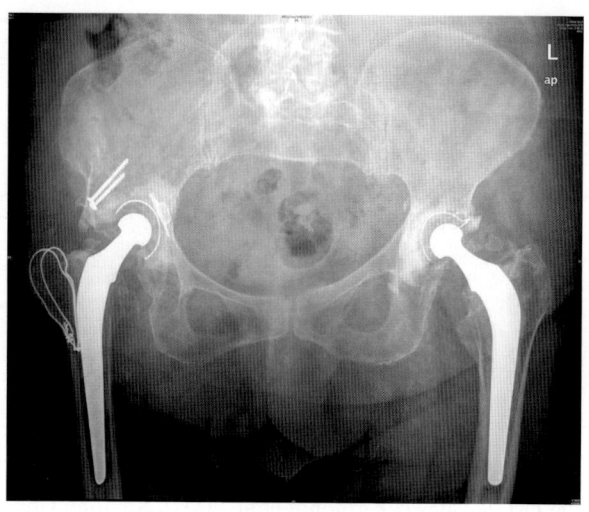

cause of THR loosening (Harris 1995). In clinical radiographs we can evaluate femoral head penetration into the PE liner by analysing wear through the years. Different methods have been used since the uniradiographic method by Charnley and the latest digitised methods, including radiostereometric analysis (RSA) (Charnley and Cupic 1973; Charnley and Halley 1975; Livermore et al. 1990; Dorr and Wan 1995; Martell and Berdia 1997; Digas et al. 2004). The validity of radiological measurement was reported later in experimental in vitro studies that determined that a fixed position of the x-ray beam reduces error in phantom studies, but in clinical radiographs, patient positioning is slightly different in each follow-up radiograph, so measurements of different clinical radiographs from the same patient are not as precise (Wan et al. 2006). Sychterz et al. reported that femoral head penetration over the years is divided into so-called bedding-in and true wear: in the 18–24 months after the operation, femoral head penetration is due to creep, the deformation of material without any loss of material, and after this period, wear, the removal of material subjected to mechanical stresses, would appear (Sychterz et al. 1999). In another comparative study, the analysis of sequential femoral head penetration into a conventional gamma sterilised-in-air PE, matched to a 28- or 32-mm metallic femoral head with uncemented hemispherical cups with good long-term fixation, was evaluated (García-Rey 2010). Measurements were done using digitised radiographs and concentric circles (Kim et al. 2001). Findings showed that wear during the early period was much higher than mean linear annual wear in every case, so we must identify this phenomenon when measuring polyethylene wear in any study.

Although different factors such as the age of the patient, diagnosis, physical activity or the position of a vertical cup with a postoperative acetabular abduction angle higher than 50° have been related to higher rates of PE wear, the type of THR and femoral head size are probably the most important. For conventional PE, cemented arthroplasties with 22- or 28-mm femoral heads produce lower wear rates than an uncemented THR with a 32-mm femoral head at a minimum follow-up of 10 years, and this is also true for the appearance of osteolysis (Oparaugo et al. 2001). A study from the Norwegian Register showed that the Charnley cup had lower

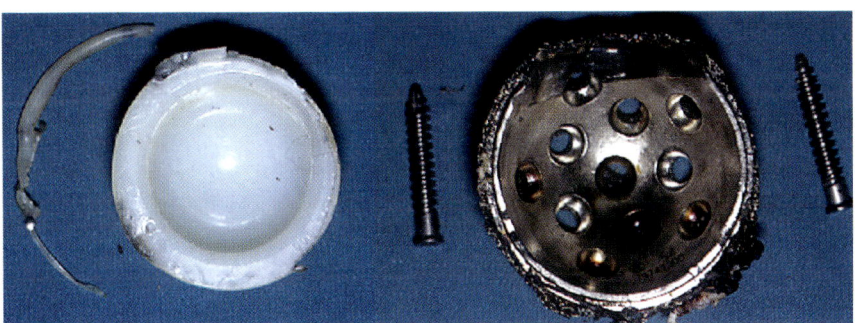

Fig. 9.2 Conventional polyethylene 32-mm liner rupture in a first-generation porous-coated uncemented cup

revision rates than other newer implants probably due to the low wear rate (Espehaug et al. 2009). However, although early loosening of the cup in cemented low-friction arthroplasty is due to a poor bone stock on the acetabular side, late loosening is due to PE wear, particularly in young patients (Garcia-Cimbrelo and Munuera 1992).

Conventional PE wear is higher in uncemented cups. Some older designs such as the cylindrical PE liners were abandoned due to the higher rates of rupture (Garcia-Rey and Garcia-Cimbrelo 2007). Thus, the use of a 32-mm femoral head with conventional PE is no longer recommended due to the high wear rates and the appearance of liner ruptures (Hallan et al. 2006; Cruz-Pardos and García-Cimbrelo 2001; Cruz-Pardos et al. 2005; Garcia-Rey and Garcia-Cimbrelo 2008) (Fig. 9.2). On the contrary, the use of a 28-mm femoral head with a conventional PE liner in uncemented cups has shown lower rates (García Rey et al. 2009). When a threaded uncemented grit-blasted titanium cup is used, wear is also related to femoral head diameter (Garcia-Cimbrelo et al. 2003). Finally, nonmodular cups seem to produce less wear due to the absence of backside wear (Young et al. 2002); nevertheless this finding has not been confirmed by other authors (González Della Valle et al. 2004).

We can summarise that conventional PE wear depends on several factors related to the patient, such as physical activity, age or weight; to surgical technique, like the placement of the cup with a high acetabular abduction angle; and to the surgeon's choice to use a large head matched to a thin PE, or maybe a modular uncemented cup.

Other PEs different from gamma sterilised in air were developed in order to improve wear performance. Some of them were sterilised in nitrogen, plasma gas or argon. These types of PEs, however, did not improve the wear rates over gamma sterilised-in-air PEs. Recently, Engh et al. reported higher wear rates for one of these types of PEs, a wear that was related to larger osteolytic lesions (2012).

9.2   Highly Cross-Linked Polyethylenes

Reducing wear debris reduced the rate of osteolysis, this phenomenon being a combination of decreased PE wear resistance with loss of mechanical properties and increased oxidation (Gómez-Barrena et al. 2008). So-called first-generation

Fig. 9.3 Radiograph of a 64-year-old female patient with an uncemented THR using remelted HXLPE matched to a 28-mm femoral head with an excellent clinical result at 10 years of follow-up

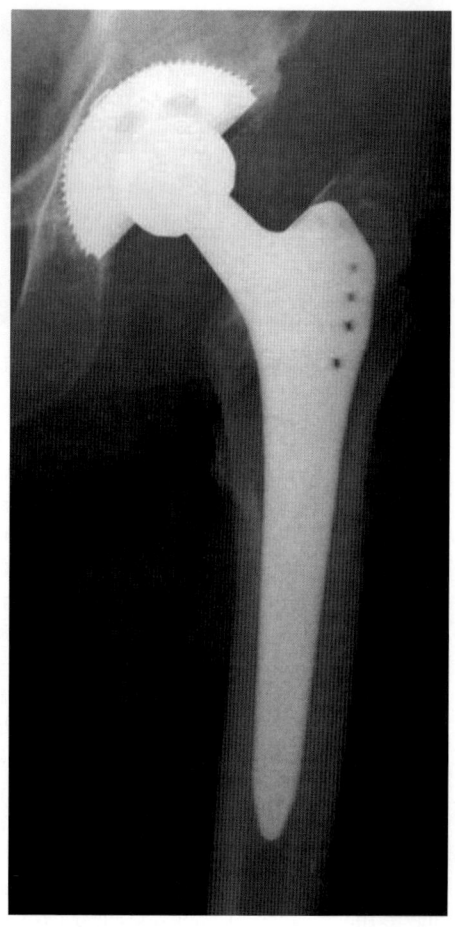

highly cross-linked polyethylenes (HXLPE) attempt to achieve this, avoiding the production of free radicals and oxidation. All HXLPE are irradiated with high doses of gamma or electron beams, a thermal treatment to anneal or remelt the PE (trying to eliminate free radicals) and a sterilisation process in the absence of air. Increased cross-linking provides decreased HXLPE wear compared to conventional PE in vitro (McKellop et al. 1999; Muratoglu et al. 2001). The early first retrieval analyses of HXLPEs showed minimal wear and the reappearance of most of the machining marks after heat treatment, and although a higher inflammatory response has been reported, there was no evidence of particle disease in the histological study (Knahr et al. 2007; Illgen et al. 2008). During the last years other clinical reports have shown reduced wear when comparing HXLPE with conventional PEs; however, we still do not know the long-term results and if these improvements result in less osteolysis and loosening (García-Rey et al. 2008; Kuzyk et al. 2011) (Fig. 9.3).

But there are still some concerns regarding HXLPEs. The mechanical properties of melted HXLPEs may be affected due to the changes in the microstructure of the polymer that could decrease toughness and fatigue resistance. To date, the annealing process does not completely eliminate free radicals (Gómez-Barrena et al. 2008). For this reason, the so-called second-generation HXLPEs have been developed in recent years. The subsequent vitamin E diffusion instead of melting after the irradiation process avoids the loss of crystallinity observed in melted HXLPE, which is one of the sources of the decreased mechanical and fatigue strength (Oral et al. 2006). The other option is sequential annealing in order to improve the oxidation resistance and decrease the appearance of free radicals without compromising mechanical properties (Dumbleton et al. 2006).

9.3 Large Femoral Heads

The improvement of wear resistance observed with HXLPEs has renewed the interest in using 32-mm-diameter or even larger femoral heads in THR. In vitro examination of large 40-mm femoral heads showed improved wear resistance compared to conventional aged PE and a higher fatigue resistance (Burroughs et al. 2006). On the other hand, fracture of the superior rim of retrieved acetabular liners observed in first-generation HXLPEs with a ring-locking mechanism suggests that a thin liner and a vertical cup alignment could be the causes of this failure (Tower et al. 2007). In another hip simulator study, the mean wear rate for a 36-mm-diameter liner was slightly higher than the rate for 28-mm liners and tended to decrease with decreasing liner thickness; they also reported a tendency for contact stress to increase as the thickness of the liner decreased in a finite element modelling; and the authors concluded that with a proper orientation, the diameter of the ball could be increased (Shen et al. 2011).

The theoretical advantages of using large femoral heads in THR are due to the increased head and neck ratio that would decrease the appearance of impingement. An improvement in the range of motion and a higher displacement of the femoral head that produce dislocation using femoral heads with a diameter larger than 32 mm has been reported in vitro (Burroughs et al. 2005). On the other hand, Sariali et al. reported that the jumping distance for dislocation decreases as the abduction angle and the head offset increases, the latter more important when using large heads (2009). The biomechanics of large heads in THR has also been assessed in finite element models to evaluate the geometry and the anatomic orientation of the cup, and although increasing the diameter of the femoral head may improve hip stability, a vertical orientation of the cup does not provide the desirable effect and also produces a maximum stress area so the durability of the PE might be altered (Crowninshield et al. 2004).

Clinical studies report a decrease in the early dislocation rate using large femoral heads compared with a 28-mm femoral head; however, the problem of dislocation increases during the following years, and wear and liner ruptures have been related to the use of these large heads combined to HXLPEs (Howie et al. 2012). Thus, they were not able to reduce the prevalence of early dislocation after primary THR in high-risk patients compared to historical controls (Lachiewicz and Soileau 2006).

Fig. 9.4 Radiograph of a
68-year-old female patient
with an uncemented THR and
vitamin E-doped PE matched
to a 32-mm femoral head
with an excellent clinical
result at 3 years of follow-up

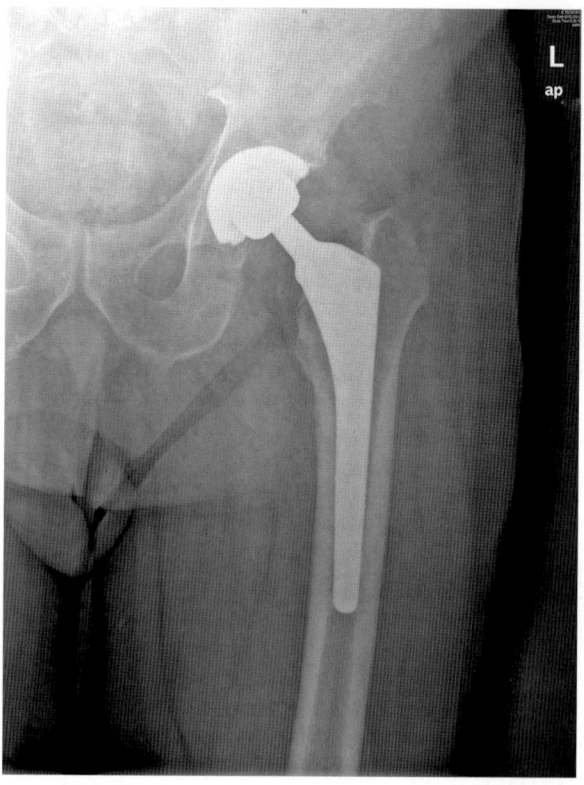

It is well known that dislocation is a multifactorial problem and large heads have not reduced the rate of instability when the abductor mechanism is absent (Kung and Ries 2007). There is also a lack of studies comparing the use of a 32-mm femoral head to a 36 mm in so far as reducing the rate of dislocation is not confirmed (Fig. 9.4).

The other variables assessed in clinical practice have been wear and range of motion. Although similar linear wear has been reported when comparing large femoral heads and 28- or 32-mm femoral heads, volumetric wear was higher in a midterm follow-up, so caution is recommended before using these implants, particularly in young patients and in those with a low risk for dislocation (Lachiewicz et al. 2009). Another study observed a similar higher volumetric wear; when range of motion was compared, equivalent results were found in contrast to in vitro studies and the risk of dislocation was not completely eliminated (Hammerberg et al. 2010). Some other clinical problems like pain due to psoas impingement when using large cup sizes have also been reported (Cobb et al. 2011).

The clinical evidence does not yet support the theoretical advantages of using femoral heads larger than 32 mm in THR combined to HXLPEs for now. The still valid concept of low-friction arthroplasty developed by Charnley must be considered before using these implants. The high-friction torque of large femoral heads in THR is a potential concern, and although there is a reduced rate of dislocation when using 36-mm femoral heads compared to 28-mm heads, the wear-related problems and the benefits of an increase in the range of motion are not substantially proven. The use of a 32-mm femoral head matched to HXLPEs can again be recommended, given the better mechanical properties of the latter, particularly in large cup sizes in primary THR.

References

Burroughs BR, Hallstrom B, Golladay GJ, Hoefffel D, Harris WH (2005) Range of motion and stability in total hip arthroplasty with 28-, 32-, 38-, and 44-mm femoral head sizes. J Arthroplasty 20:11–19

Burroughs BR, Muratoglu OK, Bragdon CR, Wannomae KK, Christensen S, Lozynsky AJ, Harris WH (2006) In vitro comparison of frictional torque and torsional resistance of aged conventional gamma-in-nitrogen sterilized polyethylene versus aged highly crosslinked polyethylene articulating against head sizes larger than 32 mm. Acta Orthop 77:710–718

Charnley J (1961) Arthroplasty of the hip: a new operation. Lancet 277(7187):1129–1132

Charnley J, Cupic Z (1973) The nine and ten year results of the low-friction arthroplasty of the hip. Clin Orthop Relat Res 95:9–25

Charnley J, Halley DK (1975) Rate of wear in total hip replacement. Clin Orthop Relat Res 112:170–179

Cobb JP, Davda K, Ahmad A, Harris SJ, Masjedi M, Hart AJ (2011) Why large-head metal-on-metal hip replacement are painful: the anatomical basis of psoas impingement on the femoral head-neck junction. J Bone Joint Surg 93:881–885

Crowninshield RD, Maloney WJ, Wentz DH, Humphrey SM, Blanchard CR (2004) Biomechanics of large heads: what they do and don't do. Clin Orthop Relat Res 429:102–107

Cruz-Pardos A, García-Cimbrelo E (2001) The Harris-Galante total hip arthroplasty: a minimum 8-year follow-up study. J Arthroplasty 16:586–597

Cruz-Pardos A, García-Cimbrelo E, Cordero-Ampuero J (2005) Porous-coated anatomic uncemented total hip arthroplasty. A 10–17-year follow-up. Hip Int 15:78–84

Digas G, Kärrholm J, Thanner J, Malchau H, Herberts P (2004) Highly cross-linked polyethylene in total hip arthroplasty: randomised evaluation of penetration rate in cemented and uncemented sockets using radiostereometric analysis. Clin Orthop Relat Res 429:6–16

Dorr LD, Wan Z (1995) Ten years of experience with porous acetabular components for revision surgery. Clin Orthop Relat Res 319:191–200

Dumbleton JH, D'Antonio JA, Manley MT, Capello WN (2006) The basis for a second-generation highly cross-linked UHMWPE. Clin Orthop Relat Res 453:265–271

Engh CA, Powers CC, Ho H, Beykirch-Padgett SE, Hopper RH Jr, Engh CA Jr (2012) The effect of poly sterilization on wear, osteolysis and survivorship of a press-fit cup at 10-year followup. Clin Orthop Relat Res 470:462–470

Espehaug B, Furnes O, Engesaeter LB, Havelin LI (2009) 18 years of results with cemented primary hip prosthesis in the Norwegian Arthroplasty Register: concerns about some newer implants. Acta Orthop 80:402–412

García Rey E, García-Cimbrelo E, Cordero Ampuero J (2009) Outcome of a hemispherical porous-coated acetabular component with a proximally hydroxyapatite-coated anatomic femoral component: a 12- to 15-year follow-up study. J Bone Joint Surg Br 91:327–332

Garcia-Cimbrelo E, Munuera L (1992) Early and late loosening of the acetabular cup after low-friction arthroplasty. J Bone Joint Surg Am 74-A:119–129

Garcia-Cimbrelo E, Cruz-Pardos A, Madero R, Ortega-Andreu M (2003) Total hip arthroplasty with use of the cementless Zweymuller Alloclassic system. A ten to thirteen-year follow-up study. J Bone Joint Surg Am 85-A:296–303

García-Rey E (2010) Bedding-in and true wear in two different generations cementless porous-coated acetabular cups. Hip Int 20(suppl 7):S86–S93

Garcia-Rey E, Garcia-Cimbrelo E (2007) Long-term results of uncemented acetabular cups with an ACS polyethylene liner. A 14-16-year follow-up study. Int Orthop 31:205–210

Garcia-Rey E, Garcia-Cimbrelo E (2008) Clinical and radiographic results and wear performance in different generations of a cementless porous-coated acetabular cup. Int Orthop 32:181–187

García-Rey E, García-Cimbrelo E, Cruz-Pardos A, Ortega-Chamarro J (2008) New polyethylenes in total hip replacement. A prospective, comparative clinical study of two types of liner. J Bone Joint Br 90-B:149–153

Gómez-Barrena E, Puertolas JA, Munuera L, Konttinen YT (2008) Update on UHMWPE research: from the bench to the bedside. Acta Orthop 79:832–840

González Della Valle A, Su E, Zoppi A, Sculco TP, Salvati EA (2004) Wear and periprosthetic osteolysis in a match-paired study of modular and nonmodular uncemented acetabular cups. J Arthroplasty 19:972–977

Hailer NP, Garellick G, Kärrholm J (2010) Uncemented and cemented primary total hip arthroplasty in the Swedish Hip Arthroplasty Register: evaluation of 170,413 operations. Acta Orthop 81(1):34–41

Hallan G, Lie SA, Havelin LI (2006) High wear rates and extensive osteolysis in 3 types of uncemented total hip arthroplasty: a review of the PCA, the Harris Galante and the Profile/Trilock Plus arthroplasties with a minimum of 12 years median follow-up in 96 hips. Acta Orthop 77:575–584

Hammerberg EM, Wan Z, Dastane M, Dorr LD (2010) Wear and range of motion of different femoral head sizes. J arthroplasty 25:839–843

Harris WH (1995) The problem is osteolysis. Clin Orthop Relat Res 311:46–53

Howie DW, Holubowycz OT, Middleton R, The Large Articulation Study Group (2012) Large femoral heads decrease the incidence of dislocation after total hip arthroplasty. A randomized controlled trial. J Bone Joint Am 94:1095–1102

Illgen RL 2nd, Forsythe TM, Pike JW, Laurent MP, Blanchard CR (2008) Highly crosslinked vs conventional polyethylene particles – an in vitro comparison of biologic activities. J Arthroplasty 23:721–731

Kim Y-H, Kim J-S, Cho S-H (2001) A comparison of polyethylene wear in hips with cobalt-chrome or zirconia heads. A prospective, randomised study. J Bone Joint Surg Br 83-B: 742–750

Knahr K, Pospischill M, Köttig P, Schneider W, Plenk H Jr (2007) Retrieval analyses of highly cross-linked polyethylene acetabular liners four and five years after implantation. J Bone Joint Surg Br 89-B:1036–1041

Kung PL, Ries MD (2007) Effect of femoral head size and abductors on dislocation after revision THA. Clin Orthop Rel Res 465:170–174

Kuzyk PR, Saccone M, Sprague S, Simunovic N, Bhandari M, Schemitsch EH (2011) Cross-linked versus conventional polyethylene for total hip replacement: a meta-analysis of randomised controlled trials. J Bone Joint Surg Br 93-B:593–600

Lachiewicz PF, Soileau ES (2006) Dislocation of primary total hip arthroplasty with 36 and 40-mm femoral heads. Clin Orthop Relat Res 453:153–135

Lachiewicz PF, Heckman DS, Soileau ES, Mangla J, Martell JM (2009) Femoral head size and wear of highly cross-linked polyethylene at 5 to 8 years. Clin Orthop Rel Res 467:3290–3296

Learmonth ID, Young C, Rorabeck C (2007) The operation of the century: total hip replacement. Lancet 370(9597):1508–1519

Livermore J, Ilstrup D, Morrey B (1990) Effect of femoral head size on wear of the polyethylene acetabular component. J Bone Joint Surg Am 72-A:518–528

Martell JM, Berdia S (1997) Determination of polyethylene wear in total hip replacements with use of digital radiographs. J Bone Joint Surg Am 79-A:1635–1641

McKellop H, Shen FW, Lu B, Campbell P, Salovey R (1999) Development of an extremely wear-resistant ultrahigh molecular weight polyethylene for total hip replacement. J Orthop Res 17:157–162

Muratoglu OK, Bragdon CR, O'Connor DO, Jasty M, Harris WH (2001) A novel method of cross-linking UHMWPE to improve wear, reduce oxidation, and retain mechanical properties. J Arthroplasty 16:149–160

Oparaugo PC, Clarke IC, Malchau H, Herberts P (2001) Correlation of wear debris-induced osteolysis and revision with volumetric wear-rates of polyethylene: a survey of 8 reports in literature. Acta Orthop 72:22–28

Oral E, Malhi A, Muratoglu O (2006) Mechanisms of decrease in fatigue crack propagation resistance in irradiated and melted UHMWPE. Biomaterials 27:917–925

Sariali E, Lazennec JY, Khiami F, Catonné Y (2009) Mathematical evaluation of jumping distance in total hip arthroplasty: influence of abduction angle, femoral head offset, and head diameter. Acta Orthop 80:277–282

Shen FW, Lu Z, Mc Kellop HA (2011) Wear versus thickness and other features of 5-Mrad cross-linked UHMWPE acetabular liners. Clin Orthop Relat Res 469:395–404

Sychterz CJ, Engh CA Jr, Yang A, Engh CA (1999) Analysis of temporal wear pattern of porous-coated acetabular components: distinguishing between true wear and so-called bedding-in. J Bone Joint Surg Am 81-A:821–830

Tower SS, Currier JH, Currier BH, Lyford KA, Van Citters DW, Mayor MB (2007) Rim cracking of the cross-linked longevity polyethylene acetabular liner after total hip arthroplasty. J Bone Joint Surg Am 89:2212–2217

Wan Z, Boutary M, Dorr LD (2006) Precision and limitation of measuring two-dimensional wear on clinical radiographs. Clin Orthop Relat Res 449:267–274

Young AM, Sychterz CJ, Hopper RH Jr, Engh CA (2002) Effect of acetabular modularity on polyethylene wear and osteolysis in total hip arthroplasty. J Bone Joint Surg Am 84-A:58–63

The Influence of Head Material on Polyethylene Wear

10

Ibrahim J. Raphael, Javad Parvizi, and Richard H. Rothman

10.1   Introduction

More than a century ago, remarkable physicians and innovators, from Themistocles Gluck to Austin Moore to Sir John Charnley, have made essential contributions to the development of hip arthroplasty procedures. Sir Charnley first introduced his modern low-friction hip prosthesis model in the early 1960s. The idea behind this concept was not only to use a small femoral head to decrease friction and therefore wear but also to allow the lubrication of bearing surfaces by native synovial fluid. Ever since, much research and effort have been invested in the fields of tribology and physics and have led to numerous improvements that make hip arthroplasty the success it is today.

In tripartite hip prostheses, the choice of adequate bearing surfaces is unique to a patient's body habitus, activity level, and physician preference. It is a decision that is made before as well as during surgery. Different combinations of metal alloys, ceramics, and plastic have been tried, and historically, some have fared much better than others. The time to failure or implant survivorship, be it due to wear, osteolysis, or prosthesis loosening, allows physicians as well as authorities to make educated decisions concerning the type of implant to be used. In a recent study, data from the National Joint Registry of England and Wales showed failure rates of 6.2 % for metal-on-metal bearings compared to 1.7 and 2.3 % for metal-on-plastic and ceramic-on-ceramic, respectively (Charnley 1961). Studying the wear properties and behavior of different materials is aimed at providing a functional and lasting prosthesis. Relatively newer combinations, more specifically ceramic heads against highly cross-linked polyethylene (HXLPE) liners look promising.

I.J. Raphael, MD (✉) • J. Parvizi, MD, FRCS • R.H. Rothman, MD, PhD
Orthopaedic Surgery Joints Division,
The Rothman Institute,
5th Floor, 925 Chestnut Street,
Philadelphia, PA 19107
e-mail: ibrahim.j.raphael@gmail.com; parvj@aol.com

K. Knahr (ed.), *Total Hip Arthroplasty*,
DOI 10.1007/978-3-642-35653-7_10, © EFORT 2013

Ceramic materials such as alumina and zirconia are nonmetallic materials made from compounds of a metal and a nonmetal. These have exceptional properties that make it an excellent implantable, permanent biomaterial. Ceramic is chemically inert; it is insusceptible to naturally occurring free radical oxidation (Smith et al. 2012). It is also extremely hard; alumina has a hardness value of around 16 gigapascals (GPa), much higher than that of cobalt-chrome (5 GPa). It is wettable, a property that allows for better lubrication diminishing friction and adhesion (Smith et al. 2012). Ceramic has minimal surface roughness; its small grain size gives it a very smooth surface, even at a microscopic scale (Smith et al. 2012). This smoothness provides better gliding and prevents debris formation and third-body wear.

HXLPE is an alternative bearing surface that was developed in an effort to achieve better implant longevity. In vitro studies have shown HXLPE liners to be better resistant to wear when compared to conventional polyethylene (Hermida et al. 2003; Muratoglu et al. 2001). Cross-linking of polyethylene is achieved by subjecting it to high doses of ionizing irradiation using gamma or electron beams followed by annealing (Rimnac and Pruitt 2008). The disadvantage of this process is the residual potential for in vivo oxidation from retained free radicals (Rimnac and Pruitt 2008; Premnath et al. 1996). In second-generation HXLPE, sterilization is achieved using sequential irradiation and annealing cycles (Dumbleton et al. 2006), some also use vitamin E stabilization to decrease the risk of future oxidation (Oral et al. 2006). A 2006 study reported a 97 and 62 % decrease in in vitro wear rates using second-generation HXLPE when compared to conventional and first-generation cross-linked polyethylene, respectively (Dumbleton et al. 2006).

Polyethylene wear debris cause osteolysis leading to aseptic loosening and eventual failure needing revision hip surgery (Amstutz et al. 1992; Devane et al. 1997; Clohisy et al. 2004; Maloney et al. 1999; Oparaugo et al. 2001; Harris 1995). Synthetic polymers such as HXLPE liners and ceramic femoral heads are reported to effectively reduce wear rates and extend implant longevity. Despite their popularity, very few studies evaluate their in vivo performance. The purpose of our study is to show that the use of ceramic femoral heads leads to a reduction of in vivo wear by around 30 % when compared to metal femoral heads against the same HXLPE acetabular component.

10.2   Materials and Methods

An Institutional Review Board (IRB) approval was initially obtained for this multi-center, retrospective study. Three institutions were involved in this project: the Rothman Institute (RI) in Philadelphia, PA, USA; the Jewish Hospital & St. Mary's HealthCare (JHSMH) in Louisville, KY, USA; and the Hospital for Special Surgery (HSS) in New York, NY, USA. A common protocol was initially drafted and followed by all parties involved.

In order to measure and reliably assess ceramic-on-polyethylene wear rate compared to metal femoral heads, we investigated the radiographic data of two main groups of patients. The target number of patients needed in the study was determined by a preliminary power analysis. The first group would consist of 250 Biolox Delta™

Table 10.1 Population demographics

	N (x-rays)	Age (years)	Head size (mm)	Follow-up (years)	Lat. cup axis angle	AP cup rotational angle
Ceramic-Crossfire™	40	63	29.6	4.5	41.0°	20.3°
Metal-Crossfire™	85	66	29.8	4.7	45.5°	16.1°
p-value	–	0.69	0.57	0.38	*0.0005*	*0.004*
Ceramic-X3™	102	59	32.6	3.8	43.1°	18.4°
Metal-X3™	171	69	33.0	3.6	44.9°	17.7°
p-value	–	*<0.0001*	0.14	0.33	0.11	0.46

(CeramTec AG, Plochingen, Germany) ceramic femoral heads articulating on X3™ (Stryker Orthopaedics, Mahwah, NJ), a second-generation HXLPE (Co2), and 250 metal femoral heads articulating on X3™ (Mo2). The second major group included 75 Biolox Delta™ ceramic femoral heads on Crossfire™ (Stryker Orthopaedics, Mahwah, NJ), a first-generation HXLPE (Co1), and 75 metal femoral heads articulating on Crossfire™ (Mo1). For patients in the X3™ group, we decided to obtain an average follow-up of 4 years. For patients who received the earlier Crossfire™ liner, we aimed for an average follow-up period of 6 years. However, at this point in time, our target sample size has not yet been reached; we present the results of our analysis on a small subset of our final patient population (Table 10.1).

We conducted a manual search in our electronic database to find available serial patient x-ray images. We looked for adequate anteroposterior (AP) pelvis radiographs taken 6 months to 1 year following primary total hip arthroplasty (THA) to account for the bedding-in period. Patients were also required to have at least another AP pelvis x-ray 4 or 6 years after index surgery. Thus, a minimum of two radiographs per patient was needed. When available, we also included any image taken between the first and last x-ray. Physical images were scanned at 300 dpi (dots per inch) and saved in the DICOM (Digital Imaging and Communications in Medicine) or TIFF (Tagged Image File Format) format. These formats are the only formats compatible with the analysis software employed. Images taken from our electronic database were directly saved as DICOM or TIFF files. All images were anonymized and labeled, and copies were securely sent to Dr. John Martell at the Weiss Memorial Hospital in Chicago, IL, USA, for analysis.

Radiographic analysis was done using the Hip Analysis Suite (HAS) version 8.0.4.0 (University of Chicago, Chicago, IL, USA). This computer-assisted edge detection method of wear measurement has been validated (Hui et al. 2003; Martell and Berdia 1997) and used repeatedly in the orthopedic literature (Garvin et al. 2008; Lachiewicz et al. 2009; Martell et al. 2003). The in vivo linear and volumetric wear rates were determined by measuring the two-dimensional change in femoral head penetration against a fixed acetabular component between the last and first x-rays. On an AP radiograph, a line connecting the two lowest points of the right and left ischial tuberosities was traced to form our reference, horizontal plane. A circle encompassing the entire femoral head was carefully traced by manually placing three points along the edges of head (Fig. 10.1). Using a comparable technique, the edges of the acetabular cup were subsequently defined. Head and cup

Fig. 10.1 Femoral head
delineation using the HAS
software

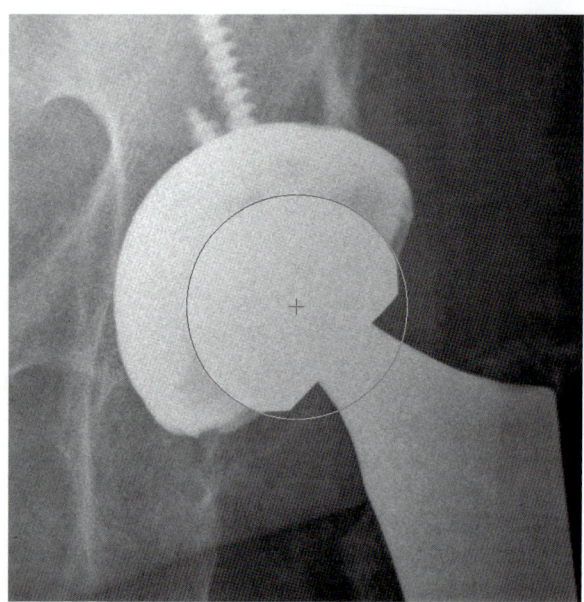

Fig. 10.2 Hip Analysis Suite
uses edge detection method

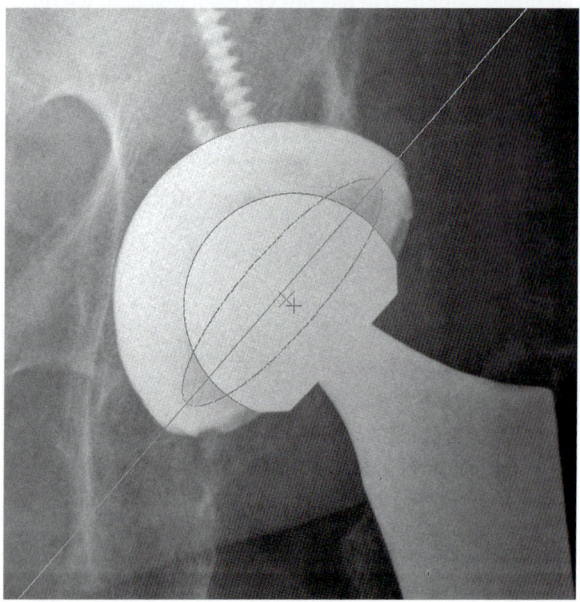

sizes were manually entered in the system. By detecting the centers of the femoral
head and the acetabular cup, the direction and magnitude of the head displacement
vector was estimated (Fig. 10.2). Cup rotation and inclination were automatically
detected. All measurements will eventually be done by two trained physicians in
order to account for interobserver reliability. One of the two physicians will also
repeat the analysis, allowing for the determination of intraobserver reliability.

Table 10.2 True linear wear rates of different bearing combinations

	Crossfire™	X3™	p-value
Ceramic	0.075 mm/year (SD=0.324)	0.075 mm/year (SD=0.324)	0.990
Metal	0.125 mm/year (SD=0.335)	0.105 mm/year (SD=0.242)	0.808
p-value	0.729	0.644	–

In addition to details of the articulating surfaces and sizes, we gathered data about age, gender, BMI, activity level (UCLA score), laterality, and date of surgery for each patient. Each patient enrolled received a unique label. A list associating labels to patient names and medical record numbers was kept as a reference with one of the authors. At the time this article was drafted, our study population included 95 patients (273 x-rays) in the X3™ group and 39 patients (125 x-rays) in the Crossfire™ group (Table 10.1). Patients are still being added to the cohort. Patients enrolled received an American Express™ gift card as a token of appreciation for participating in the study and as reimbursement for travel expenses. This strategy contributes to a steady increase in the number of patients joining the study.

10.3   Results

As previously mentioned, our total sample size consisted of 134 patients (398 images), still far from our target total number of 650 patients. There was no statistical difference in the average head sizes used in the four groups (Table 10.1). The average age for patients in group Co2 was 59 years of age and 69 years for those in the Mo2 group (Table 10.1). We found the difference in age to be statistically significant within the X3™ group ($p < 0.001$). We also reported the mean cup axis and rotational angles (Table 10.1). The true linear wear, which excludes the bedding-in period, for all four groups can be found in Table 10.2.

10.4   Discussion

Wear is the loss of surface material usually due to friction, abrasion, or erosion that occurs between two surfaces in relative motion. In THA, tribology is the science that measures the interaction of implant-bearing surfaces, notably the acetabular cup liner and femoral head. Tribology plays a fundamental role in the success of arthroplasty. We are continuously attempting to improve implant survivorship by making it more impervious to the unforgiving mechanical and biochemical stresses the human body inflicts. Instability/dislocation, aseptic loosening, and infection are the three most common causes for revision surgery following primary THA (Bozic et al. 2009; Jafari et al. 2010). Liner wear can lead to osteolysis and subsequent loosening; it could also be an independent reason for revision (Yamauchi et al. 2001; Bozic et al. 2009; Jafari et al. 2010; Sundfeldt et al. 2006). Dowd et al. report that osteolysis is inevitable with wear rates greater than 0.3 mm/year; this risk becomes negligible with rates smaller than 0.1 mm/year (Dowd et al. 2000).

Since its FDA approval in 1998, HXLPE has become a frequently used alternative bearing surface in THA (McKellop et al. 1999). Biomaterial science and modern manufacturing have made tremendous progress in terms of maximizing polyethylene durability. Several papers in the literature evaluate the wear rates of different forms of polyethylene liners. First-generation HXLPE liners are reported to have up to 72 % reduction in wear when compared to earlier conventional polyethylene (Lachiewicz et al. 2009; Martell et al. 2003; D'Antonio et al. 2005; Digas et al. 2004; Kurtz et al. 2011; Lee et al. 2011; Orradre Burusco et al. 2011; Ranawat et al. 2012; Thomas et al. 2011). In contrast, because it is relatively new, fewer studies assess second-generation HXLPE liner wear rates. In a prospective study by D'Antonio et al., the wear rate of X3™ liners was reported to be 0.015 mm/year, a 58 % decrease in wear rate compared to Crossfire™ liners (0.036 mm/year) (D'Antonio et al. 2012). By sequential irradiation and annealing, second-generation liners have been developed in an effort to reduce liner fractures and in vivo oxidation, two major defects of their antecedents (Dumbleton et al. 2006).

This study is unique in that it simultaneously evaluates the in vivo wear of first- and second-generation HXLPE liners. Contrary to other studies, we do not rely on previously reported wear values in the medical literature as our control population. The rates we obtained are slightly different to the values reported in the literature; however, we believe this number will be more reliable once patient collection is complete. We observed a wear reduction of 40 % with Crossfire™ and 28 % with X3™ liners. With both liners, wear rates were more pronounced with metal (cobalt-chrome alloy) femoral heads.

Large-diameter femoral heads decrease the risk of dislocation and impingement and allow for a greater range of motion in the hip joint (Burroughs et al. 2005; Berry et al. 2005). It is still unclear whether femoral head size contributes to the degree of polyethylene wear. In some studies, larger femoral heads have been found to have a higher wear rate than smaller heads (Kesteris et al. 1996; Livermore et al. 1990; Tarasevicius et al. 2008; Kabo et al. 1993); in others, no clear difference could be detected (Lachiewicz et al. 2009; Bragdon et al. 2007).

According to the Nationwide Inpatient Sample (NIS) data, more than 200,000 THA were performed in the USA in 2005 (Kurtz et al. 2007). Kurtz et al. project that the demand for THA will exceed half a million surgeries in 2030, a 174 % increase compared with the year 2005 (Kurtz et al. 2007). The hip revision burden is expected to reach 14.5 % in 2030 (Kurtz et al. 2007). As the demand for arthroplasty increases, the absolute number of revisions is bound to rise. Innovative ways to increase implant survivorship are needed, possibly by developing more stable and resistant alternative bearing surfaces.

References

Amstutz HC, Campbell P, Kossovsky N, Clarke IC (1992) Mechanism and clinical significance of wear debris-induced osteolysis. Clin Orthop 276:7–18

Berry DJ, von Knoch M, Schleck CD, Harmsen WS (2005) Effect of femoral head diameter and operative approach on risk of dislocation after primary total hip arthroplasty. J Bone Joint Surg Am 87(11):2456–2463

Bozic KJ, Kurtz SM, Lau E et al (2009) The epidemiology of revision total hip arthroplasty in the United States. J Bone Joint Surg Am 91(1):128–133

Bragdon CR, Greene ME, Freiberg AA, Harris WH, Malchau H (2007) Radiostereometric analysis comparison of wear of highly cross-linked polyethylene against 36- vs 28-mm femoral heads. J Arthroplasty 22(6 Suppl 2):125–129

Burroughs BR, Hallstrom B, Golladay GJ, Hoeffel D, Harris WH (2005) Range of motion and stability in total hip arthroplasty with 28-, 32-, 38-, and 44-mm femoral head sizes. J Arthroplasty 20(1):11–19

Charnley J (1961) Arthroplasty of the hip. A new operation. Lancet 1(7187):1129–1132

Clohisy JC, Calvert G, Tull F, McDonald D, Maloney WJ (2004) Reasons for revision hip surgery: a retrospective review. Clin Orthop Relat Res 429:188–192

D'Antonio JA, Manley MT, Capello WN et al (2005) Five-year experience with Crossfire highly cross-linked polyethylene. Clin Orthop Relat Res 441:143–150

D'Antonio JA, Capello WN, Ramakrishnan R (2012) Second-generation annealed highly cross-linked polyethylene exhibits low wear. Clin Orthop Relat Res 470(6):1696–1704

Devane PA, Robinson EJ, Bourne RB et al (1997) Measurement of polyethylene wear in acetabular components inserted with and without cement. A randomized trial. J Bone Joint Surg 79A:682–689

Digas G, Kärrholm J, Thanner J, Malchau H, Herberts P (2004) The Otto Aufranc Award. Highly cross-linked polyethylene in total hip arthroplasty: randomized evaluation of penetration rate in cemented and uncemented sockets using radiostereometric analysis. Clin Orthop Relat Res 429:6–16

Dowd JE, Sychterz CJ, Young AM, Engh CA (2000) Characterization of long-term femoral-head-penetration rates: association with and prediction of osteolysis. J Bone Joint Surg Am 82:1102–1107

Dumbleton JH, D'Antonio JA, Manley MT, Capello WN, Wang A (2006) The basis for a second-generation highly cross-linked UHMWPE. Clin Orthop Relat Res 453:265–271

Garvin KL, Hartman CW, Mangla J, Murdoch N, Martell JM (2008) Wear analysis in THA utilizing oxidized zirconium and crosslinked polyethylene. Clin Orthop Relat Res 467(1):141–145

Harris W (1995) The problem is osteolysis. Clin Orthop Relat Res 311:46–53

Hermida JC, Bergula A, Chen P, Colwell CW Jr, D'Lima DD (2003) Comparison of the wear rates of twenty-eight and thirty-two-millimeter femoral heads on cross-linked polyethylene acetabular cups in a wear simulator. J Bone Joint Surg Am 85-A(12):2325–2331

Hui AJ, McCalden RW, Martell JM et al (2003) Validation of two and three-dimensional radiographic techniques for measuring polyethylene wear after total hip arthroplasty. J Bone Joint Surg Am 85-A(3):505–511

Jafari SM, Coyle C, Mortazavi SMJ, Sharkey PF, Parvizi J (2010) Revision hip arthroplasty: infection is the most common cause of failure. Clin Orthop Relat Res 468(8):2046–2051

Kabo JM, Gebhard JS, Loren G, Amstutz HC (1993) In vivo wear of polyethylene acetabular components. J Bone Joint Surg Br 75(2):254–258

Kesteris U, Ilchmann T, Wingstrand H, Onnerfalt R (1996) Polyethylene wear in Scanhip arthroplasty with a 22 or 32 mm head: 62 matched patients followed for 7–9 years. Acta Orthop Scand 67(2):125–127

Kurtz S, Ong K, Lau E, Mowat F, Halpern M (2007) Projections of primary and revision hip and knee arthroplasty in the United States from 2005 to 2030. J Bone Joint Surg Am 89(4):780–785

Kurtz SM, Gawel HA, Patel JD (2011) History and systematic review of wear and osteolysis outcomes for first-generation highly crosslinked polyethylene. Clin Orthop Relat Res 469(8):2262–2277

Lachiewicz PF, Heckman DS, Soileau ES, Mangla J, Martell JM (2009) Femoral head size and wear of highly cross-linked polyethylene at 5 to 8 years. Clin Orthop Relat Res 467(12):3290–3296

Lee J-H, Lee BW, Lee B-J, Kim S-Y (2011) Midterm results of primary total hip arthroplasty using highly cross-linked polyethylene: minimum 7-year follow-up study. J Arthroplasty 26(7):1014–1019

Livermore J, Ilstrup D, Morrey B (1990) Effect of femoral head size on wear of the polyethylene acetabular component. J Bone Joint Surg Am 72(4):518–528

Maloney WJ, Galante JO, Anderson M, Goldberg V, Harris WH, Jacobs J, Kraay M, Lachiewicz P, Rubash HE, Schutzer S, Woolson ST (1999) Fixation, polyethylene wear, and pelvic osteolysis in primary total hip replacement. Clin Orthop Relat Res 369:157–164

Martell JM, Berdia S (1997) Determination of polyethylene wear in total hip replacements with use of digital radiographs. J Bone Joint Surg Am 79(11):1635–1641

Martell JM, Verner JJ, Incavo SJ (2003) Clinical performance of a highly cross-linked polyethylene at two years in total hip arthroplasty: a randomized prospective trial. J Arthroplasty 18(Supplement(0)):55–59

McKellop H, Shen FW, Lu B, Campbell P, Salovey R (1999) Development of an extremely wear-resistant ultra high molecular weight polyethylene for total hip replacements. J Orthop Res 17:157–167

Muratoglu OK, Bragdon CR, O'Connor DO, Jasty M, Harris WH (2001) A novel method of cross-linking ultra-high-molecular-weight polyethylene to improve wear, reduce oxidation, and retain mechanical properties. Recipient of the 1999 HAP Paul Award. J Arthroplasty 16(2):149–160

Oparaugo PC, Clarke IC, Malchau H et al (2001) Correlation of wear debris-induced osteolysis and revision with volumetric wear-rates of polyethylene: a survey of 8 reports in the literature. Acta Orthop Scand 72:22–28

Oral E, Christensen SD, Malhi AS, Wannomae KK, Muratoglu OK (2006) Wear resistance and mechanical properties of highly cross-linked, ultrahigh–molecular weight polyethylene doped with vitamin E. J Arthroplasty 21(4):580–591

Orradre Burusco I, Romero R, Brun M, López Blasco JJ (2011) Cross-linked ultra-high-molecular weight polyethylene liner and ceramic femoral head in total hip arthroplasty: a prospective study at 5 years follow-up. Arch Orthop Trauma Surg 131(12):1711–1716

Premnath V, Harris WH, Jasty M, Merrill EW (1996) Gamma sterilization of UHMWPE articular implants: an analysis of the oxidation problem. Ultra High Molecular Weight Poly Ethylene. Biomaterials 17(18):1741–1753

Ranawat AS, Tsailis P, Meftah M et al (2012) Minimum 5-year wear analysis of first-generation highly cross-linked polyethylene in patients 65 years and younger. J Arthroplasty 27(3):354–357

Rimnac C, Pruitt L (2008) How do material properties influence wear and fracture mechanisms? J Am Acad Orthop Surg 16(Suppl 1):S94–S100

Smith AJ, Dieppe P, Vernon K, Porter M, Blom AW (2012) Failure rates of stemmed metal-on-metal hip replacements: analysis of data from the National Joint Registry of England and Wales. Lancet. doi:10.1016/S0140-6736(12)60353-5

Sundfeldt M, Carlsson LV, Johansson CB, Thomsen P, Gretzer C (2006) Aseptic loosening, not only a question of wear: a review of different theories. Acta Orthop 77(2):177–197

Tarasevicius S, Robertsson O, Kesteris U, Kalesinskas RJ, Wingstrand H (2008) Effect of femoral head size on polyethylene wear and synovitis after total hip arthroplasty: a sonographic and radiographic study of 39 patients. Acta Orthop 79(4):489–493

Thomas GER, Simpson DJ, Mehmood S et al (2011) The seven-year wear of highly cross-linked polyethylene in total hip arthroplasty: a double-blind, randomized controlled trial using radiostereometric analysis. J Bone Joint Surg Am 93(8):716–722

Yamauchi K, Hasegawa Y, Iwasada S et al (2001) Head penetration into Hylamer acetabular liner sterilized by gamma irradiation in air and in a nitrogen atmosphere. J Arthroplasty 16(4):463–470

Basic Science and Longtime Results of Different Polyethylene Articulations

11

Stephan M. Röhrl and Robert M. Streicher

11.1 Background

Today polyethylene is the most commonly used bearing surface in hip prostheses. After discouraging attempts with prostheses with polytetrafluoroethylene (Teflon), John Charnley used ultra-high-molecular-weight polyethylene (UHMWPE) with cement as fixation, starting in 1962. Up until recently, with small modifications only, identical material has been used in total hip arthroplasty. PE can be found in everyday life, for instance, cutting boards and gliding surfaces of skis and snowmobiles because of low wear and excellent gliding qualities.

UHMWPE is an outstanding material for orthopaedic applications with excellent abrasion resistance, low coefficient of friction, high-impact resistance, self-lubricating surface, negligible water absorption, good chemical resistance, energy absorption and sound damping properties. These properties are maintained in the temperature range between −269 and 90 °C (Stein 1999).

11.1.1 Modifications and Failures

However, modifications of the original polyethylene may change its mechanical properties to either enhanced or deteriorated clinical performance. Many attempts to improve the qualities of UHMWPE have been made in the past. The evolution of

S.M. Röhrl, MD, PhD (✉)
Department of Surgery and Neurosciences, Oslo University Hospital,
Orthopaedic, Ullevål, Kirkeveien 166, N-0407 Oslo, Norway
e-mail: s.m.rohrl@medisin.uio.no

R.M. Streicher, PhD
Dr. Streicher GmbH, Leutschenstrassse 41, Freienbach, Switzerland
e-mail: robert@dr-streicher.com

K. Knahr (ed.), *Total Hip Arthroplasty*,
DOI 10.1007/978-3-642-35653-7_11, © EFORT 2013

Table 11.1 Evolution of UHMWPE for joint implants

Method/technology	Name/example	Reported year of introduction
Conventional PE		
UHMWPE	RCH-100, Chirulen	1962
Gamma irradiation sterilisation (air)		1968
Carbon fibre reinforcement	Poly 2	1970
Pioneer highly cross-linked PE		
Non-stabilised highly cross-linked		1972–1978
Modern PE		
Higher purity, better consolidation, manufacturing in clean room	Medical grade	1985
Quality without Ca stearate	GUR 402/405	1985
Gamma sterilisation in inert gas	Sulene	1986
High-pressure remelted	Hylamer, Hylamer M	1987
Surface heat polishing	PCA	1989
Gamma inert gas sterilisation/annealing	Duration	1996
Highly cross-linked PE		
First-generation highly cross-linked, annealed	Crossfire	1998
First-generation highly cross-linked, remelted	Durasul, Longevity, Marathon	1999–2001
Second-generation sequentially highly cross-linked, annealed	X3	2005
Second-generation vitamin E-doped highly cross-linked, annealed	E1	2007

PE in orthopaedics is shown in Table 11.1. Some material modifications have proven to be clinical failures. Carbon fibre reinforcement intended to give better strength and a lower wear rate. The experimental results with the so-called Poly 2 were promising (Fruh and Willmann 1998). But the in vivo results were devastating (Kilgus et al. 1992). It appeared that fatigue strength was lower than in normal UHMWPE resulting in delamination and clinical failures (Korkala and Syrjanen 1998). Hylamer was another attempt to improve UHMWPE. Through high pressure and temperature, the crystallinity was increased, and material properties were enhanced, confirmed by in vitro studies. Thousands of prostheses were implanted worldwide without a randomised clinical study performed verifying the in vivo performance. Hylamer implants show high failure rates because of increased wear in clinical series (Scott et al. 2000; Sychterz et al. 2000), probably due to its reduced toughness and the influence of irradiation sterilisation. Another attempt to improve UHMWPE was heat pressing the surface to reduce its roughness, but already after 4 years the inserts showed extreme delamination (Bloebaum et al. 1991).

11.1.2 Technical Advances: Between Assumptions and Facts

Engineers around the world try to simulate biological conditions in laboratory experiments; however, the biological processes are so complex that even excellent experimental data cannot guarantee corresponding clinical results. Still new materials pass the strict regulations of, for example, FDA, CE, TÜV, and ASTM and are declared safe for in vivo use. Changes often address a certain problem in earlier versions such as fixation or wear. The new implants conquer the market with promises to improve longevity and function for the patient.

However, doctors with only the best intentions for their patients are stuck in an *inevitable dilemma between the possible benefits of improved implants and the fact that they lack clinical evidence.* You cannot use the newest technology and at the same time have longtime documentation. It is therefore of imminent importance to introduce new materials and technology under controlled conditions (Malchau 2000; Nelissen et al. 2011).

11.2   What Methods to Look At?

Hip arthroplasty is a well-documented procedure. The search term "longtime results", however, reduces the number of available articles to roughly above 100. Most articles are from retrospective cohorts and only few are designed as prospective study and provide longtime follow-up (Bruzzone et al. 2009). Nevertheless, it is shown that implant wear leads through a biological reaction to aseptic loosening (Sochart 1999); hence, wear is accepted as an indicator for longtime performance. As regards precision and accuracy for wear measurements, radiostereometry is the golden standard (Borlin et al. 2006; Valstar et al. 2005). The final answer about clinical in vivo performance however is given by large numbers of patients operated by different surgeons. Respective data can be obtained by registries as they are common in the Scandinavian countries and meanwhile also in many other countries (New Zealand, Australia, England and many more). One of the disadvantages with registry data is that the data lags behind. This has in recent years become evident by the metal-on-metal (MoM) bearing issue worldwide. The early warning signs from the Australian registry (Buergi and Walter 2007) came after thousands of patients already had received this implant. Still, registry data offers survival data on implants in a high number of patients, confounders are eliminated, and they have a hard end point (Ranstam and Robertsson 2010).

With regard to the definition of longtime data, the authors performed an arbitrary decision. Up to 2 years data is considered as short-term, 2–9 years as midterm, and 10 years and longer as long-term data.

11.3 What Articulations Are There?

An articulation of an artificial hip joint essentially consists of the acetabular side and the head on the femoral stem. Each side has gone through changes during the meanwhile 60-year-old success story of Sir John Charnley – the inventor of the low-friction hip arthroplasty (Charnley and Halley 1975; Learmonth et al. 2007).

11.3.1 Polyethylene

PE is a linear homopolymer consisting of repeating $-CH_2-$ units with very long and entangled molecular chains. Table 11.1 outlines the major chronological PE families. It is a biphasic polymer consisting of crystalline domains in an amorphous matrix. The unique arrangement of ultra-high-molecular-weight PE with chains to be randomly part of crystallites, responsible for strength and stiffness; the amorphous matrix, responsible for toughness; and the entanglements, acting as pseudo-cross-links, result in the specific properties of this type of PE. The strong chemical intramolecular bonding and the weak physical intermolecular bonding of the PE molecules make PE sensitive to out of plane cross-shear motion, which is the normal kinematics in the hip joint and to a certain extent in the knee joint (TKR), especially in deeper flexion.

The particle of the powder determines the so-called resin. GUR 1050 is the most commonly used resin for orthopaedic implants today. The initial step in processing implants of PE can be in two different ways. Compression moulding includes discontinuously pressing the powder under temperatures over the melting point into sheets. Ram extrusion stands for continuously pressing and heating the powder into cylindrical bars. Both semi-fabricates are then machined into the final implant component. Ram extrusion is currently the most common way of fabrication. The main impact on wear and performance has been attributed to the sterilisation and cross-linking process (McKellop et al. 1999).

11.3.2 Sterilisation of Implants

Chemical disinfection was used for PE acetabular components in the early 1960s due to its thermolabile structure, and by the late 1960s gamma sterilisation to nominal 25 kGy was routinely used. This enabled the components to be sterilised in packaged form. Gamma sterilisation in air containing packaging was the predominant method of sterilisation until the early 1980s, when questions arose regarding oxidation of components due to the reaction between oxygen and free radicals created during radiation sterilisation. Molecular changes are induced during irradiation sterilisation causing chain scission, cross-linking and oxidation, depending on the absorbed dose and the atmosphere in which irradiation takes place. In 1986 the environment for gamma sterilisation of UHMWPE implant components was changed from ambient air to inert gas (Sulene®, Sulzer) or sterilisation with ethylene

Table 11.2 Hip simulator wear rates for UHMWPE following irradiation

Radiation dose (kGy)	Wear rate (mm³/million cycles)
0	140
30	50
50	30
75	10
100	5

oxide (EtO) (Reflection, Smith & Nephew). The former was the first attempt to use the energy of the irradiation sterilisation treatment for intentionally cross-linking of the PE and showed an in vitro reduction in wear rate of 30 % and reduced dramatic fatigue and delamination wear of TKR. This sterilisation method was adapted only after 1991 in the USA, and most major implant manufacturers introduced their variation of this method since then. The latter was an attempt to preserve the excellent mechanical properties of UHMWPE. Additional stabilisation of UHMWPE components by a thermal method after sterilisation was introduced in 1996 (Duration®, Howmedica).

11.3.3 Cross-Linked Polyethylene

HXLPE is already in clinical use since 1976 and has shown in anecdotal reports superior wear resistance. Pioneers such as Oonishi, Grobbelar (Grobbelaar et al. 1978) and Wroblewski tried to enhance wear behaviour by cross-linking polyethylene by different means. Extended cross-linking is accomplished by gamma or electron-beam irradiation of PE bars or sheets with cumulating irradiation doses. As the radiation dose is increased, the wear resistance is increased (Table 11.2) until an asymptote is reached at about 100 kGy absorbed.

Further increase in irradiation does not show any benefit in wear reduction, while the mechanical properties, especially the toughness of HXLPE, degrade. A subsequent process, either annealing (below the melt temperature) or remelting (above the melt temperature), can reduce or eliminate free radicals from the high-energy irradiation process that might else induce oxidation of HXLPE in the long term. This is then followed by a final machining, packaging and sterilisation process. The sterilisation is generally performed by gas or gas-plasma or conventional gamma sterilisation in inert environment.

11.3.3.1 Wear
HXLPE demonstrates a dramatic reduction in wear in simulator testing compared to conventionally produced and in inert environment irradiation-sterilised PE components, and laboratory data from various research groups and institutes have shown a reduction in wear of 90 % more or less (Wang et al. 2003). The amount of particles is dramatically reduced, but their size and morphology for some of the HXLPEs are not altered, an important aspect for any histiocytic response. Moreover, independent studies have shown HXLPE to be more resistant to wear, even after accelerated

ageing or when exposed to foreign body debris. This generation of HXLPE has been widely used in clinical practice for THR but also with restrictions for TKR components.

Simulator studies have also shown that due to the direction independence of the HXLPEs in contrary to non-cross-linked PE the wear of artificial hip joints becomes independent on the head size and thickness of the cup/insert components (Herrera et al. 2007). This in consequence may allow the use of larger heads and thinner components, which address anatomical situation and increasing dislocation and subluxation incidences, being a major course for early failure of THRs. A larger head will also increase the ROM and consequently reduce implant/implant impingement. Studies have also shown an enhanced stability sensation with such restored hip joint and consequently enhanced patient satisfaction. Studies, which were conducted to confirm the theoretical advantages of the cross-linking, have been conducted by producing various cup inserts made from HXLPE and machining various internal diameters into cups of various outer diameters. The resulting PE thickness ranged from 1.8 to 7.9 mm, and the inserts were tested up to five million cycles at various inclination angels in standard hip joint simulators (Streicher and Thomsen 2003). Similar tests with similar components have been conducted in other laboratories with deviating test protocols (Kelly et al. 2010). All laboratory results confirm that this HXLPE produces similar low wear rates independent on head size and liner thickness even in impingement mode.

11.3.3.2 Mechanical Integrity

Despite the well-documented advantages of cross-linking and subsequent thermal processes for achieving a dramatic wear reduction, other issues with this category of polymers have been demonstrated or raised. In general changes in its morphology will compromise the mechanical behaviour of HXLPEs, such as ductility and toughness. While in the irradiation source, if ^{60}Co or electron beam has shown no different effect, the post-irradiation treatment definitely has. Annealing affects the toughness and mechanical resistance to a much lesser extent than remelting, as the PE microstructure is modified to a lesser amount and, therefore, the relationship between crystalline and amorphous phases not changed while some clinical fractures of remelted liners have been reported (Tower et al. 2007; Waewsawangwong and Goodman 2012). Some post-treatments also affect the dimensions of the crystallites which are key for the mechanical response of the HXLPE. This reduction of the mechanical resistance has been addressed by several companies by either using lower irradiation doses for HXLPE for THR and TKR or only for TKR.

11.3.3.3 Oxidation

On the other hand, annealing does not eliminate the free radicals completely while remelting does. Although oxidation does not seem to be a limiting factor for THR in the midterm and also oxidising HXLPE (Willie et al. 2006) did not exhibit any implant failure until more than 10 years in vivo (Capello et al. 2011), there is concern about long-term results. Because oxidation of UHMWPE takes months or years to reach appreciable levels at ambient or body temperature, thermal ageing techniques have been developed to accelerate the oxidation of UHMWPE, with the expectation that the mechanical behaviour after accelerated ageing will be comparable to naturally aged material (Edidin et al. 2000). The mechanical behaviour of UHMWPE evolves during natural (shelf) ageing after gamma irradiation in air, but the kinetics and characteristics of mechanical degradation remain poorly understood, largely due to previous emphasis on indirect measurement techniques. Furthermore, while it is recognised that ageing at elevated temperatures will accelerate the oxidation of air-irradiated UHMWPE, the clinical relevance of such a thermally degraded material remains uncertain, particularly if fatigue or joint simulator testing is to be performed after ageing. This is even more so in view of the fact that THR does not exhibit increasing wear rates with time, nor is the wear rate well correlated with the shelf ageing time. Such an observation suggests that accelerated ageing of hip inserts may not reflect either the chemical or clinical pathway actually taken by such inserts, and recent results of oxidising remelted HXLPE support this (Duffy et al. 2009).

11.3.4 Femoral Heads

Also the femoral side offers a large diversity caused by different sizes and materials. Head sizes vary from 22 mm in early and up to 40 mm in the later years. With regard to head material, there are three groups. The first is metal heads represented by steel and CoCr, and the second is ceramic heads. The latter includes pure alumina or zirconia heads and newer ceramics, which are compound materials. The third group combines a hybrid material with a metal core and a ceramic-like surface (Oxinium, L-fit) (Kadar et al. 2012).

11.3.5 Complexity of Articulations

Considering that companies have separate manufacturing procedures, different virgin materials and quality assurance during the production process, it becomes obvious that options for an articulation are numerous and complex. This renders prediction about clinical performance almost impossible.

The lessons of the past are that in vitro results cannot be extrapolated uncritically to the in vivo performance of implants. To start, small well-controlled randomised in vivo studies are therefore needed before a new implant, after having passed through the laboratory tests, may be used on a big scale (Malchau 2000; Nelissen et al. 2011).

Finally, the articulation has to pass the *ultimate test: longtime performance in patients*. The next paragraph shows some longtime results for the major polyethylene families as long as there is in vivo data available. The results do not claim to be a comprehensive presentation of literature available but rather try to illustrate some lessons learned on the way.

Fig. 11.1 Kaplan-Meier survivorship curve with accompanying 95 % confidence intervals for the end point of revision for any reason and for the cup (Callaghan et al. 2009)

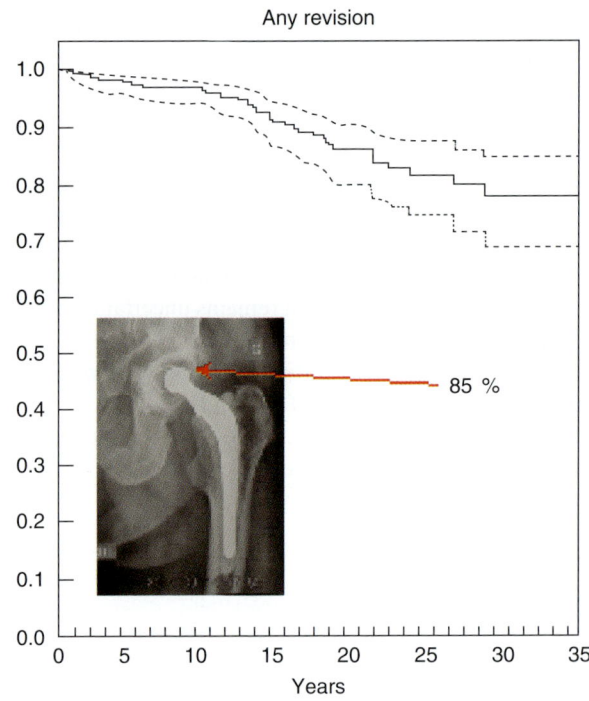

11.4   What Longtime Data Is There?

11.4.1 Conventional PE

The benchmark for all modern hip implants is of course the low-friction arthroplasty by Sir John Charnley with UHMWPE gamma sterilised in air and a 22-mm head. Callaghan (Callaghan et al. 2009) presented a follow-up at a minimum of 35 years of 262 patients (330 hips). Twelve patients (15 hips) were alive and one was lost to follow-up. Survivorship (and 95 % confidence interval) at 35 years was 78 % ± 8 % for any reason and 85 % ± 7 % because of aseptic acetabular loosening (Fig. 11.1).

Buckwalter measured in the earlier 30-year follow-up of the same cohort a wear rate of 0.13 mm annually (Buckwalter et al. 2006). Mean rate for revised components was 0.213 mm/year and 0.098 mm/year for stable ones. This is in accordance with Dumbleton who found in a meta-analysis that osteolysis is rarely observed at a wear rate of <0.1 mm/year. Dumbleton and his co-authors suggest that a practical wear rate threshold of 0.05 mm/year would eliminate the risk for osteolysis (Dumbleton et al. 2002). At a mean follow-up of 22 years (20–30), 94 % out of 320 arthroplasties in 261 patients considered the procedure with the original Charnley stem as successful (Wroblewski et al. 1999a).

Tarasevicius and colleagues followed a cohort of 1,720 cemented hip prosthesis (ScanHip) operated at Lund University Hospital in Sweden for 20 years. The cohort consisted of 308 patients with a 22-mm and 1,412 with a 32-mm CoCr head (Tarasevicius et al. 2006). They found a 3 times higher revision rate with 32-mm heads against conventional UHMWPE (sterilised in air). The wear rate was 0.18 mm/year for these cups. But another factor to consider is activity. Not only the time implanted also the use of the implants is decisive for wear and implant survival (Zahiri et al. 1998). Younger patients usually are more demanding and have a higher level of activity. In a cohort of 118 patients (144 hips) younger than 50 years, Teusig and colleagues measured a wear rate of 0.19 mm annually. This led to poor survival of only 60 % in the cementless pressfit cups after 10–18 years (Teusink et al. 2012).

In one of our own cohorts with 32-mm ceramic (alumina) heads against conventional UHMWPE in uncemented cups, we measured a wear rate of 0.1 mm/year (Rohrl et al. 2006). After 12 years all cups were stable but showed cystic osteolysis in relation to screw holes of the cup (Fig. 11.2).

One of the downsides with UHMWPE is that the material degrades over time when exposed to oxygen. On the shelf the cups are oxidised and lose their mechanical properties (Kurtz et al. 2005). In vivo the articulating surfaces of polyethylene components are exposed to joint fluid containing proteins, lipids, oxygen and free reactive oxygen radicals (Treuhaft and MCCarty 1971).

However, Kurtz and colleagues found in retrieved cups that the weight-bearing part of the inner diameter was not oxidised. The most severe oxidation was observed at the rim, suggesting that the femoral head inhibits access of oxygen-containing body fluids to the bearing surface (Kurtz et al. 2006). They speculate that this could be a reason why material degeneration is not seen as a clinical problem for hip joints up to date.

11.4.2 Modern PE

Modern UHMWPE aims to improve the preservation of mechanical properties by sterilisation in inert atmosphere or ethylene oxide. Concise longtime data is scarce because it is often not clear when manufacturers did switch to the new process during the 1990s of the last century. The Swedish hip registry compares the survival of cups from 1979 to 1991 (69,469 hips) to cups implanted in the period from 1992 to 2007 (125,110 hips) (Fig. 11.3). After 16 years they found a tendency to better performance of these newer cups with modern UHMWPE (Garellick et al. 2011).

Dahl et al. measured wear in 87 patients with cemented modern cups comparing 28-mm CoCr to ceramic heads. After 10 years he found a wear rate of 0.09 mm/year for CoCr and 0.04 for ceramic. They did not observe a clinical difference in survival yet but found radiologically more osteolysis in the CoCr group (Dahl et al. 2012).

The question is whether these RSA data can predict longtime outcome. In 2003 Digas et al. measured increased wear of EtO sterilised PE in cemented and uncemented cups (Digas et al. 2003). The wear rate was 0.2 mm/year and hereby far above the save zone of 0.05 mm/year (Dumbleton et al. 2002). Six years later

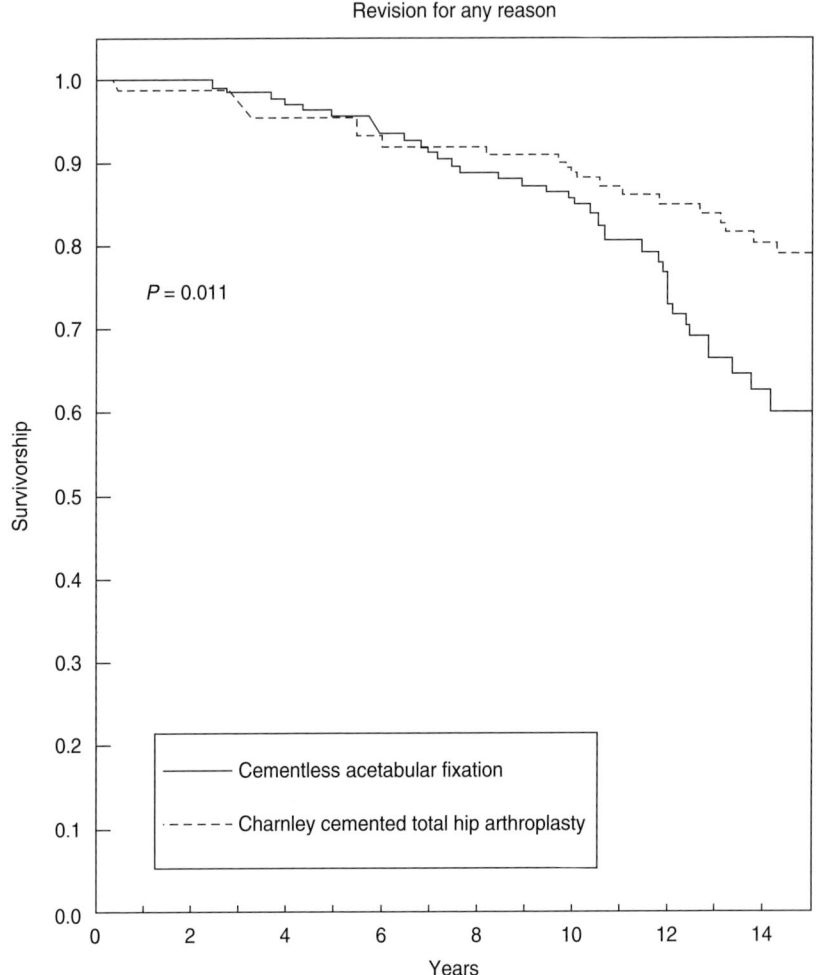

Fig. 11.2 Survivorship curve with revision of the acetabular and/or femoral component for any reason as the end point (Teusink et al. 2012)

Espehaug and colleagues published survival data from the Norwegian arthroplasty register of 62,305 primary hips. Arthroplasties with EtO PE cups had a 2.4 higher risk for revision after a follow-up time between 11 and 20 years (Fig. 11.4). The cup was sterilised with EtO, hence not moderately cross-linked with gamma radiation. This led inevitably to an increased wear rate and subsequently to a higher failure rate (Espehaug et al. 2009).

Additional stabilisation of UHMWPE components by annealing after sterilisation (Duration®, Howmedica) has now reached more than 10 years. Clinical results show a significant reduction in wear rate of 35 % compared to identical but in air irradiation-sterilised PE components (Geerdink et al. 2009).

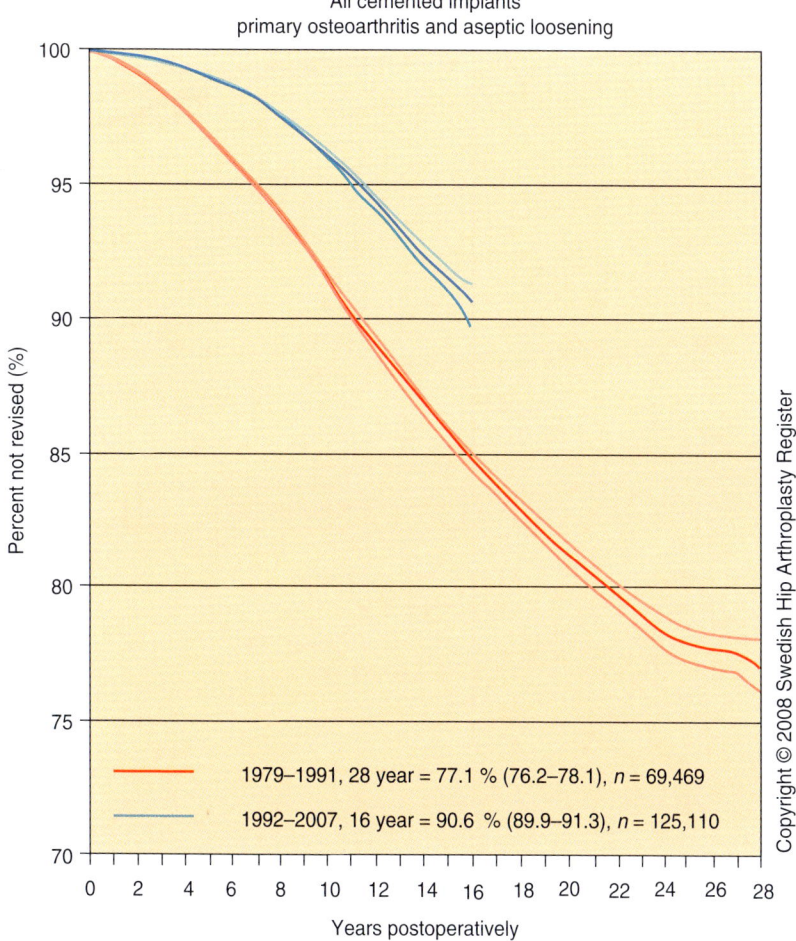

Fig. 11.3 Kaplan-Meier survival of all cemented implants from the Swedish hip registry. Implants from 1979 to 1991 with conventional UHMPE gamma sterilised in air has a higher revision rate than later UHMWPE mainly sterilised and packed in inert atmosphere

11.4.3 Highly Cross-Linked Polyethylene

This leads us to the last group of PE with at least 10 years observation time: highly cross-linked PE.

11.4.3.1 Pioneer Highly Cross-Linked Polyethylene

Three versions of intentionally highly cross-linked PE have been used as cemented cups of THR in the late 1970s; one of those historic types has been chemically cross-linked while the other two were cross-linked using high doses of irradiation, the primary and most reliable means of creating cross-linked PE. None of them

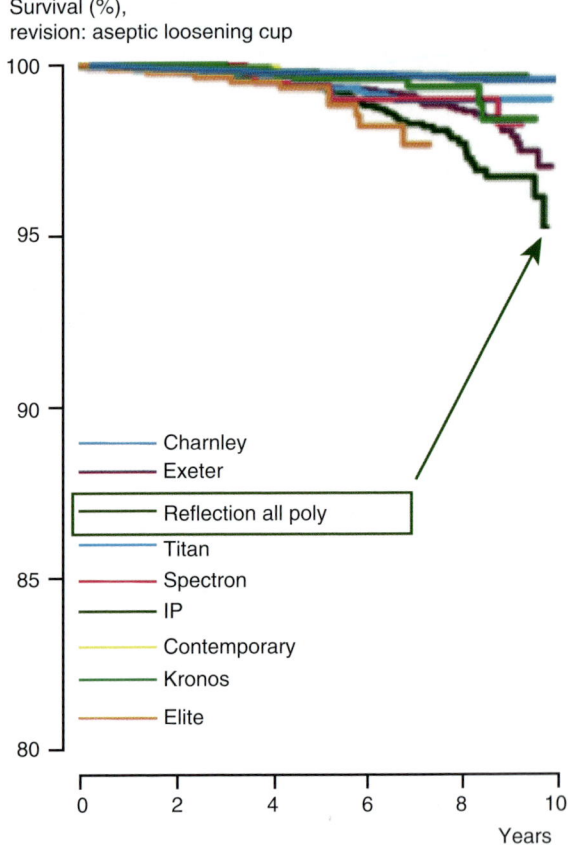

Fig. 11.4 Prosthesis survival with revision of cup due to aseptic loosening (Espehaug et al. 2009)

used any post-treatment to avoid post-oxidation. Retrospective wear measurement and results of >10 years are available: Wroblewski (Wroblewski et al. 1999b) reports in his 10-year data a wear rate of 0.037 mm/year and a reduction of 75 % versus conventionally sterilised PE, and Oohnishi (Oonishi et al. 1997) as well as Grobbelaar (Grobbelaar 1999) report 20-year results with similar reduction in wear rate.

11.4.3.2 First-Generation Highly Cross-Linked Polyethylene

Few 10-year reports on modern HXLPE have been published recently. All of them show reduced wear compared to conventional PE irradiated in air and in inert atmosphere. The wear reduction is independent of the post-radiation treatment (submelt annealed or remelted). In a case series Röhrl et al. followed eight patients with cemented submelt annealed PE for 10 years. They found an extremely (Fig. 11.5) low wear rate of 2 μm/year after a creep phase of approximately 3 months (Rohrl et al. 2012). Johanson et al. looked in a randomised study of 60 patients with cemented cups on the wear rate of remelted HXLPE (Johanson et al. 2012). The wear rate was as well extremely low (Fig. 11.6). However, they did not find any clearly

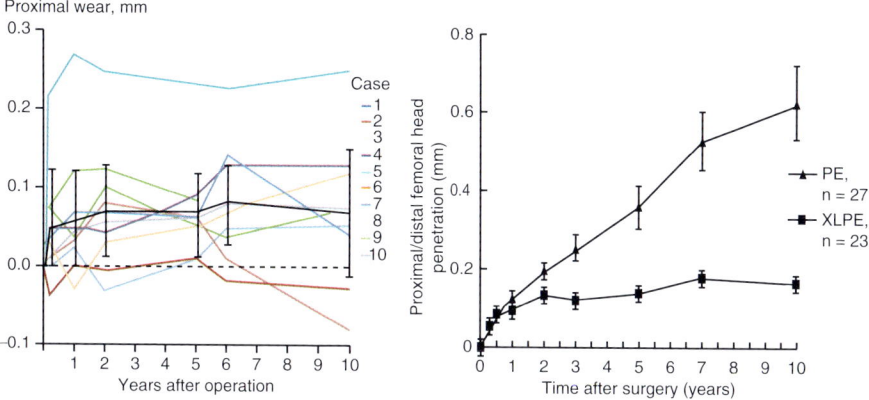

Fig. 11.5 *Left* and *right*. *Left*: Proximal penetration/wear for the individual patients (coloured lines and the mean (*black line*) with 95 % CI (whiskers)) (Rohrl et al. 2012). *Right*: Mean ± SD of the proximal penetration rate between 2 and 10 years was lower ($p < 0.001$) in XLPE (remelted) than in the conventional PE group (Johanson et al. 2012)

beneficial effects on implant fixation, radiolucencies, bone mineral density loss, function or implant survival.

The main question remains whether the lower wear of HXLPE will also improve the clinical outcome. The Scandinavian arthroplasty registries cannot provide sufficient data because of too short follow-up periods and low patient numbers so far. The Australian registry is the first to publish 10-year survival data with first-generation HXLPE. Their data suggests better survival of arthroplasties with HXLPE (pink line) (Fig. 11.6). The lowest revision rate is seen for HXLPE on cera-mised metal heads. Personal communication, however, suggests caution so far because these data consists of few cases and are mainly operated by specialised surgeons (purple line) (Graves 2011).

11.4.3.3 Second-Generation HXLPE

The history of second-generation HXLPE is still too young. The newest second-generation of HXLPE has been introduced in 2005/2007 to address the deficiencies of the previous generation by usage of enhanced technologies to minimise the com-promise made with fist-generation materials. Almost all new generation HXLPEs are now irradiated by gamma rays instead of electron beam. To retain the mechani-cal properties, the annealing procedure is used for almost all materials on the mar-ket, while for the quenching of the free radicals 2 different methods are use. One uses a sequential irradiation/annealing process repeated 3 times (X3, Stryker); oth-ers incorporate vitamin E as radical scavenger in various amounts and processes into the HXLPE (e.g. E1®, Biomet; ECIMA®, Corin; Vitamys®, Mathys).

Both methods are still compromises – the annealing due to the thermodynamics at the temperature chosen to maintain the mechanical properties does not completely eliminate all radicals and some oxidation is still possible, although much below the values achieved with historic HXLPEs.

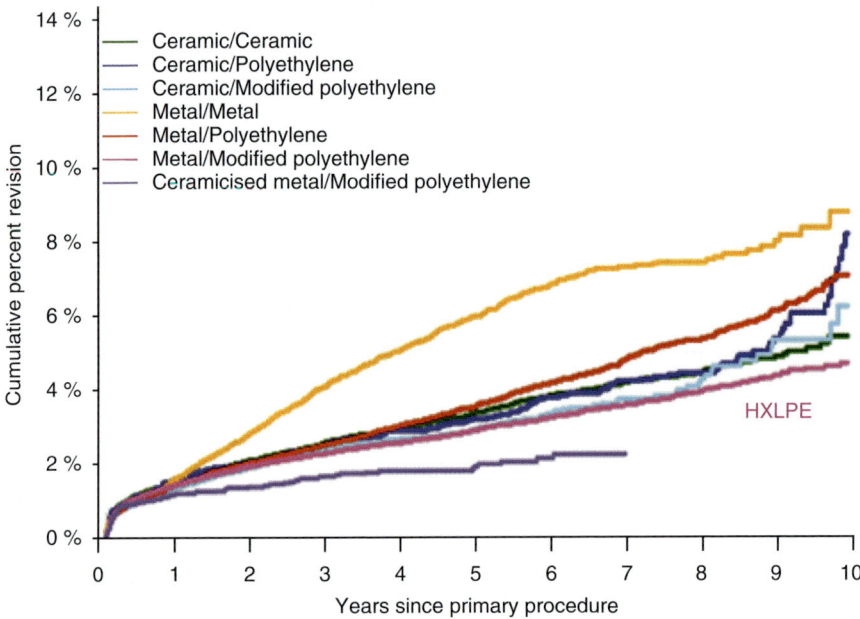

Fig. 11.6 10-year survival data for HXLPE from the Australian arthroplasty register

The other method applied for the production of third-generation HXLPEs is the addition of vitamin E or other radical scavengers (King et al. 2009) adopted from the chemical and polymer processing industry, introduced to orthopaedics since 2007. Several methods have been introduced to blend the antioxidants with PE (Oral and Muratoglu 2011; Oral et al. 2007). Some blend vitamin E with the polymer powder before the consolidation process to produce sheets or bars and cross-link and anneal them, while others diffuse and homogenise the antioxidant using a temperature treatment after cross-linking PE. The sterilisation then can be by irradiation or nonirradiation. Both manufacturing methods consume already substantial amounts of the antioxidant during either cross-linking or final sterilisation.

Several concerns with this new technology have been voiced. PE is a paraffin and inclusions or other substances agglomerate at its grain boundaries and consequently will affect the mechanical properties, the reason to have eliminated Ca stearate. Comparative laboratory data has shown that the addition of, for example, vitamin E to the virgin PE degrades its strength (Yau et al. 2009). The other concern is about the antioxidant itself: the optimum method to achieve homogeneity is not clear yet. The ideal amount of antioxidant has not been established yet, and it is a nonrenewable resource, so it may not be sufficient to last for the lifetime of the patient. Although, for example, vitamin E is biocompatible by itself, this is not evident for any of the reaction products produced during quenching radicals created by the irradiation.

Still, early clinical results up to 2 years for one of those vitamin E-doped HXLPEs look encouraging (Lindalen et al. 2012). In a randomised controlled trial, there was no difference between 32-mm and 36-mm ceramic heads. Clinical experience will show if this doped HXLPEs will come up to expectations in the long term.

11.5   What Have We Learned?

Patient's demographics are changing and their expectations are rising. This has a major impact on the bearings used in total joint replacement. Wear and subsequent osteolysis can jeopardise the long-term survival and the best articulation design and materials need to be applied to reduce or avoid its incidence.

Survival data from registers and wear measurements of cohorts with high-precision methods can give valuable information, though the ultimate proof is the documentation of longtime in vivo performance.

Ultra-high-molecular-weight polyethylene has been used as a bearing surface in arthroplasty for 60 years and the metal-/ceramic-on-PE articulation is the gold standard for hip and knee joint implants. Gamma irradiation sterilisation of PE in inert gas was introduced more than 25 years ago, yielded significantly enhanced wear resistance and reduced ageing issue as evident from long-term clinical experience. Ceramic heads reduced wear in articulations with conventional PE compared with CoCr heads. The introduction of first-generation HXLPE more than 10 years ago has proven a further reduction in wear rates and yielded positive clinical results. Two methods to reduce free radicals generated during the cross-linking process are commonly used, but up to 10 years there is no difference in wear rates between these methods. Highly cross-linked PE is a powerful material to reduce the amount of the wear particles to a sub-risk level and improve the chance for better long-term results of artificial joint prostheses. Careful and diligent follow-up in their clinical application is needed to determine their ultimate success.

References

Bloebaum RD, Nelson K, Dorr LD, Hofmann AA, Lyman DJ (1991) Investigation of early surface delamination observed in retrieved heat-pressed tibial inserts. Clin Orthop Relat Res 269:120–127

Borlin N, Rohrl SM, Bragdon CR (2006) RSA wear measurements with or without markers in total hip arthroplasty. J Biomech 39:1641–1650

Bruzzone M, La Russa M, Garzaro G, Ferro A, Rossi P, Castoldi F, Rossi R (2009) Long-term results of cementless anatomic total hip replacement in dysplastic hips. Chir Organi Mov 93:131–136

Buckwalter AE, Callaghan JJ, Liu SS, Pedersen DR, Goetz DD, Sullivan PM, Leinen JA, Johnston RC (2006) Results of Charnley total hip arthroplasty with use of improved femoral cementing techniques. a concise follow-up, at a minimum of twenty-five years, of a previous report. J Bone Joint Surg Am 88:1481–1485

Buergi ML, Walter WL (2007) Hip resurfacing arthroplasty: the Australian experience. J Arthroplasty 22:61–65

Callaghan JJ, Bracha P, Liu SS, Piyaworakhun S, Goetz DD, Johnston RC (2009) Survivorship of a Charnley total hip arthroplasty. A concise follow-up, at a minimum of thirty-five years, of previous reports. J Bone Joint Surg Am 91:2617–2621

Capello WN, D'Antonio JA, Ramakrishnan R, Naughton M (2011) Continued improved wear with an annealed highly cross-linked polyethylene. Clin Orthop Relat Res 469:825–830

Charnley J, Halley DK (1975) Rate of wear in total hip replacement. Clin Orthop Relat Res 112:170–179

Dahl J, Soderlund P, Nivbrant B, Nordsletten L, Rohrl SM (2012) Less wear with aluminium-oxide heads than cobalt-chrome heads with ultra high molecular weight cemented polyethylene cups: a ten-year follow-up with radiostereometry. Int Orthop 36:485–490

Digas G, Thanner J, Nivbrant B, Rohrl S, Strom H, Karrholm J (2003) Increase in early polyethylene wear after sterilization with ethylene oxide: radiostereometric analyses of 201 total hips. Acta Orthop Scand 74:531–541

Duffy GP, Wannomae KK, Rowell SL, Muratoglu OK (2009) Fracture of a cross-linked polyethylene liner due to impingement. J Arthroplasty 24(158):e115–e159

Dumbleton JH, Manley MT, Edidin AA (2002) A literature review of the association between wear rate and osteolysis in total hip arthroplasty. J Arthroplasty 17:649–661

Edidin AA, Jewett CW, Kalinowski A, Kwarteng K, Kurtz SM (2000) Degradation of mechanical behavior in UHMWPE after natural and accelerated aging. Biomaterials 21:1451–1460

Espehaug B, Furnes O, Engesaeter LB, Havelin LI (2009) 18 years of results with cemented primary hip prostheses in the Norwegian Arthroplasty Register: concerns about some newer implants. Acta Orthop 80:402–412

Fruh HJ, Willmann G (1998) Tribological investigations of the wear couple alumina-CFRP for total hip replacement. Biomaterials 19:1145–1150

Garellick G, Kärrholm J, Rogmark C, Herberts P (2011) Swedish hip arthroplasty register annual report 2010. In Register, SHA (ed). Göteborg, Sweden

Geerdink CH, Grimm B, Vencken W, Heyligers IC, Tonino AJ (2009) Cross-linked compared with historical polyethylene in THA: an 8-year clinical study. Clin Orthop Relat Res 467:979–984

Graves S (2011) Australian Orthopaedic Association National Joint Replacement Registry. In: AOA (ed) Annual report, Adelaide, http://www.aoa.org.au

Grobbelaar CJ (1999) Longterm results with crosslinked PE. In: Knahr K (ed) Tribology in Total Hip Arthroplasty, EFORT reference in orthopaedics and traumatology, Chapter 5

Grobbelaar CJ, du Plessis TA, Marais F (1978) The radiation improvement of polyethylene prostheses. A preliminary study. J Bone Joint Surg Br 60-B:370–374

Herrera L, Lee R, Longaray J, Essner A, Wang A (2007) Hip simulator evaluation of the effect of femoral head size on sequentially cross-linked acetabular liners. Wear 263:1034–1037

Johanson PE, Digas G, Herberts P, Thanner J, Karrholm J (2012) Highly crosslinked polyethylene does not reduce aseptic loosening in cemented THA 10-year findings of a randomized study. Clin Orthop Relat Res 470(11):3083–3093

Kadar T, Furnes O, Aamodt A, Indrekvam K, Havelin LI, Haugan K, Espehaug B, Hallan G (2012) The influence of acetabular inclination angle on the penetration of polyethylene and migration of the acetabular component: a prospective, radiostereometric study on cemented acetabular components. J Bone Joint Surg Br 94:302–307

Kelly NH, Rajadhyaksha AD, Wright TM, Maher SA, Westrich GH (2010) High stress conditions do not increase wear of thin highly crosslinked UHMWPE. Clin Orthop Relat Res 468:418–423

Kilgus DJ, Funahashi TT, Campbell PA (1992) Massive femoral osteolysis and early disintegration of a polyethylene-bearing surface of a total knee replacement. A case report. J Bone Joint Surg Am 74:770–774

King R, Narayan VS, Ernsberger C, Hanes M (2009) Characterization of gamma-irradiated UHMWPE stabilized with a hindered-phenol antioxidant. In: Trans 55th Annual Meeting of the Orthopaedic Research Society, Las Vegas, NV, Vol 19

Korkala O, Syrjanen KJ (1998) Intrapelvic cyst formation after hip arthroplasty with a carbon fibre-reinforced polyethylene socket. Arch Orthop Trauma Surg 118:113–115

Kurtz SM, Hozack WJ, Purtill JJ, Marcolongo M, Kraay MJ, Goldberg VM, Sharkey PF, Parvizi J, Rimnac CM, Edidin AA (2006) 2006 Otto Aufranc Award Paper: significance of in vivo degradation for polyethylene in total hip arthroplasty. Clin Orthop Relat Res 453:47–57

Kurtz SM, Rimnac CM, Hozack WJ, Turner J, Marcolongo M, Goldberg VM, Kraay MJ, Edidin AA (2005) In vivo degradation of polyethylene liners after gamma sterilization in air. J Bone Joint Surg Am 87:815–823

Learmonth ID, Young C, Rorabeck C (2007) The operation of the century: total hip replacement. Lancet 370:1508–1519

Lindalen E, Lindalen E, Hovik O, Rohrl SM (2012) Low wear of E-vitamin infused highly cross-linked polyethylene using 32 and 36 mm ceramic heads – a prospective randomized controlled trial using markerless radiostereometry. European hip society, Milano (e-poster)

Malchau H (2000) Introducing new technology: a stepwise algorithm. Spine 25:285

McKellop H, Shen FW, Lu B, Campbell P, Salovey R (1999) Development of an extremely wear-resistant ultra high molecular weight polyethylene for total hip replacements. J Orthop Res 17:157–167

Nelissen RG, Pijls BG, Karrholm J, Malchau H, Nieuwenhuijse MJ, Valstar ER (2011) RSA and registries: the quest for phased introduction of new implants. J Bone Joint Surg Am 93(Suppl 3):62–65

Oonishi H, Kuno M, Tsuji E, Fujisawa A (1997) The optimum dose of gamma radiation-heavy doses to low wear polyethylene in total hip prostheses. J Mater Sci Mater Med 8:11–18

Oral E, Muratoglu OK (2011) Vitamin E diffused, highly crosslinked UHMWPE: a review. Int Orthop 35:215–223

Oral E, Wannomae KK, Rowell SL, Muratoglu OK (2007) Diffusion of vitamin E in ultra-high molecular weight polyethylene. Biomaterials 28:5225–5237

Ranstam J, Robertsson O (2010) Statistical analysis of arthroplasty register data. Acta Orthop 81:10–14

Rohrl SM, Nivbrant B, Nilsson KG (2012) No adverse effects of submelt-annealed highly crosslinked polyethylene in cemented cups: an RSA study of 8 patients 10 years after surgery. Acta Orthop 83:148–152

Rohrl SM, Nivbrant B, Snorrason F, Karrholm J, Nilsson KG (2006) Porous-coated cups fixed with screws: a 12-year clinical and radiostereometric follow-up study of 50 hips. Acta Orthop 77:393–401

Scott DL, Campbell PA, McClung CD, Schmalzried TP (2000) Factors contributing to rapid wear and osteolysis in hips with modular acetabular bearings made of hylamer. J Arthroplasty 15:35–46

Sochart DH (1999) Relationship of acetabular wear to osteolysis and loosening in total hip arthroplasty. Clin Orthop Relat Res 363:135–150

Stein HL (1999) Ultra high molecular polyethylene (UHMWPE). Engineered Materials Handbook, Vol 2: Engineering Plastics, ASM International, USA

Streicher RM, Thomsen M (2003) Polyethylene as an implant material. Orthopade 32:23–31

Sychterz CJ, Young AM, McAuley JP, Engh CA (2000) Comparison of head penetration into Hylamer and Enduron polyethylene liners: a follow-up report. J Arthroplasty 15: 372–374

Tarasevicius S, Kesteris U, Robertsson O, Wingstrand H (2006) Femoral head diameter affects the revision rate in total hip arthroplasty: an analysis of 1,720 hip replacements with 9–21 years of follow-up. Acta Orthop 77:706–709

Teusink MJ, Callaghan JJ, Warth LC, Goetz DD, Pedersen DR, Johnston RC (2012) Cementless acetabular fixation in patients 50 years and younger at 10 to 18 years of follow-up. J Arthroplasty 27(1316–1323):e1312

Tower SS, Currier JH, Currier BH, Lyford KA, Van Citters DW, Mayor MB (2007) Rim cracking of the cross-linked longevity polyethylene acetabular liner after total hip arthroplasty. J Bone Joint Surg Am 89:2212–2217

Treuhaft PS, MCCarty DJ (1971) Synovial fluid pH, lactate, oxygen and carbon dioxide partial pressure in various joint diseases. Arthritis Rheum 14:475–484

Valstar ER, Gill R, Ryd L, Flivik G, Borlin N, Karrholm J (2005) Guidelines for standardization of radiostereometry (RSA) of implants. Acta Orthop 76:563–572

Waewsawangwong W, Goodman SB (2012) Unexpected failure of highly cross-linked polyethylene acetabular liner. J Arthroplasty 27(323):e321–e324

Wang A, Manley MT, Serekian P (2003) Wear and structural fatigue simulation of crosslinked ultra-high molecular weight polyethylene for hip and knee bearing applications. ASTM STP 1445:151–168

Willie BM, Bloebaum RD, Ashrafi S, Dearden C, Steffensen T, Hofmann AA (2006) Oxidative degradation in highly cross-linked and conventional polyethylene after 2 years of real-time shelf aging. Biomaterials 27:2275–2284

Wroblewski BM, Fleming PA, Siney PD (1999a) Charnley low-frictional torque arthroplasty of the hip. 20-to-30 year results. J Bone Joint Surg Br 81:427–430

Wroblewski BM, Siney PD, Fleming PA (1999b) Low-friction arthroplasty of the hip using alumina ceramic and cross-linked polyethylene. A ten-year follow-up report. J Bone Joint Surg Br 81:54–55

Yau S, Le K-P, Wang A (2009) Doping vitamin E by diffusion deteriorates properties of cross-linked UHMWPE: verified by experiments. In: Trans 55th Annual Meeting of the Orthopaedic Research Society, Las Vegas, NV, Vol 458

Zahiri CA, Schmalzried TP, Szuszczewicz ES, Amstutz HC (1998) Assessing activity in joint replacement patients. J Arthroplasty 13:890–895

Part IV

Large Diameter Heads

Head Size and Metal-on-Metal Bearings

12

Henri Migaud, Charles Berton, Sophie Putman,
Antoine Combes, Alexandre Blairon, Gregory Kern,
and Julien Girard

12.1 Introduction

The reintroduction of metal-on-metal (M-M) bearing components in total hip arthroplasty (THA) occurred with small-diameter heads (28–32 mm) in the late 1980s and gave excellent results up to 15 years of follow-up (Dastane et al. 2011; Grübl et al. 2007; Migaud et al. 2011). Shortly thereafter, M-M hip resurfacing (SRA) resurged, and favorable outcomes are currently reported at follow-up exceeding 12 years (Amstutz et al. 2010; Coulter et al. 2012; Treacy et al. 2011). From this rapid overview of the literature on metallic articulations, one may erroneously conclude that bearing diameter has no influence on survival of M-M articulations. Currently, there is growing controversy regarding M-M bearings considering adverse reactions to metallic debris (ARMD) and concerns about blood ion elevation (Engh et al. 2010; Glyn-Jones et al. 2009; Hart et al. 2012; Heneghan et al. 2012). In fact, these side effects were rare at the time small M-M bearings were reintroduced: Rising metallic ion levels in blood were low (Grübl et al. 2007), and aseptic lymphocytic vasculitis-associated lesions (ALVAL) were extremely

H. Migaud, MD (✉) • C. Berton, MD • S. Putman, MD • A. Combes, MD
A. Blairon, MD • G. Kern, MD
Department of Orthopaedic Surgery, Roger Salengro Hospital,
University of Lille, 2 avenue Oscar Lambret, 59037, Lille France
e-mail: hemigaud@nordnet.fr; charles.berton@gmail.com;
sophie.putman@wanadoo.fr; antoinecombes@yahoo.fr;
alexandreblairon@yahoo.fr; gregorykern@hotmail.com

J. Girard, MD, PhD
Department of Orthopaedic Surgery, Roger Salengro Hospital,
University of Lille, 2 avenue Oscar Lambret, 59037 Lille, France

Department of Sports Medicine,
University of Lille 2,
Lille, France
e-mail: j_girard_lille@yahoo.fr

K. Knahr (ed.), *Total Hip Arthroplasty*,
DOI 10.1007/978-3-642-35653-7_12, © EFORT 2013

uncommon (<1/15,000) with small M-M (Willert et al. 2005) while pseudotumors were marginal (1/100,000) (Gruber et al. 2007). Looking back, controversy mainly emerged after large M-M bearings were launched in the late 1990s, particularly after the introduction of large-diameter head (LDH) THA and after dissemination of SRA (Heneghan et al. 2012). The goal of this chapter is to assess if these concerns apply equally to different diameters of M-M articulations.

12.2   Material and Methods

A search of the PubMed database identified articles reporting the influence of bearing diameter on outcomes (survival, adverse effects, reasons for failure) of M-M hip replacement. The key words were "hip prosthesis" and "metal-on-metal" "diameter" with the following conditions: English language, publication date limited to 10 years, and case reports excluded. Of the 169 papers selected, 93 were discarded because they did not directly relate to M-M bearings, leaving 76 articles that are the basis of this chapter. In parallel, articles were added after a complementary search of PubMed for papers on the results of M-M bearings (small diameter and SRA) after minimum 7 years follow-up (18 papers labeled by * in the Reference list) and papers relating to specific complications of M-M (14 papers labeled by ◊). Finally, eight meta-analyses or reports on M-M from registers were also added (eight papers labeled by †).

All these papers were screened to answer the following questions: (1) Do small and large M-M articulations have specific complications (impingement, instability, groin pain)? (2) Are small and large M-M articulations equal regarding blood ion concentrations? (3) Is there any advantage of large over small M-M articulations? (4) Is ARMD related to the diameter of M-M articulations? (5) Do survival and reason for reoperation differ according to M-M bearing diameter? (6) Do all small-diameter M-M function equally?

12.3   Results

12.3.1 Do Small and Large M-M Articulations Have Specific Complications (Impingement, Instability, Groin Pain)?

The rate of dislocation is extremely low with SRA and LDH THAs. Most LDH series report rates equal to zero or below 0.5 % (Berton et al. 2010; Cicek et al. 2010; Lavigne et al. 2011a, b; Stuchin 2008; Zhang et al. 2010). Similarly, SRA is associated with comparable rates of dislocation, mostly equal to zero (Amstutz et al. 2010; Coulter et al. 2012; Shimmin et al. 2010; Smith et al. 2010). In contrast, delayed dislocation after SRA or LDH THAs may indicate synovial reactions to metallic debris and should alert surgeons (Langton et al. 2011b; Pandit et al. 2008; Theruvil et al. 2011). The rate of dislocation with small-diameter M-M is in line with the results of large M-M bearings and below the ranges reported for conventional

THA: no dislocation noted in many series (Grübl et al. 2007; Migaud et al. 2011), rates below 1 % in a few series (Randelli et al. 2012) but usually lower rates than with conventional THA (Cuckler et al. 2004; Lombardi et al. 2011; Migaud et al. 2011). If some series with small-diameter M-M record higher dislocation rates, it is because femoral stems do not reproduce proximal femoral anatomy and abductor lever arm (Herman et al. 2011; Randelli et al. 2012).

Prevention of impingement and dislocation was the main reason for promoting the introduction of large-diameter M-M in the late 1990s (Cuckler et al. 2004; Peters et al. 2007; Smith et al. 2005). In fact, the rate of impingement with small-diameter M-M is almost 50 % in retrieval studies (Marchetti et al. 2011), but is rarely the reason for revision (Grübl et al. 2007; Hwang et al. 2011; Migaud et al. 2011), except when it favors instability (Randelli et al. 2012). Impingement is rarely seen after SRA (Hart et al. 2012; Lavigne et al. 2011b), even if it is suspected to be a factor promoting neck narrowing (Spencer et al. 2008) or increased blood ion levels (Hart et al. 2011; Langton et al. 2011b), and particularly edge loading (Underwood et al. 2012).

There is general agreement on a high rate of groin pain with large M-M heads (LDH or SRA) (Berton et al. 2010; Browne et al. 2010, 2011; Lavigne et al. 2011b), although a few series argue that it is comparable to conventional THA (Meding et al. 2012). In contrast, low rates of anterior groin pain are reported with small M-M articulations – none by Migaud et al. (2011) and Eswaramoorthy et al. (2008) and only 1 out of 105 by Grubl et al. (2007) – but correlate with higher cobalt (Co) concentrations and suspected synovial reactions. In contrast, some series have recorded almost 20 % groin pain after LDH THA or SRA (Berton et al. 2010; Lavigne et al. 2011b), and even 35 % according to Lardanchet et al. (2012), who compared three designs of LDH THAs. These higher rates could be attributed to increased socket inclination (Berton et al. 2010), favoring anterior cup overhang and iliopsoas irritation as well as greater wear and synovial reactions (De Haan et al. 2008; Lardanchet et al. 2012). Moreover, residual anterior pain may be related to failure of osteointegration that is observed with some LDH designs (Berton et al. 2010; Long et al. 2010; Matthies et al. 2011). On the other hand, independently of socket orientation, excessive LDH extent may promote iliopsoas irritation and favor a high rate of anterior groin pain with large M-M articulations (Cobb et al. 2011). One should keep in mind that residual anterior groin pain after LDH or SRA may indicate synovial reactions to metallic debris, advocating complementary investigations (magnetic resonance imaging (MRI), ultrasound, and blood ion measurement) (Hauptfleisch et al. 2012; Kwon et al. 2011).

12.3.2 Are Small and Large M-M Articulations Equal Regarding Blood Ion Concentrations?

Large M-M articulations were introduced to theoretically reduce wear and, consequently, blood ion production (Affatato et al. 2007, 2008, 2011; Dowson et al. 2004a; Leslie et al. 2008; Rieker et al. 2005). This was confirmed by many randomized series comparing SRA and small-diameter M-M: Vendittoli et al. (2010b) noted similar concentrations with Metasul™ 28 mm (Co 1.62 μg/L) versus SRA (1.58 μg/L) at 2-year follow-up. Smolders et al. (2011) discerned similar Co concentrations at 2-year follow-up comparing M-M THA and SRA (0.9 μg/L vs. 1.2 μg/L). The historical non-randomized series of Clarke et al. (2003) established that ion concentrations with SRA increased by 57 % versus small-diameter M-M. In another non-randomized study, Daniel et al. (2006, 2008) obtained comparable 1-year concentrations for Birmingham SRA (2.3 μg/L) versus Metasul™ 28 mm (1.7 μg/L). Similarly, Moroni et al. (2008) reported non-different Co rates at 15 months (1.17 μg/L for Birmingham SRA and 1.35 for Metasul™ 28-mm THA).

The results were dramatically different with LDH M-M THA: Lavigne et al. (2011a) observed Co levels ranging from 0.65 μg/L (Biomet Magnum THA) to 2.68 μg/L (Durom LDH) at 2-year follow-up, and Vendittoli et al. (2011) recorded Co levels of 2.7 μg/L with Durom™ LDH. All reports on ion concentrations after LDH underlined the deleterious effects of modularity (modular sleeves and open geometry of LDH design) that strongly increase ion concentrations from bearings (Lavigne et al. 2011a; Vendittoli et al. 2011). Similarly, Langton et al. (2011a) found that 26 % of patients who received ASR™ LDH had Co concentrations exceeding 7 μg/L, with significant damage to the trunnion-taper interface, again indicating the adverse effects of modularity in LDH THA. In another randomized study, Garbuz et al. (2010) reported 1-year Co concentration with SRA to be 0.51 μg/L vs. 5.09 μg/L for LDH THA with the same bearing component (Durom™). Finally, comparing SRA and LDH THAs, Maurer-Ertl et al. (2012) observed that Co levels were fourfold higher for LDH versus SRA with no effect of socket inclination.

In contrast, blood Co levels are virtually comparable from one study to another and very low with small-diameter M-M (Grübl et al. 2007; Migaud et al. 2011), suggesting that, for this design, wear is poorly impacted by extrinsic factors, particularly surgery. On the other hand, large M-M articulations are strongly influenced by surgical variables of SRA and LDH THA: De Haan et al. (2008) and Desy et al. (2011) underlined that high concentrations are associated with significant socket inclination and the small diameter of resurfacing articulations. As mentioned previously for LDH THA, the open geometry of LDH and complex modularity markedly elevate blood ion concentrations (Garbuz et al. 2010; Lardanchet et al. 2012; Lavigne et al. 2011a). On the other hand, articulation diameter has limited influence on Co levels with small M-M articulations: Engh et al. (2009), in a randomized study at 1-year follow-up, observed no difference in Co concentrations comparing 28-mm (0.77 μg/L) to 36-mm (0.73 μg/L) M-M bearings. Moreover, Bernstein et al. (2011) found no difference in a case–control study of 28- and 36-mm heads (Co 2.34 μg/L) vs. 40- and 44-mm heads (Co 2.22 μg/L) at 1-year follow-up. In this series, the larger heads (40 and 44 mm) had 180° articulating surfaces that were significantly different from LDH hip replacements that included sockets from resurfacing limited bearing surfaces (±165° according to diameter). The latter feature may cause runaway wear and make these large M-M articulations more sensitive to malposition (De Haan et al. 2008; Griffin et al. 2010; Langton et al. 2008, 2010). The sensitivity of large M-M to malposition has also been postulated in vitro (Angadji et al. 2009). Excessive production of debris from modularity and trunnion-taper junction, the weak point of LDH THA, was not implicated in in vitro studies (Flanagan et al. 2010; Hu et al. 2011) but was finally identified on retrievals (Bolland et al. 2011; Langton ct al. 2010). LDH THA and SRA are sensitive to malposition considering that the arc of coverage (De Haan et al. 2008) is reduced as these cups have an opening angle below 180° (usually ±165°). This result advocates inclining these sockets from resurfacing lower than is usually estimated for conventional THA (Jeffers et al. 2009), particularly for small-diameter LDH and SRA that have a very limited arc of coverage (Amstutz et al. 2012; Angadji et al. 2009; Corten and MacDonald 2010; Langton et al. 2011b).

One should keep in mind that Co elevation indicates high wear of articulating surfaces or excessive production from modularity junctions and should warrant investigations to ascertain indications of revision (Langton et al. 2011b). In contrast, ARMD may occur with or without blood ion elevation (Co is the main marker), showing the importance of complementary assessment (ultrasound or MRI) in symptomatic (Donell et al. 2010; Hauptfleisch et al. 2012) or asymptomatic (Williams et al. 2011) patients, particularly if high serum metal ion levels are observed. Usually, metal ion levels decrease after revision of M-M articulations performed because of ARMD or metallosis (Ebreo et al. 2011). One should also consider the limitations of ion levels: (1) Current baseline values do not take into account the influence of either activity or exercise (Khan et al. 2006). (2) Co levels are a vital issue in blood (De Haan et al. 2008; Grübl et al. 2007; Khan et al. 2006), so pathological values should be investigated (EFORT consensus statement 2012). (3) Intra-articular Co levels should be quantified, as they may be more predictive than blood levels in precisely assessing bearing function (Davda et al. 2011).

12.3.3   Is There Any Advantage of Large over Small M-M Articulations?

Independent studies and meta-analyses support the view that functioning improves after SRA versus small M-M or conventional THA (Smith et al. 2010; Vendittoli et al. 2010a). Better function is not related to bone preservation by SRA but to the effect of LDH on gait and function parameters (Zhou et al. 2009). Gait speed and postural balance after SRA and LDH THAs were similar in a randomized study reported by Lavigne et al. (2010), confirming that the effect of large heads on bone preservation explains the better results usually achieved by SRA over conventional THA (Vendittoli et al. 2010a).

12.3.4   Is ARMD Related to the Diameter of M-M Articulations?

ARMD is marginal with small-diameter M-M, particularly forged high-carbide alloys (Grübl et al. 2007; Migaud et al. 2011). To the our best knowledge, only one case of limited pseudotumor-like lesions has been reported with small M-M of forged high-carbide Co-Cr (Cobalt-Chromium) alloys (Gruber et al. 2007). Likewise, ALVAL are very rare with small-diameter M-M. Willert et al. (2005) estimated the rate to be 1/10,000. In contrast, pseudotumors are more frequent with large-diameter M-M: The rate ranges from 0.1 to 3 % after hip resurfacing (Beaulé et al. 2011; Pandit et al. 2008), and higher values, from 2 to 69 %, have been observed after LDH THA (Malviya et al. 2011; Matthies et al. 2012). Pseudotumors are more frequent with LDH and are specific to this design: (a) They may occur without blood ion elevation (Hart et al. 2012; Kwon et al. 2011; Langton et al. 2011b); (b) while socket malorientation strongly influences their incidence, they could also develop with adequately oriented components (Hart et al. 2012); (c) pseudotumors emerge earlier with LDH design (Hart et al. 2012); and finally (d) they are not necessarily correlated to bearing dysfunction but rather to modularity failure (Lardanchet et al. 2012; Mertl et al. 2010; Smith et al. 2012).

12.3.5 Do Survival and Reason for Reoperation Differ According to M-M Bearing Diameter?

The main reasons for small-diameter M-M revisions are instability and loosening, even if metallurgy (clearance, high-carbide content, and forged Cr-Co) is adequate (Dowson et al. 2004a, b; Girard et al. 2010, 2007). In contrast, low-carbide and/or cast Cr-Co small M-M are revised in a large proportion of patients because of osteolysis (Park et al. 2005), ARMD, and unexplained pain (Donell et al. 2010). If the SRA reoperation rate is slightly higher than conventional THA, the main reasons are technical errors (femoral neck fracture, heterotopic ossifications, inadequate socket settlement) that usually decrease with learning curve evolution (Amstutz et al. 2010; Corten and MacDonald 2010; Jiang et al. 2011; Shimmin et al. 2010; Smith et al. 2010; Treacy et al. 2011). In contrast, LDH THAs are mainly revised because of unexplained pain (mostly groin pain), ARMD, and instability secondary to synovial effusion and muscle destruction (Lardanchet et al. 2012; Malviya et al. 2011; Mertl et al. 2010).

Design and metallurgy have a strong influence on the reoperation rate and reasons for revision. In an Australian register (de Steiger et al. 2011), the DePuy ASR system (SRA and LDH) was revised at rates significantly higher than any small M-M bearing, and the reasons for revision were mainly ARMD and osteolysis. This is quite different from other SRA systems that are revised after longer follow-up and mainly because of femoral neck fracture, loosening, and pain related to malposition (Amstutz et al. 2010; Hart et al. 2012; Jiang et al. 2011). Reduced clearance and limited arc of coverage were the main factors that explained ASR failures as well as cast Co-Cr with low-carbide content (Dowson et al. 2004a, b; Jameson et al. 2010; Kretzer et al. 2009).

Components are usually smaller in female patients, worsening the results of SRA as well as LDH THAs (Amstutz et al. 2011; de Steiger et al. 2011; van der Weegen et al. 2011). Gender is probably a confounding factor. It appeared to exacerbate the results among 1,589 THAs with small-diameter M-M, the revision rates being respectively 8.2 % in women versus 2.7 % in men (Latteier et al. 2011).

Squeaking is rarely reported to be a reason for reoperation of M-M bearings, particularly small-diameter M-M (Graves et al. 2011; Grübl et al. 2007; Migaud et al. 2011). A few cases with large M-M have been observed (Cicek et al. 2010), but not on a large scale in registries (Jiang et al. 2011; Shimmin et al. 2010; Smith et al. 2012). In fact, squeaking is probably related to errors in component design that increase clearance and reduce lubrication (Brockett et al. 2008).

Reasons for reoperation differ with respect to diameter: Small-diameter M-M (28–32 mm) were mainly revised because of instability, and few because of osteolysis (Eswaramoorthy et al. 2008; Grübl et al. 2007; Randelli et al. 2012). In contrast to the small M-M group with hemispherical sockets, larger bearings (36–44 mm) were mainly revised because of ARMD (Smith et al. 2012) that included metallosis, pseudotumors, and ALVAL, which is also the main reason for reoperation after LDH THAs (Barrett et al. 2012).

The majority of small M-M series with 10-year survival exceeded 98 % (Grübl et al. 2007; Hwang et al. 2011; Rieker et al. 2005), except when inadequate options were used for M-M articulation (Donell et al. 2010; Korovessis et al. 2006; Milosev et al. 2006). In contrast, the majority of LDH THA series had lower survival rates at 5 years: 92 % with Durom™ (Berton et al. 2010), 89 % with different designs (Bolland et al. 2011), and 89 % for hips with acetabular components smaller than 56-mm ASR (Jameson et al. 2010). SRA clearly affords better survival when high-volume centers are considered: 88.5 % at 10 years according to Amstutz et al. (2010) and 100 % in hips that had a femoral component larger than 46 mm. Treacy et al. (2011) reported 95.5 % survival without revision because of infection at 10 years. At 10 years, Coulter et al. (2012) obtained rates of 89 % in women and 97 % in men. Holland et al. (2012) recorded 92 % survival at 10 years with 94.6 % in male and 84.6 % in female patients. The results appear to be worse in females than in males, making gender a confounding factor, but survival is identical in men and in women when the femoral component is ≥48 mm (Amstutz et al. 2011). Obviously, SRA diameter has a definitive influence on survivorship, more than metallurgy or design, but at similar levels as surgical features (position, impingement).

To summarize, SRA warrants careful selection to exceed 90 % 10-year survival based on NICE (National Institute for Health and Clinical Excellence) criteria that are rarely reached by resurfacing, even in high-volume centers (Smith et al. 2012). In contrast, obesity, which is usually a factor in failure of conventional THAs in young and active patients, appears to be favorable to SRA survival in parallel with increased articulation diameter (Le Duff et al. 2007).

12.3.6 Do All Small-Diameter M-M Function Equally?

The historical design of Metasul™ (forged high-carbide Co-Cr alloy) has now reached 15 years of follow-up, and the majority of studies report favorable results, with survival ranging from 94 to 100 % (Eswaramoorthy et al. 2008; Girard et al.

2010; Grübl et al. 2007; Hwang et al. 2011; Migaud et al. 2011). Embedding of Metasul™ into polyethylene improved lubrication in vitro combined with low clearance (Liu et al. 2004, 2006, 2007). In contrast, forged high-carbide Lubrimet™ with metal insert directly fixed into the metal back (without polyethylene interposition) had only 93 % 10-year survival (Neumann et al. 2010). The latter series divulged cases of metallosis, but unfortunately, the authors incorporated components from different manufacturers and did not report blood ion concentrations that could be elevated because of modularity (different manufacturers, additional M-M trunnion-taper junction on the acetabular side) (Neuerburg et al. 2012). Surprisingly, Neuerburg et al. (2012) obtained lower results with Metasul™, with only 90 % 10-year survivorship. Again, this series mixed components from different manufacturers, which could have produced metallic wear debris, and did not assess blood ion levels despite obvious metallic debris reactions in 20 of 63 revised hips (Neuerburg et al. 2012). Using Metasul™ with homogenous components from the same manufacturer, Randelli et al. (2012) recorded only 94 % survival, but at 14 years of follow-up, dislocation became the major reason for revision, with only one revision related to M-M bearing wear. Holloway et al. (2009) reported a limited Metasul™ series (27 cases) at 8.5 years follow-up and observed one revision because of acetabular osteolysis but did not assess blood ion levels, while analysis of histological tissue harvested at revision did not favor ARMD. Hwang et al. (2011) observed 98.7 % survival at 14 years in 78 Metasul™, with only one revision related to osteolysis with lymphocyte infiltration but with Co 0.57 μg/L. Finally, Saito et al. (2010) reported only 94.4 % survival at 12 years with Metasul™, but the majority of revisions were attributed to recurrent dislocation, and no patient had ARMD.

In summary, Metasul™ appears to be a viable option, particularly in young and active patients, as suggested by favorable results at follow-up exceeding 12 years and as long as there is no mixed modularity option (i.e. all components should be provided by the same manufacturer).

In contrast, Ultima™ (cast on forged Co-Cr alloy low carbide) has clearly lower results: 13.8 % revision after 4–11 years of follow-up (Donell et al. 2010) and 6 % osteolysis at 2 years follow-up (Park et al. 2005). A few studies related to cast on forged high-carbide small M-M have reported favorable results but usually after follow-up that did not exceed 7 years, which is half of the follow-up of forged on forged high carbide (i.e. Metasul™) (Kindsfater et al. 2012). If some reports on Metasul™ underline abnormal failures rates at follow-up exceeding 10 years, they are related to non-osteointegration of poorly coated Wagner cups (Maezawa et al. 2006), loosening of poorly designed cups (Saito et al. 2010), or instability (Randelli et al. 2012), but not to the bearing itself (Migaud et al. 2011) or a marginal rate (Grübl et al. 2007). In contrast, after shorter follow-up of 7 years, Milosev et al. (2006) obtained lower survival (91 %) and a high number of osteolysis with low-carbide content Sikomet™. Using the same bearing, Korovesis et al. (2006) observed 93 % survival at 9 years but an osteolysis rate uncommon with Metasul™ articulation: 1 out of 42 hips at a mean of 13 years (Migaud et al. 2011), 1 out of 105 at a minimum of 10 years (Grübl et al. 2007), and 2 out of 78 hips at a mean of 12.5 years (Hwang et al. 2011).

12.4 Discussion

These data confirm that the implant design, component position, metallurgy, and tribological properties of M-M bearings are major issues for obtaining long-term results. M-M articulation diameter is not the only key factor for success. Some strongly argue that LDH THAs are subject to high rates of complications and reoperation, particularly because of significant sensitivity to component malorientation. SRAs are also sensitive to malposition, and impingement is probably underestimated despite being one of the main issues related to surgical technique as well as socket inclination. The latter underline the technical difficulties in correctly performing SRA and advocate these arthroplasties only in selected high-volume centers. More than bearing diameter, surgical and metallurgical factors appear to be determinants of M-M bearing success: Besides component alignment, prevention of impingement, selection of adequate metal (wear resistance of forged instead of cast alloys, favorable effect of high-carbide content), avoidance of excessive modularity (LDH is the major concern), and adequate coupling design (arc of coverage, ample clearance) are key factors.

Whatever the bearing diameter, some issues are encouraging regarding M-M articulations: (1) Correctly designed, small-diameter M-M have endured for 10 years (Grübl et al. 2007) and have almost reached 15 years of follow-up (Hwang et al. 2011; Migaud et al. 2011) although they were mainly implanted in young and active patients. (2) There is no risk of rupture with M-M, the rate of squeaking is marginal, and they can be applied in case of acetabular reconstruction, in contrast to ceramic-on-ceramic bearings (Girard et al. 2010; Parmaksizoglu et al. 2009). (3) LDH THA is a highly demanding technical and surgical procedure that does not forgive even slight errors (in design, clearance, and orientation) that would be acceptable in conventional THA. LDH THAs require cumbersome surveys, and because of previously mentioned concerns (residual groin pain, ion production, risk of ARMD), they will probably be abandoned progressively. The risk of ARMD and excessive ion production annihilate the slight functional advantage of LDH over small-diameter M-M. (4) SRA is adequate in young and active patients, and M-M bearings are the only viable option for resurfacing. SRA bearing diameter appears to be the key to success of this design, as those below 48 mm are cause for concern. However, for these small-size articulations, other options such as ceramic-on-ceramic also raise concerns, particularly in young and active patients who may require hard bearings. SRA also is an unforgiving, technically demanding procedure that should probably be done in select high-volume centers (a threshold should be precisely determined but a minimum of 70–100 SRAs/year appear to be a reasonable recommendation). To avoid smaller diameters (46 mm or below) and prevent impingement, head-neck ratio may drive the selection of larger-diameter heads and increase acetabular bone resection (Loughead et al. 2006), even while this issue is still being discussed (Vendittoli et al. 2010a). SRA is a viable option if it is well oriented with adequate clearance and metallurgy, producing highly resistant articulations for young and active patients (male or female with femoral heads $\geq$46 mm).

12.5   Recommendations Regarding the Use of M-M Bearings According to Diameter

On behalf of EFORT, a group of experts detailed an adequate survey of M-M bearings according to diameter (EFORT consensus statement 2012). In summary, the use of small M-M (≤32 mm) should follow the recommendations of conventional THA. LDH THAs should be assessed annually, including blood ion levels, X-rays, and clinical evaluations. SRA assessment should track LDH THA up to the fifth year and conventional THA thereafter. In case of symptoms and/or Co elevation, ultrasound or MRI should be performed (EFORT consensus statement 2012). If M-M bearings become symptomatic and/or present Co >7 μg/L, closer follow-up should be implemented (every 6 months, with clinical-biological examination and ultrasound or MRI), particularly if any pejorative factor is present, such as small diameter for SRA of LDH or step cup inclination.

Conflict of Interest   Henri Migaud is an occasional consultant to Zimmer and Tornier. Julien Girard is an occasional consultant for education and research to Zimmer, Smith and Nephew and Wright Medical Technology.

Charles Berton, Sophie Putman, Antoine Combes, Alexandre Blairon and Gregory Kern have no conflict of interest to report.

References

Affatato S, Leardini W, Jedenmalm A, Ruggeri O, Toni A (2007) Larger diameter bearings reduce wear in metal-on-metal hip implants. Clin Orthop Relat Res 456:153–158

Affatato S, Spinelli M, Zavalloni M, Leardini W, Viceconti M (2008) Predictive role of the lambda ratio in the evaluation of metal-on-metal total hip replacement. Proc Inst Mech Eng H 222:617–628

Affatato S, Traina F, Ruggeri O, Toni A (2011) Wear of metal-on-metal hip bearings: metallurgical considerations after hip simulator studies. Int J Artif Organs 34:1155–1164

Amstutz HC, Le Duff MJ, Campbell PA, Gruen TA, Wisk LE (2010) Clinical and radiographic results of metal-on-metal hip resurfacing with a minimum ten-year follow-up. J Bone Joint Surg Am 92:2663–2671, *

Amstutz HC, Wisk LE, Le Duff MJ (2011) Sex as a patient selection criterion for metal-on-metal hip resurfacing arthroplasty. J Arthroplasty 26:198–208, *

Amstutz HC, Le Duff MJ, Johnson AJ (2012) Socket position determines hip resurfacing 10-year survivorship. Clin Orthop Relat Res 470(11):3127–3133, Epub ahead of print

Angadji A, Royle M, Collins SN, Shelton JC (2009) Influence of cup orientation on the wear performance of metal-on-metal hip replacements. Proc Inst Mech Eng H 223:449–457

Barrett WP, Kindsfater KA, Lesko JP (2012) Large-diameter modular metal-on-metal total hip arthroplasty: incidence of revision for adverse reaction to metallic debris. J Arthroplasty 27:976–983, *

Beaulé PE, Kim PR, Powell J, Canadian Hip Resurfacing Study Group (2011) A survey on the prevalence of pseudotumors with metal-on-metal hip resurfacing in Canadian academic centers. J Bone Joint Surg Am 93:118–121, ◊

Bernstein M, Walsh A, Petit A, Zukor DJ, Huk OL, Antoniou J (2011) Femoral head size does not affect ion values in metal-on-metal total hips. Clin Orthop Relat Res 469:1642–1650

Berton C, Girard J, Krantz N, Migaud H (2010) The Durom large diameter head acetabular component: early results with a large-diameter metal-on-metal bearing. J Bone Joint Surg Br 92:202–208

Bolland BJ, Culliford DJ, Langton DJ, Millington JP, Arden NK, Latham JM (2011) High failure rates with a large-diameter hybrid metal-on-metal total hip replacement: clinical, radiological and retrieval analysis. J Bone Joint Surg Br 93:608–615

Brockett CL, Harper P, Williams S, Isaac GH, Dwyer-Joyce RS, Jin Z, Fisher J (2008) The influence of clearance on friction, lubrication and squeaking in large diameter metal-on-metal hip replacements. J Mater Sci Mater Med 19:1575–1579

Browne JA, Bechtold CD, Berry DJ, Hanssen AD, Lewallen DG (2010) Failed metal-on-metal hip arthroplasties: a spectrum of clinical presentations and operative findings. Clin Orthop Relat Res 468:2313–2320

Browne JA, Polga DJ, Sierra RJ, Trousdale RT, Cabanela ME (2011) Failure of larger-diameter metal-on-metal total hip arthroplasty resulting from anterior iliopsoas impingement. J Arthroplasty 26:978.e5–978.e8

Cicek H, Kilicarslan K, Yalcin N, Arslan E, Dogramaci Y, Yildirim H (2010) Primary metal-on-metal total hip arthroplasty with large-diameter femoral heads: a clinical trial of 59 hips. Acta Orthop Belg 76:758–765

Clarke MT, Lee PT, Arora A, Villar RN (2003) Levels of metal ions after small- and large-diameter metal-on-metal hip arthroplasty. J Bone Joint Surg Br 85:913–917

Cobb JP, Davda K, Ahmad A, Harris SJ, Masjedi M, Hart AJ (2011) Why large-head metal-on-metal hip replacements are painful: the anatomical basis of psoas impingement on the femoral head-neck junction. J Bone Joint Surg Br 93:881–885

Corten K, MacDonald SJ (2010) Hip resurfacing data from national joint registries: what do they tell us? What do they not tell us? Clin Orthop Relat Res 468:351–357

Coulter G, Young DA, Dalziel RE, Shimmin AJ (2012) Birmingham hip resurfacing at a mean of ten years: results from an independent centre. J Bone Joint Surg Br 94:315–321, *

Cuckler JM, Moore KD, Lombardi AV Jr, McPherson E, Emerson R (2004) Large versus small femoral heads in metal-on-metal total hip arthroplasty. J Arthroplasty 19(8 suppl 3):41–44

Daniel J, Ziaee H, Salama A, Pradhan C, McMinn DJ (2006) The effect of the diameter of metal-on-metal bearings on systemic exposure to cobalt and chromium. J Bone Joint Surg Br 88:443–448

Daniel J, Ziaee H, Pradhan C, McMinn DJ (2008) Systemic metal exposure in large- and small-diameter metal-on-metal total hip replacements. Orthopedics 31(12 Suppl 2), pii: orthosupersite.com/view.asp?rID=37189

Dastane M, Wan Z, Deshmane P, Long WT, Dorr LD (2011) Primary hip arthroplasty with 28-mm Metasul articulation. J Arthroplasty 26:662–664

Davda K, Lali FV, Sampson B, Skinner JA, Hart AJ (2011) An analysis of metal ion levels in the joint fluid of symptomatic patients with metal-on-metal hip replacements. J Bone Joint Surg Br 93:738–745, *

De Haan R, Campbell PA, Su EP, De Smet KA (2008) Revision of metal-on-metal resurfacing arthroplasty of the hip: the influence of malpositioning of the components. J Bone Joint Surg Br 90:1158–1163

de Steiger RN, Hang JR, Miller LN, Graves SE, Davidson DC (2011) Five-year results of the ASR XL acetabular system and the ASR hip resurfacing system: an analysis from the Australian Orthopaedic Association National Joint Replacement Registry. J Bone Joint Surg Am 93:2287–2293, †

Desy NM, Bergeron SG, Petit A, Huk OL, Antoniou J (2011) Surgical variables influence metal ion levels after hip resurfacing. Clin Orthop Relat Res 469:1635–1641

Donell ST, Darrah C, Nolan JF, Wimhurst J, Toms A, Barker TH, Case CP, Tucker JK, Norwich Metal-on-Metal Study Group (2010) Early failure of the Ultima metal-on-metal total hip replacement in the presence of normal plain radiographs. J Bone Joint Surg Br 92:1501–1508

Dowson D, Hardaker C, Flett M, Isaac GH (2004a) A hip joint simulator study of the performance of metal-on-metal joints: Part I: the role of materials. J Arthroplasty 19(8 suppl 3):118–123

Dowson D, Hardaker C, Flett M, Isaac GH (2004b) A hip joint simulator study of the performance of metal-on-metal joints. Part II: design. J Arthroplasty 19(8 suppl 3):124–130

Ebreo D, Khan A, El-Meligy M, Armstrong C, Peter V (2011) Metal ion levels decrease after revision for metallosis arising from large-diameter metal-on-metal hip arthroplasty. Acta Orthop Belg 77:777–781

EFORT consensus statement (2012) Current evidence on the management of metal-on-metal bearings. http://www.rpa.spot.pt/getdoc/a8aef145-61d9-4377-8d7b-524df9382aa5/Consensus-Statement_Metal_on_Metal_120416-(1).aspx, accessed 15 September 2012[†]

Engh CA Jr, MacDonald SJ, Sritulanondha S, Thompson A, Naudie D, Engh CA (2009) 2008 John Charnley award: metal ion levels after metal-on-metal total hip arthroplasty: a randomized trial. Clin Orthop Relat Res 467:101–111,[*]

Engh CA Jr, Ho H, Engh CA (2010) Metal-on-metal hip arthroplasty: does early clinical outcome justify the chance of an adverse local tissue reaction? Clin Orthop Relat Res 468:406–412

Eswaramoorthy V, Moonot P, Kalairajah Y, Biant LC, Field RE (2008) The Metasul metal-on-metal articulation in primary total hip replacement: clinical and radiological results at ten years. J Bone Joint Surg Br 90:1278–1283,[*]

Flanagan S, Jones E, Birkinshaw C (2010) In vitro friction and lubrication of large bearing hip prostheses. Proc Inst Mech Eng H 224:853–864

Garbuz DS, Tanzer M, Greidanus NV, Masri BA, Duncan CP (2010) The John Charnley Award: Metal-on-metal hip resurfacing versus large-diameter head metal-on-metal total hip arthroplasty: a randomized clinical trial. Clin Orthop Relat Res 468:318–325

Girard J, Bocquet D, Autissier G, Fouilleron N, Fron D, Migaud H (2010) Metal-on-metal hip arthroplasty in patients thirty years of age or younger. J Bone Joint Surg Am 92:2419–2426

Glyn-Jones S, Pandit H, Kwon YM, Doll H, Gill HS, Murray DW (2009) Risk factors for inflammatory pseudotumour formation following hip resurfacing. J Bone Joint Surg Br 91:1566–1574,[◊]

Graves SE, Rothwell A, Tucker K, Jacobs JJ, Sedrakyan A, Suppl 3 (2011) A multinational assessment of metal-on-metal bearings in hip replacement. J Bone Joint Surg Am 93(suppl 3):43–47,[†]

Griffin WL, Nanson CJ, Springer BD, Davies MA, Fehring TK (2010) Reduced articular surface of one-piece cups: a cause of runaway wear and early failure. Clin Orthop Relat Res 468:2328–2332

Gruber FW, Bock A, Trattnig S, Lintner F, Ritschl P (2007) Cystic lesion of the groin due to metallosis: a rare long-term complication of metal-on-metal total hip arthroplasty. J Arthroplasty 22:923–927,[◊]

Grübl A, Marker M, Brodner W, Giurea A, Heinze G, Meisinger V, Zehetgruber H, Kotz R (2007) Long-term follow-up of metal-on-metal total hip replacement. J Orthop Res 25:841–848, [*]

Hart AJ, Skinner JA, Henckel J, Sampson B, Gordon F (2011) Insufficient acetabular version increases blood metal ion levels after metal-on-metal hip resurfacing. Clin Orthop Relat Res 469:2590–2597

Hart AJ, Matthies A, Henckel J, Ilo K, Skinner J, Noble PC (2012) Understanding why metal-on-metal hip arthroplasties fail: a comparison between patients with well-functioning and revised birmingham hip resurfacing arthroplasties. AAOS exhibit selection. J Bone Joint Surg Am 94:e22

Hauptfleisch J, Pandit H, Grammatopoulos G, Gill HS, Murray DW, Ostlere S (2012) A MRI classification of periprosthetic soft tissue masses (pseudotumours) associated with metal-on-metal resurfacing hip arthroplasty. Skeletal Radiol 41:149–155

Heneghan C, Langton D, Thompson M (2012) Ongoing problems with metal-on-metal hip implants. BMJ 344:e1349. doi:10.1136/bmj.e1349,[†]

Herman KA, Highcock AJ, Moorehead JD, Scott SJ (2011) A comparison of leg length and femoral offset discrepancies in hip resurfacing, large head metal-on-metal and conventional total hip replacement: a case series. J Orthop Surg Res 6:65

Holland JP, Langton DJ, Hashmi M (2012) Ten-year clinical, radiological and metal ion analysis of the Birmingham Hip Resurfacing: from a single, non-designer surgeon. J Bone Joint Surg Br 94:471–476

Holloway I, Walter WL, Zicat B, Walter WK (2009) Osteolysis with a cementless second generation metal-on-metal cup in total hip replacement. Int Orthop 33:1537–1542,[*]

Hu XQ, Wood RJ, Taylor A, Tuke MA (2011) The tribological behaviour of different clearance MOM hip joints with lubricants of physiological viscosities. Proc Inst Mech Eng H 225:1061–1069

Hwang KT, Kim YH, Kim YS, Choi IY (2011) Cementless total hip arthroplasty with a metal-on-metal bearing in patients younger than 50 years. J Arthroplasty 26:1481–1487,[*]

Jameson SS, Langton DJ, Nargol AV (2010) Articular surface replacement of the hip: a prospective single-surgeon series. J Bone Joint Surg Br 92:28–37

Jeffers JR, Roques A, Taylor A, Tuke MA (2009) The problem with large diameter metal-on-metal acetabular cup inclination. Bull NYU Hosp Jt Dis 67:189–192

Jiang Y, Zhang K, Die J, Shi Z, Zhao H, Wang K (2011) A systematic review of modern metal-on-metal total hip resurfacing vs standard total hip arthroplasty in active young patients. J Arthroplasty 26:419–426,[†]

Khan M, Takahashi T, Kuiper JH, Sieniawska CE, Takagi K, Richardson JB (2006) Current in vivo wear of metal-on-metal bearings assessed by exercise-related rise in plasma cobalt level. J Orthop Res 24:2029–2035

Kindsfater KA, Sychterz Terefenko CJ, Gruen TA, Sherman CM (2012) Minimum 5-year results of modular metal-on-metal total hip arthroplasty. J Arthroplasty 27(4):545–550, Epub 9 Sept 2011

Korovessis P, Petsinis G, Repanti M, Repantis T (2006) Metallosis after contemporary metal-on-metal total hip arthroplasty. Five- to nine-year follow-up. J Bone Joint Surg Am 88:1183–1191,[*]

Kretzer JP, Kleinhans JA, Jakubowitz E, Thomsen M, Heisel C (2009) A meta-analysis of design- and manufacturing-related parameters influencing the wear behavior of metal-on-metal hip joint replacements. J Orthop Res 27:1473–1480

Kwon YM, Ostlere SJ, McLardy-Smith P, Athanasou NA, Gill HS, Murray DW (2011) "Asymptomatic" pseudotumors after metal-on-metal hip resurfacing arthroplasty: prevalence and metal ion study. J Arthroplasty 26:511–518,[◊]

Langton DJ, Jameson SS, Joyce TJ, Webb J, Nargol AV (2008) The effect of component size and orientation on the concentrations of metal ions after resurfacing arthroplasty of the hip. J Bone Joint Surg Br 90:1143–1151,[◊]

Langton DJ, Jameson SS, Joyce TJ, Hallab NJ, Natu S, Nargol AV (2010) Early failure of metal-on-metal bearings in hip resurfacing and large-diameter total hip replacement: a consequence of excess wear. J Bone Joint Surg Br 92:38–46

Langton DJ, Jameson SS, Joyce TJ, Gandhi JN, Sidaginamale R, Mereddy P, Lord J, Nargol AV (2011a) Accelerating failure rate of the ASR total hip replacement. J Bone Joint Surg Br 93:1011–1016

Langton DJ, Joyce TJ, Jameson SS, Lord J, Van Orsouw M, Holland JP, Nargol AV, De Smet KA (2011b) Adverse reaction to metal debris following hip resurfacing: the influence of component type, orientation and volumetric wear. J Bone Joint Surg Br 93:164–171,[◊]

Lardanchet JF, Taviaux J, Arnalsteen D, Gabrion A, Mertl P (2012) One-year prospective comparative study of three large-diameter metal-on-metal total hip prostheses: serum metal ion levels and clinical outcomes. Orthop Traumatol Surg Res 98:265–274

Latteier MJ, Berend KR, Lombardi AV Jr, Ajluni AF, Seng BE, Adams JB (2011) Gender is a significant factor for failure of metal-on-metal total hip arthroplasty. J Arthroplasty 26(6 suppl):19–23,[◊]

Lavigne M, Therrien M, Nantel J, Roy A, Prince F, Vendittoli PA (2010) The John Charnley Award: the functional outcome of hip resurfacing and large-head THA is the same: a randomized, double-blind study. Clin Orthop Relat Res 468:326–336

Lavigne M, Belzile EL, Roy A, Morin F, Amzica T, Vendittoli PA (2011a) Comparison of whole-blood metal ion levels in four types of metal-on-metal large-diameter femoral head total hip arthroplasty: the potential influence of the adapter sleeve. J Bone Joint Surg Am 93(suppl 2): 128–136

Lavigne M, Laffosse JM, Ganapathi M, Girard J, Vendittoli P (2011b) Residual groin pain at a minimum of two years after metal-on-metal THA with a twenty-eight-millimeter femoral head,

THA with a large-diameter femoral head, and hip resurfacing. J Bone Joint Surg Am 93 (suppl 2):93–98

Le Duff MJ, Amstutz HC, Dorey FJ (2007) Metal-on-metal hip resurfacing for obese patients. J Bone Joint Surg Am 89:2705–2711

Leslie I, Williams S, Brown C, Isaac G, Jin Z, Ingham E, Fisher J (2008) Effect of bearing size on the long-term wear, wear debris, and ion levels of large diameter metal-on-metal hip replacements – an in vitro study. J Biomed Mater Res B Appl Biomater 87:163–172

Liu F, Wang FC, Jin ZM, Hirt F, Rieker C, Grigoris P (2004) Steady-state elastohydrodynamic lubrication analysis of a metal-on-metal hip implant employing a metallic cup with an ultra-high molecular weight polyethylene backing. Proc Inst Mech Eng H 218:261–270

Liu F, Jin Z, Roberts P, Grigoris P (2006) Importance of head diameter, clearance, and cup wall thickness in elastohydrodynamic lubrication analysis of metal-on-metal hip resurfacing prostheses. Proc Inst Mech Eng H 220:695–704

Liu F, Jin Z, Roberts P, Grigoris P (2007) Effect of bearing geometry and structure support on transient elastohydrodynamic lubrication of metal-on-metal hip implants. J Biomech 40:1340–1349

Lombardi AV Jr, Skeels MD, Berend KR, Adams JB, Franchi OJ (2011) Do large heads enhance stability and restore native anatomy in primary total hip arthroplasty? Clin Orthop Relat Res 469:1547–1553

Long WT, Dastane M, Harris MJ, Wan Z, Dorr LD (2010) Failure of the Durom Metasul acetabular component. Clin Orthop Relat Res 468:400–405

Loughead JM, Starks I, Chesney D, Matthews JN, McCaskie AW, Holland JP (2006) Removal of acetabular bone in resurfacing arthroplasty of the hip: a comparison with hybrid total hip arthroplasty. J Bone Joint Surg Br 88:31–34

Malviya A, Ramaskandhan JR, Bowman R, Hashmi M, Holland JP, Kometa S, Lingard E (2011) What advantage is there to be gained using large modular metal-on-metal bearings in routine primary hip replacement? A preliminary report of a prospective randomised controlled trial. J Bone Joint Surg Br 93:1602–1609

Maezawa K, Nozawa M, Matsuda K, Yuasa T, Shitoto K, Kurosawa H (2006) Early failure of modern metal-on-metal total hip arthroplasty using a Wagner standard cup. J Arthroplasty 21:522–526

Marchetti E, Krantz N, Berton C, Bocquet D, Fouilleron N, Migaud H, Girard J (2011) Component impingement in total hip arthroplasty: frequency and risk factors. A continuous retrieval analysis series of 416 cups. Orthop Traumatol Surg Res 97:127–133,◊

Matthies AK, Henckel J, Skinner JA, Hart AJ (2011) A retrieval analysis of explanted Durom metal-on-metal hip arthroplasties. Hip Int 21:724–731

Matthies AK, Skinner JA, Osmani H, Henckel J, Hart AJ (2012) Pseudotumors are common in well-positioned low-wearing metal-on-metal hips. Clin Orthop Relat Res 470:1895–1906,◊

Maurer-Ertl W, Friesenbichler J, Sadoghi P, Pechmann M, Trennheuser M, Leithner A (2012) Metal ion levels in large-diameter total hip and resurfacing hip arthroplasty – preliminary results of a prospective five year study after two years of follow-up. BMC Musculoskelet Disord 13:56

Meding JB, Meding LK, Keating EM, Berend ME (2012) Low incidence of groin pain and early failure with large metal articulation total hip arthroplasty. Clin Orthop Relat Res 470:388–394

Mertl P, Boughebri O, Havet E, Triclot P, Lardanchet JF, Gabrion A (2010) Large diameter head metal-on-metal bearings total hip arthroplasty: preliminary results. Orthop Traumatol Surg Res 96:14–20

Migaud H, Putman S, Krantz N, Vasseur L, Girard J (2011) Cementless metal-on-metal versus ceramic-on-polyethylene hip arthroplasty in patients less than fifty years of age: a comparative study with twelve to fourteen-year follow-up. J Bone Joint Surg Am 93(Suppl 2):137–142

Milosev I, Trebse R, Kovac S, Cör A, Pisot V (2006) Survivorship and retrieval analysis of Sikomet metal-on-metal total hip replacements at a mean of seven years. J Bone Joint Surg Am 88:1173–1182,*

Moroni A, Savarino L, Cadossi M, Baldini N, Giannini S (2008) Does ion release differ between hip resurfacing and metal-on-metal THA? Clin Orthop Relat Res 466:700–707

Neuerburg C, Impellizzeri F, Goldhahn J, Frey P, Naal FD, von Knoch M, Leunig M, von Knoch F (2012) Survivorship of second-generation metal-on-metal primary total hip replacement. Arch Orthop Trauma Surg 132:527–533,*

Neumann DR, Thaler C, Hitzl W, Huber M, Hofstädter T, Dorn U (2010) Long-term results of a contemporary metal-on-metal total hip arthroplasty: a 10-year follow-up study. J Arthroplasty 25:700–708,*

Pandit H, Glyn-Jones S, McLardy-Smith P (2008) Pseudotumours associated with metal-on-metal hip resurfacings. J Bone Joint Surg Br 90:847–851,◊

Park YS, Moon YW, Lim SJ, Yang JM, Ahn G, Choi YL (2005) Early osteolysis following second-generation metal-on-metal hip replacement. J Bone Joint Surg Am 87:1515–1521,◊

Parmaksizoglu AS, Ozkaya U, Bilgili F, Basilgan S, Kabukcuoglu Y (2009) Large diameter metal-on-metal total hip arthroplasty for Crowe IV developmental dysplasia of the hip. Hip Int 19:309–314

Peters CL, McPherson E, Jackson JD, Erickson JA (2007) Reduction in early dislocation rate with large-diameter femoral heads in primary total hip arthroplasty. J Arthroplasty 22(6 Suppl 2): 140–144

Randelli F, Banci L, D'Anna A, Visentin O, Randelli G (2012) Cementless Metasul metal-on-metal total hip arthroplasties at 13 years. J Arthroplasty 27:186–192,*

Rieker CB, Schön R, Konrad R, Liebentritt G, Gnepf P, Shen M, Roberts P, Grigoris P (2005) Influence of the clearance on in-vitro tribology of large diameter metal-on-metal articulations pertaining to resurfacing hip implants. Orthop Clin North Am 36:135–142

Saito S, Ishii T, Mori S, Hosaka K, Ootaki M, Tokuhashi Y (2010) Long-term results of metasul metal-on-metal total hip arthroplasty. Orthopedics 33(8). doi:10.3928/01477447-20100625-11,*

Shimmin AJ, Walter WL, Esposito C (2010) The influence of the size of the component on the outcome of resurfacing arthroplasty of the hip: a review of the literature. J Bone Joint Surg Br 92:469–476,†

Smith AJ, Dieppe P, Vernon K, Porter M, Blom AW, National Joint Registry of England and Wales (2012) Failure rates of stemmed metal-on-metal hip replacements: analysis of data from the National Joint Registry of England and Wales. Lancet 379:1199–1204

Smith TM, Berend KR, Lombardi AV Jr, Emerson RH Jr, Mallory TH (2005) Metal-on-metal total hip arthroplasty with large heads may prevent early dislocation. Clin Orthop Relat Res 441:137–142

Smith TO, Nichols R, Donell ST, Hing CB (2010) The clinical and radiological outcomes of hip resurfacing versus total hip arthroplasty: a meta-analysis and systematic review. Acta Orthop 81:684–695,†

Smolders JM, Hol A, Rijnberg WJ, van Susante JL (2011) Metal ion levels and functional results after either resurfacing hip arthroplasty or conventional metal-on-metal hip arthroplasty. Acta Orthop 82:559–566

Spencer S, Carter R, Murray H, Meek RM (2008) Femoral neck narrowing after metal-on-metal hip resurfacing. J Arthroplasty 23:1105–1109

Stuchin SA (2008) Anatomic diameter femoral heads in total hip arthroplasty: a preliminary report. J Bone Joint Surg Am 90(suppl 3):52–56

Theruvil B, Vasukutty N, Hancock N, Higgs D, Dunlop DG, Latham JM (2011) Dislocation of large diameter metal-on-metal bearings an indicator of metal reaction? J Arthroplasty 26:832–837,◊

Treacy RB, McBryde CW, Shears E, Pynsent PB (2011) Birmingham hip resurfacing: a minimum follow-up of ten years. J Bone Joint Surg Br 93:27–33,*

Underwood RJ, Zografos A, Sayles RS, Hart A, Cann P (2012) Edge loading in metal-on-metal hips: low clearance is a new risk factor. Proc Inst Mech Eng H 226:217–226

van der Weegen W, Hoekstra HJ, Sijbesma T, Bos E, Schemitsch EH, Poolman RW (2011) Survival of metal-on-metal hip resurfacing arthroplasty: a systematic review of the literature. J Bone Joint Surg Br 93:298–306,†

Vendittoli PA, Ganapathi M, Roy AG, Lusignan D, Lavigne M (2010a) A comparison of clinical results of hip resurfacing arthroplasty and 28 mm metal on metal total hip arthroplasty: a randomised trial with 3–6 years follow-up. Hip Int 20:1–13,*

Vendittoli PA, Roy A, Mottard S, Girard J, Lusignan D, Lavigne M (2010b) Metal ion release from bearing wear and corrosion with 28 mm and large-diameter metal-on-metal bearing articulations: a follow-up study. J Bone Joint Surg Br 92:12–19

Vendittoli PA, Amzica T, Roy AG, Lusignan D, Girard J, Lavigne M (2011) Metal Ion release with large-diameter metal-on-metal hip arthroplasty. J Arthroplasty 26:282–288

Willert HG, Buchhorn GH, Fayyazi A, Flury R, Windler M, Köster G, Lohmann CH (2005) Metal-on-metal bearings and hypersensitivity in patients with artificial hip joints. A clinical and histomorphological study. J Bone Joint Surg Am 87:28–36,◊

Williams DH, Greidanus NV, Masri BA, Duncan CP, Garbuz DS (2011) Prevalence of pseudotumor in asymptomatic patients after metal-on-metal hip arthroplasty. J Bone Joint Surg Am 93:2164–2171,◊

Zhang X, Xu W, Li J, Fang Z, Chen K (2010) Large-diameter metal-on-metal cementless total hip arthroplasty in the elderly. Orthopedics 33:872

Zhou YX, Guo SJ, Liu Q, Tang J, Li YJ (2009) Influence of the femoral head size on early postoperative gait restoration after total hip arthroplasty. Chin Med J (Engl) 122:1513–1516

Aseptic Loosening of Metal-on-Metal (MOM) Total Hip Arthroplasties (THA) with Large-Diameter Heads

13

Christoph H. Lohmann, G. Singh, G. Goldau, T. Müller, B. Feuerstein, M. Rütschi, and H. Meyer

Large-diameter metal-on-metal (MOM) bearing surfaces evolved directly from the success of hip surface replacement using MOM bearing surfaces. In cases of failed femoral components with well-fixed acetabular components, large-diameter bearing surfaces served well as revision implants compatible with standard stems to avoid cup revision. Reduced dislocation rates with large-diameter bearings and potentially reduced wear (Lombardi et al. 2011) due to increased fluid-film lubrication prompted their use in primary THA. However, unacceptably high revision rates, early aseptic loosening, adverse tissue reactions and pseudotumour formation and increased metal ion release have been observed in large-diameter MOM THAs (Smith et al. 2012; Bolland et al. 2011; Langton et al. 2010; Barrett et al. 2012; Hasegawa et al. 2012; Bosker et al. 2012; Berton et al. 2010; Matthies et al. 2011). The possible reasons for this phenomenon are failure to achieve optimum fluid-film lubrication, edge loading and impingement, increased torque from the large head as

C.H. Lohmann (✉) • G. Goldau • T. Müller • H. Meyer
Department of Orthopaedic Surgery,
Otto-von-Guericke-University, Magdeburg, Germany
e-mail: lohmannch@t-online.de

G. Singh
Department of Orthopaedic Surgery, Otto-von-Guericke-University,
Magdeburg, Germany

University Orthopaedics, Hand and Reconstructive Microsurgery Cluster,
National University Health System, Singapore, Singapore

B. Feuerstein
Institute for Mechanical Engineering, Magdeburg-Stendal
University of Applied Sciences, Magdeburg, Germany

M. Rütschi
Department of Orthopaedic Surgery, Loretto Hospital,
Freiburg, Germany

K. Knahr (ed.), *Total Hip Arthroplasty*,
DOI 10.1007/978-3-642-35653-7_13, © EFORT 2013

well as corrosion and wear at the cone-taper interface leading to deposition of large amounts of metal wear debris in the periprosthetic tissues.

13.1 Evolution of Large-Diameter Metal-on-Metal Bearing Surfaces

The use of metal-on-metal (MOM) bearing surfaces in total hip arthroplasty (THA) is not a new phenomenon. The McKee-Farrar (Brown et al. 2002; Howie et al. 2005) and Ring (Bryant et al. 1991) implants had MOM bearing surfaces in the 1960s. The subsequent advent of the Charnley hip (Jacobsson et al. 1996) in the 1970s led to a frameshift in clinical practice, with early promising results leading to most surgeons abandoning MOM bearing surfaces for metal-on-polyethylene (MOP). Advances in the understanding of osteolysis secondary to polyethylene wear particles coupled with the phenomenon of younger patients with higher activity demands undergoing THA surgery led to a quest for hard-on-hard bearing surfaces and the reintroduction of MOM hips in the late 1980s. Second-generation MOM with high-carbon cobalt-chrome alloy bearing surfaces were developed and the first of these was introduced into clinical practice by Weber in 1988 (Weber 1992). These were thought to have low-wear profiles and therefore increased implant longevity especially in the young patient. Large-diameter MOM heads (36-mm diameter or larger) evolved directly from the success of hip surface replacement as salvage implants which were compatible with standard stems in cases of failed femoral components with well-fixed acetabular components, in an attempt to avoid cup revision. Large-diameter bearings then gained popularity in an attempt to reduce the dislocation risk in revision as well as primary THA. They were also shown to increase the stability and reduce the risk of dislocation of THA (Lombardi et al. 2011) by increasing the distance the prosthetic head has to travel to dislocate. The risk of impingement was also thought to be reduced with large heads, thus theoretically reducing metallic wear debris in MOM hips (Fig. 13.1).

MOM bearing surfaces were not without problems, the main concerns being elevated metal ions in blood, urine and solid organs, potential hypersensitivity including pseudotumour formation and aseptic lymphocyte-dominated vasculitis-associated lesion (ALVAL) reactions, potential carcinogenesis, teratogenicity and early aseptic loosening (Smith et al. 2012; Bozic et al. 2012; Morrey et al. 2011; Catelas and Wimmer 2011; Delaunay et al. 2010; Browne et al. 2010; Mann et al. 2012; Haddad et al. 2011; Shetty and Villar 2006; MacDonald 2004; Amstutz and Grigoris 1996; Fabi et al. 2012; Gonzalez et al. 2011). Large-diameter heads, which theoretically should increase fluid-film lubrication and reduce wear in addition to increasing stability, had paradoxically higher revision rates and failed earlier in the context of MOM hips (Smith et al. 2012). Smith et al. (2012) reported an analysis of 400,000 primary THA procedures (out of which 31,171, 8 %, had stemmed MOM hips) from the National Joint Registry of England and Wales, which showed that larger head sizes increased implant failure rates for MOM hips. Overall 5-year revision rate for MOM prostheses was 6.2 % and 5-year MOM revision rates for 28-mm and 52-mm heads in men aged 60 years were 3.2 and 5.1 %, respectively. In contrast, they reported that ceramic-on-ceramic bearing surfaces with large heads

Fig. 13.1 Plain anteroposterior radiograph of a patient with large-diameter MOM THA with osteolysis at the greater trochanter

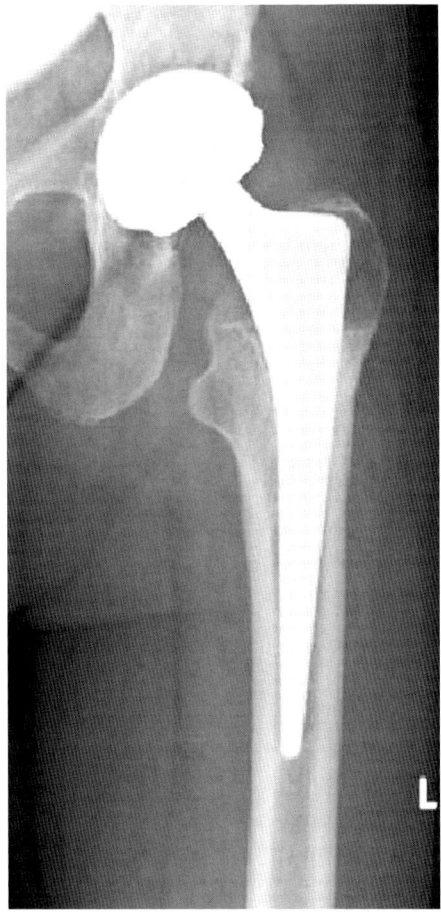

did better than conventional 28-mm head sizes. Potential reasons for this rather surprising observation include failure to achieve optimum fluid-film lubrication, edge loading, increased torque from the large head or corrosion and wear at the cone-taper interface (head-neck junction). Perhaps these phenomena represent inevitable adverse consequences of modularity superimposed on a simple exchange of the conventional MOP bearing on a stem for a large MOM bearing.

Certain MOM designs such as the ASR hip (Bernthal et al. 2012) have had unacceptably high revision rates and have been withdrawn from the market. This has perhaps led to the assumption among some that the failure of MOM hips is exclusively an implant-specific phenomenon. Alison Smith and colleagues (2012) reported that large-head MOM failure is a class effect and is not implant specific. We believe that both phenomena prevail-implant-specific failures in addition to an overall class effect, as exemplified by the ASR hip. Despite the data that has recently emerged, MOM bearing surfaces are still being used rather extensively. In 2009, 35 % of THA surgeries in the United States had MOM bearings. At present, there are more than 500,000 patients with implanted MOM hips in the USA and more than 40,000 in the UK (Smith et al. 2012).

13.2   Modularity in Large-Diameter MOM THA

In general, modular THA implant designs confer distinct advantages such as increased intraoperative flexibility, adjustment of leg length and offset via the head-neck taper and femoral anteversion via the neck-stem taper. This potentially leads to optimal restoration of soft tissue tension and biomechanics of the replaced hip. Other advantages of modularity include decreased implant inventory and the ability to remove the femoral head at revision surgery to improve exposure or change head size without component removal (Srinivasan et al. 2012). However, multiple modular junctions represent additional sites for implant failure through fretting and crevice corrosion and release of metal particles. This may lead to instability and, in the worst-case scenario, dissociation at the modular interface (Jacobs et al. 1995). Retrieval studies have demonstrated that even with modern taper designs and corrosion-resistant materials, fretting movement and corrosion may result at modular interfaces. This is especially so when mixed metals are used, i.e. acetabular cup and head components made from cobalt-chrome alloys coupled with titanium stems (Kop and Swarts 2009). Malviya et al. (2011) reported an increase in whole blood metal ion levels in patients with large-diameter metal-on-metal hip arthroplasties and suggested that this phenomenon may be due to micromotion at the head-neck junction or excess stem micromotion (Malviya et al. 2011).

In the context of large-diameter MOM hip arthroplasties, exchanging the bearing couple from MOP to MOM and subsequently increasing the head size results in an increased sliding distance of the bearing couple and moment arm from the cone-taper to the joint line. The behaviour of the stem may also be affected as there are documented differences in the frictional torque of MOM and MOP bearing surfaces, with MOM bearings having increased torque on the trunnion. Edge-loading, low clearance and psoas impingement are other problems which have been described in the context of large diameter MoM hips (Underwood et al. 2012, Brockett et al. 2008, Browne et al. 2011, Cobb et al. 2011). Superimposed on these complex alterations in biomechanics are the inherent problems of modular interfaces, as discussed above.

13.3   Corrosion at the Cone-Taper Interface

Modular mixed-metal THA designs allow combination of the wear resistance of cobalt-chrome femoral heads with the flexibility of titanium stems. Collier and colleagues (1992) studied the cone-taper interface of 139 retrieved modular hip arthroplasties sent by 87 surgeons and found that in mixed-metal systems there was evidence of time-dependent corrosion at the taper interface whereas there was no evidence of corrosion among the implants which had components made from the same alloy. In an earlier study, Collier et al. (1991) discussed that the crevice provided between the head and neck will function as a corrosion site if it is wide enough to allow aqueous intrusion but sufficiently narrow to maintain a stagnant zone. As corrosion progresses in this zone, oxygen is depleted, resulting in an excess of positively charged metal ions in the aqueous environment of the crevice. This is then balanced by the migration of negatively charged chloride ions resulting in the

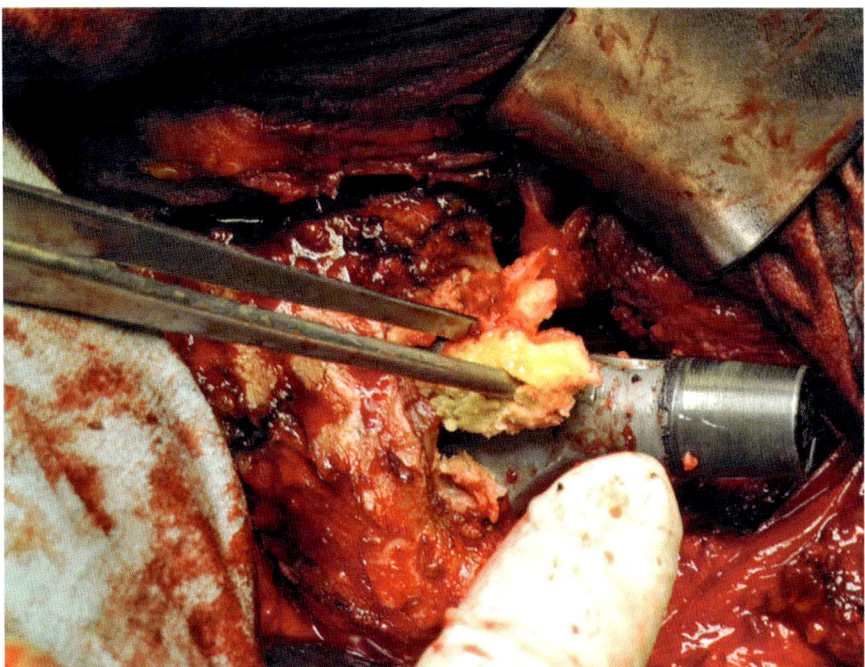

Fig. 13.2 Intraoperative photograph showing corrosion of the taper and necrotic periprosthetic tissue resembling thick pus in gross appearance. Cultures were sterile

production of hydrochloric acid which is capable of dissolving both the otherwise stable cobalt and titanium alloys (Collier et al. 1992; Collier et al. 1991).

A mixed-alloy combination has been thought to be resistant to galvanically accelerated crevice corrosion in the context of hip arthroplasty. However, (Collier et al. 1992) reported that in a detailed examination of the results of some these studies, there were indications for the potential for corrosion. Although titanium and its alloys reportedly develop a protective layer by passivation, it is evident that a combination of different metals like iron and cobalt-chrome or titanium and cobalt-chrome produces an electrochemical potential. Willert et al. (2005) reported that the passivation layer of the alloy safely protects the release of ions and may inhibit electrochemical conduction. However, micromotion may damage and initiate electrochemical dissolution of the protective layer leading to galvanic corrosion in the context of mixed metals. Wear as well as corrosion debris may be released from the surface as a result of continued fretting corrosion and oscillating micromotion (Fig. 13.2).

It has been shown that corrosion occurs at the cone-taper interface but most of the studies in the literature are focussed on implants using conventional 28-mm heads (Gill et al. 2012; Cook et al. 1994; Huber et al. 2009). The authors believe that corrosion occurring at the cone-taper interfaces of large-diameter MOM THAs leads to instability at the cone-taper junction, deposition of metal wear and corrosion debris in the periprosthetic tissues and consequent early aseptic loosening and failure. In the authors' series of 114 revisions of large-diameter MOM THAs with a mean duration

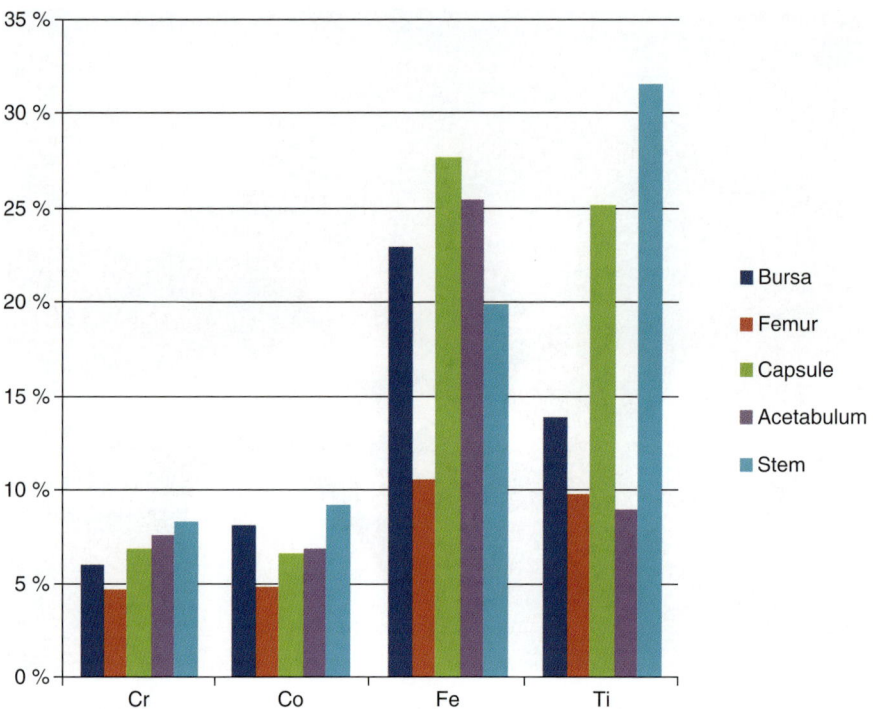

Fig. 13.3 Element analysis showing the relative proportions of different metals in the periprosthetic tissue samples

of implantation of 46 months, 107 retrieved implants (94 %) had corrosion as well as gross instability at the cone-taper interface (the heads were loose on the taper). Electrochemical studies on the stem and head adapter showed an open circuit potential in normal saline suggesting galvanic corrosion. Periprosthetic tissues were processed by routine histology and immunological responses to metal wear debris were examined. Periprosthetic tissue metal content was also analysed, and titanium as well as iron was detected at higher levels compared with cobalt and chromium. This is most likely due to abrasive wear at the failed cone-taper junction. Head size did not correlate with periprosthetic tissue metal content (Meyer et al. 2012) (Fig. 13.3).

13.4 Tissue Responses in Failed Large-Diameter MOM THAs

Immune responses to particulate wear debris are the subject of much controversy and not fully understood. There appears to be a complex interplay of immunological processes which contribute to periprosthetic osteolysis, metal hypersensitivity and aseptic loosening of endoprostheses. Most of the current literature (Barrett et al. 2012; Goodman 2007; Lohmann et al. 2007; Ng et al. 2011) emphasises two key responses – a nonspecific macrophage-mediated granulomatous response which lacks immunological memory and is also seen in foreign body granulomatous reactions (e.g. suture

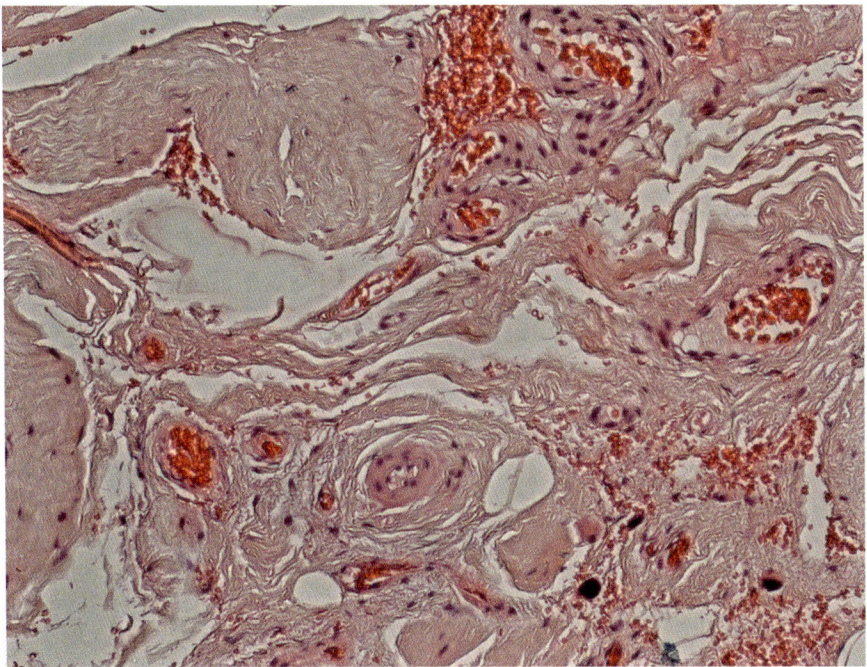

Fig. 13.4 Histology slide of retrieval tissue demonstrating vasculitis and haemorrhage

material) and a T-cell-mediated type IV hypersensitivity reaction which involves diffuse and perivascular lymphocytic infiltrates. This latter type of response involves a specific antigen, co-stimulatory molecules, an antigen presenting cell and T lymphocytes. The lymphocyte-dominated response is adaptive and has immunological memory and is also seen in several autoimmune disease processes (Goodman 2007; Lohmann et al. 2007). Histologic findings common to both types of responses include vasculitis with perivascular and intramural lymphocytic infiltration of the postcapillary vessels, swelling of the vascular endothelium, recurrent localised bleeding and necrosis. A host of inflammatory cytokines such as interleukin-6 (IL-6), prostaglandin E_2 (PGE$_2$) and tumour necrosis factor alpha (TNFα) have been implicated in the pathways leading to periprosthetic osteolysis (Fig. 13.4).

Lymphocyte-dominated responses have been seen in failed 28-mm MOM hips. In our histological analysis of periprosthetic tissue specimens taken from 114 revision large-diameter MOM hips, there were only nine cases which displayed a lymphocyte-dominated type of response (Meyer et al. 2012). All other cases had a predominantly foreign body type of response and areas of necrosis with macrophages being the most numerous cell type. This may be attributed to the fact that in the studies with 28-mm heads, the cone-taper interfaces were more stable, resulting in a different profile of released particulate wear debris (Fig. 13.5).

Immunological reactions to metal wear debris can result in early aseptic loosening and, if not recognised, may result in devastating necrosis of surrounding muscle and bone. Barrett et al. (2012) suggested that MOM THA with second-generation

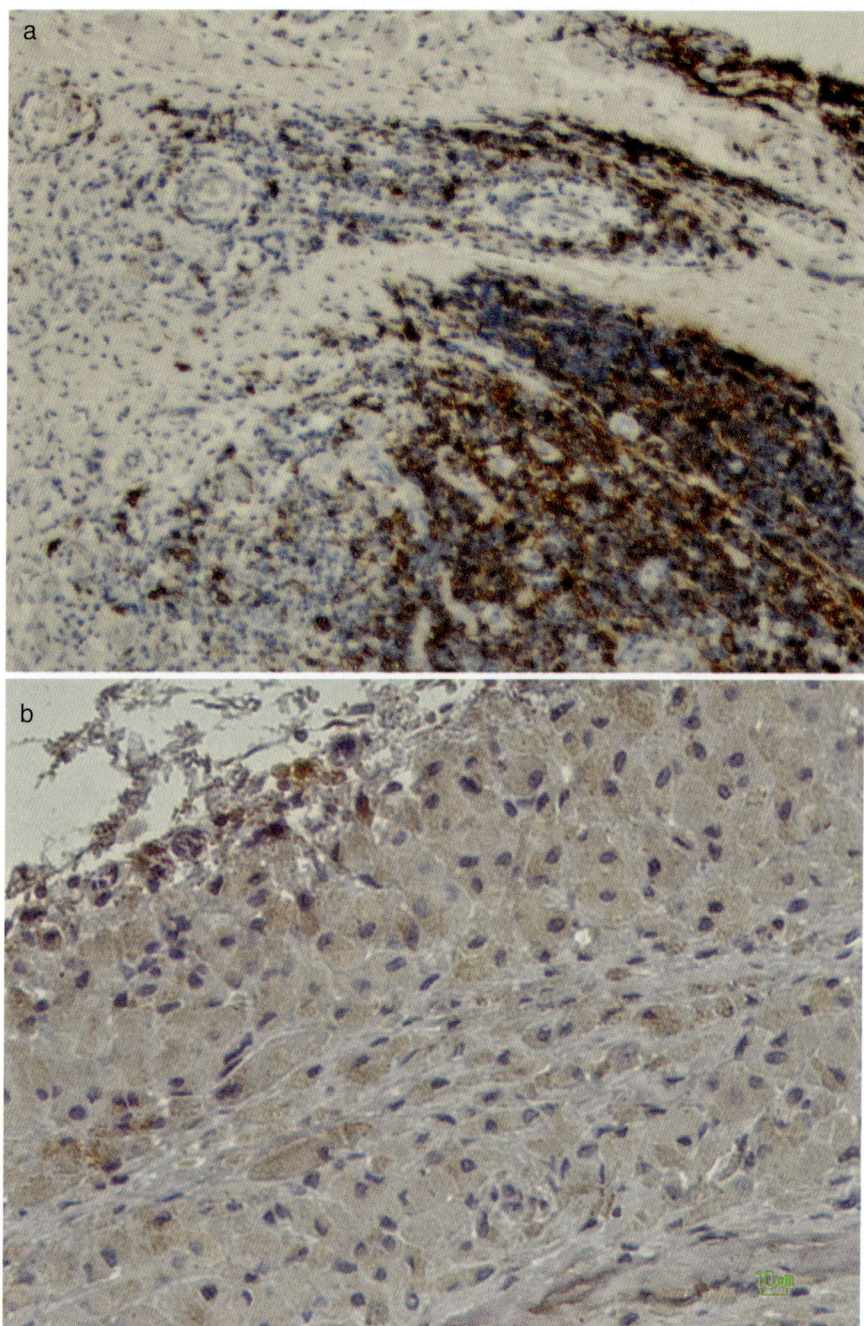

Fig. 13.5 Immunohistochemistry of retrieval tissue (**a**) CD20 antibody staining for B cells, 10 ×
magnification, and (**b**) CD68 antibody staining for cells of the monocyte-macrophage lineage, 20
× magnification

modular designs is a reasonable choice for selected patients, but surgeons using these implants must be aware of the potential for adverse reaction to metallic debris (ARMED). This includes metallosis, pseudotumours and ALVAL. Further research is necessary to better characterise the immunological reactions to metal particles and wear debris. The authors are of the view that large-diameter MOM THA should not be used in primary THA, given the potential problems and high revision rates secondary to aseptic loosening.

13.5   Summary

In summary, large-diameter MOM bearing surfaces have a significantly higher revision rate and early failure due to aseptic loosening. The key mechanisms contributing to this are likely to be failure to achieve optimum fluid-film lubrication, edge loading and impingement, increased torque forces and corrosion at the cone-taper interface leading to instability and loosening as well as deposition of large amounts of metal particulate debris in the periprosthetic tissues. Immunological responses to metal wear debris are still a subject of ongoing research, and at present, the authors do not recommend the use of large-diameter MOM bearing surfaces for primary THA.

References

Amstutz HC, Grigoris P (1996) Metal on metal bearings in hip arthroplasty. Clin Orthop Relat Res 329 (Suppl.):S11–S34(Review)

Barrett WP, Kindsfater KA, Lesko JP (2012) Large-diameter modular metal-on-metal total hip arthroplasty: incidence of revision for adverse reaction to metallic debris. J Arthroplasty 27(6):976.e1–983.e1

Bernthal NM, Celestre PC, Stravrakis AI, Ludington JC, Oakes DA (2012) Disappointing short-term results with the Depuy ASR XL metal-on-metal total hip arthroplasty. J Arthroplasty 27(4):539–544, Epub 13 Oct 2011

Berton C, Girard J, Krantz N, Migaud H (2010) The Durom large diameter head acetabular component: early results with a large diameter metal-on-metal bearing. J Bone Joint Surg Br 92-B:202–208

Bolland BJRF, Culliford DJ, Langton DJ, Millington JPS, Arden NK, Latham JM (2011) High failure rates with a large diameter hybrid metal-on-metal total hip replacement: clinical radiological and retrieval analysis. J Bone Joint Surg Br 93(5):608–615

Bosker BH, Ettema HB, Boomsma MF, Kollen BJ, Maas M, Verheyen CCPM (2012) High incidence of pseudotumour formation after large-diameter metal-on-metal total hip replacement: a prospective cohort study. J Bone Joint Surg Br 94-B:755–761

Bozic KJ, Browne J, Dangles CJ, Manner PA, Yates AJ Jr, Weber KL, Boyer KM, Zemaitis P, Woznica A, Turkelson CM, Wies JL (2012) Modern metal-on-metal hip implants. J Am Acad Orthop Surg 20(6):402–406, Review

Brockett CL, Harper P, Williams S, Isaac GH, Dwyer-Joyce RS, Jin Z, Fisher J (2008) The influence of clearance on friction, lubrication and squeaking in large diameter metal-on-metal hip replacements. J Mater Sci Mater Med 19(4):1575–1579

Brown SR, Davies WA, DeHeer DH, Swanson AB (2002) Long-term survival of McKee-Farrar total hip prostheses. Clin Orthop Relat Res (402):157–163

Browne JA, Bechtold CD, Berry DJ, Hanssen AD, Lewallen DG (2010) Failed metal-on-metal hip arthroplasties: a spectrum of clinical presentations and operative findings. Clin Orthop Relat Res 468:2313–2320

Browne JA, Polga DJ, Sierra RJ, Trousdale RT, Cabanela ME (2011) Failure of larger-diameter metal-on-metal total hip arthroplasty resulting from anterior iliopsoas impingement. J Arthroplasty 26(6):978.e5–e8

Bryant MJ, Mollan RA, Nixon JR (1991) Survivorship analysis of the ring hip arthroplasty. J Arthroplasty 6(Suppl.):S5–S10

Catelas I, Wimmer MA (2011) New insights into wear and biological effects of metal-on-metal bearings. J Bone Joint Surg Am 93(suppl 2):76–83

Cobb JP, Davda K, Ahmad A, Harris SJ, Masjedi M, Hart AJ (2011) Why large-head metal-on-metal hip replacements are painful: the anatomical basis of psoas impingement on the femoral head-neck junction. J Bone Joint Surg Br 93(7):881–885

Collier JP, Suprenant VA, Jensen RE, Mayor MB (1991) Corrosion at the interface of cobalt-alloy heads on titanium-alloy stems. Clin Orthop Relat Res 271:305–312

Collier JP, Suprenant VA, Jensen RE, Mayor MB, Suprenant HP (1992) Corrosion between the components of modular femoral hip prostheses. J Bone Joint Surg Br 74-B:511–517

Cook SD, Barrack RL, Clemow AJT (1994) Corrosion and wear at the modular interface of uncemented femoral stems. J Bone Joint Surg Br 76-B:68–72

Delaunay C, Petit I, Learmonth ID, Oger P, Vendittoli PA (2010) Metal-on-metal bearings total hip arthroplasty: the cobalt and chromium ions release concern. Orthop Traumatol Surg Res 96:894–904

Fabi D, Levine B, Paprosky W, Della Valle C, Sporer S, Klein G, Levine H, Hartzband M (2012) Metal-on-metal total hip arthroplasty: causes and high incidence of early failure. Orthopedics 35(7):e1009–e1016

Gill IPS, Webb J, Sloan K, Beaver RJ (2012) Corrosion at the neck-stem junction as a cause of metal ion release and pseudotumour formation. J Bone Joint Surg Br 94-B:895–900

Gonzalez MH, Carr R, Walton S, Mihalko WM (2011) The evolution and modern use of metal-on-metal bearings in total hip arthroplasty. Instr Course Lect 60:247–255

Goodman SB (2007) Wear particles, periprosthetic osteolysis and the immune system. Biomaterials 28:5044–5048

Haddad FS, Thakrar RR, Hart AJ, Skinner JA, Nargol AV, Nolan JF, Gill HS, Murray DW, Blom AW, Case CP (2011) Metal-on-metal bearings: the evidence so far. J Bone Joint Surg Br 93(5):572–579, Review

Hasegawa M, Yoshida K, Wakabayashi H, Sudo A (2012) Cobalt and chromium ion release after large-diameter metal-on-metal total hip arthroplasty. J Arthroplasty 27(6):990–996, Epub 8 Feb 2012

Howie DW, McCalden RW, Nawana NS, Costi K, Pearcy MJ, Subramanian C (2005) The long-term wear of retrieved McKee-Farrar metal-on-metal total hip prostheses. J Arthroplasty 20(3):350–357

Huber M, Reinisch G, Trettenhahn G, Zweymuller K, Lintner F (2009) Presence of corrosion products and hypersensitivity-associated reactions in periprosthetic tissue after aseptic loosening of total hip replacements with metal bearing surfaces. Acta Biomater 5:172–180

Jacobs JJ, Urban RM, Gilbert JL, Skipor AK, Black J, Jasty M, Galante JO (1995) Local and distant products from modularity. Clin Orthop Relat Res 319:94–105

Jacobsson SA, Djerf K, Wahlström O (1996) Twenty-year results of McKee-Farrar versus Charnley prosthesis. Clin Orthop Relat Res 329:S60–S68

Kop AM, Swarts E (2009) Corrosion of a hip stem with a modular neck taper junction. A retrieval study of 16 cases. J Arthroplasty 24(7):1019–1023

Langton DJ, Jameson SS, Joyce TJ, Hallab NJ, Natu S, Nargol AVF (2010) Early failure of metal-on-metal bearings in hip resurfacing and large-diameter total hip replacement: a consequence of excess wear. J Bone Joint Surg Br 92-B:38–46

Lohmann CH, Nuechtern JV, Willert HG, Junk-Jantsch S, Ruether W, Pflueger G (2007) Hypersensitivity reactions in total hip arthroplasty. Orthopedics 30(9):760–761

Lombardi AV Jr, Skeels MD, Berend KR, Adams JB, Franchi OJ (2011) Do large heads enhance stability and restore native anatomy in primary total hip arthroplasty? Clin Orthop Relat Res 469(6):1547–1553

MacDonald SJ (2004) Metal-on-metal total hip arthroplasty: the concerns. Clin Orthop Relat Res 429:86–93 (Review)

Malviya A, Ramaskandhan JR, Bowman R, Kometa S, Hashmi M, Lingard E, Holland JP (2011) What advantage is there to be gained by using large modular metal-on-metal bearings in routine primary hip replacement? A preliminary report of a prospective randomized controlled trial. J Bone Joint Surg Br 93 B:1602–1609

Mann BS, Whittingham-Jones PM, Shaerf DA, Nawaz ZS, Harvie P, Hart AJ, Skinner JA (2012) Metal-on-metal bearings, inflammatory pseudotumours, and their neurological manifestations. Hip Int 22(2):129–136

Matthies AK, Henckel J, Skinner JA, Hart AJ (2011) A retrieval analysis of explanted Durom metal-on-metal hip arthroplasties. Hip Int 21(6):724–731

Meyer H, Mueller T, Goldau G, Chamaon K, Ruetschi M, Lohmann CH (2012) Corrosion at the cone-taper interface leads to failure of large-diameter metal-on-metal total hip arthroplasties. Clin Orthop Relat Res 470(11):3101–3108

Morrey BF, Berry DJ, An K, Kitaoka HB, Pagnano MW (2011) Joint replacement arthroplasty basic science, hip, knee and ankle. In: Fourth Centennial Edition, Vol II. Wolters Klumer Health, Philadelphia, p 510–514

Ng VY, Lombardi AV, Berend KR, Skeels MD, Adams JB (2011) Perivascular lymphocytic infiltration is not limited to metal-on-metal bearings. Clin Orthop Relat Res 469:523–529

Shetty VD, Villar RN (2006) Development and problems of metal-on-metal hip arthroplasty. Proc Inst Mech Eng H 220(2):371–377 (Review)

Smith AJ, Dieppe P, Vernon K, Porter M, Blom AW (2012) Failure rates of stemmed metal-on-metal hip replacements: analysis of data from the National Joint Registry of England and Wales. Lancet 379:1199–1204

Srinivasan A, Jung E, Levine BR (2012) Modularity of the femoral component in total hip arthroplasty. J Am Acad Orthop Surg 20(4):214–222

Underwood RJ, Zografos A, Sayles RS, Hart A, Cann P (2012) Edge loading in metal-on-metal hips: low clearance is a new risk factor. Proc Inst Mech Eng H 226(3):217–226

Weber BG (1992) Metal-metal total prosthesis of the hip joint: back to the future. Z Orthop Ihre Grenzgeb 130(4):306–309 (Article in German)

Willert HG, Buchhorn GH, Fayyazi A, Flury R, Windler M, Köster G, Lohmann CH (2005) Metal-on-metal bearings and hypersensitivity in patients with artificial hip joints. A clinical and histomorphological study. J Bone Joint Surg Am 87(1):28–36

Large Head Articulations: Benefits and Drawbacks

14

Robert M. Streicher

14.1 Introduction

Approximately 22 % of all total hip arthroplasty (THA) revisions in the USA are due to dislocation, 6.9 % due to periprosthetic osteolysis, and 5 % due to bearing surface wear. In Asian countries where the activities of daily living include squatting, dislocations and impingement are generally more frequent than in the western world. Also younger patients who have a longer life expectancy and a higher activity level require more durable and stable THAs and a larger range of movement (ROM).

It has been shown that all these conditions correlate with the size of the prosthesis articulation, the material of the acetabular inserts, and the femoral head. Therefore, new prostheses with new bearing materials are constantly being developed to find the best compromise between different clinical needs such as a better joint stability versus the wear rate of the bearing. The ideal prosthesis for THA should have almost no wear of the bearing's surface and allow for a head size that minimises impingement and dislocation, providing the highest possible ROM. This chapter does not comment on metal-on-metal large-diameter bearings as they have shown unacceptable clinical failures and are discussed in another chapter of this book.

14.2 Historical Evolution of the Head Size

Originally, large head diameters (48 mm) metal-on-metal bearings were used, but these caused friction problems and loosening due to clearance incompatibilities.

In the 1960s, Sir John Charnley, after having started with TEFLON and 48 mm heads, introduced low-friction prostheses with a small head diameter (22.2 mm) and

R.M. Streicher, PhD
Dr. Streicher GmbH,
Leutschenstrasse 41, Freienbach, Switzerland
e-mail: robert@dr-streicher.com

K. Knahr (ed.), *Total Hip Arthroplasty*,
DOI 10.1007/978-3-642-35653-7_14, © EFORT 2013

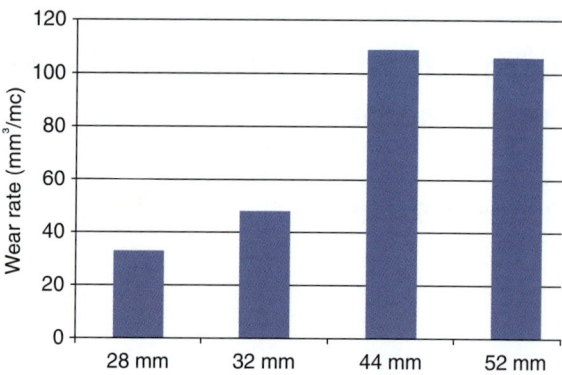

Fig. 14.1 Volumetric wear rate vs. diameter of the femoral head in articulations with conventional polyethylene acetabular cup liners

an ultrahigh molecular weight polyethylene (PE) acetabular cup as the low-friction arthroplasty. His expectations that with a smaller head the friction and thus the wear of the bearing would be reduced were confirmed later. It has been demonstrated that smaller heads produce less volumetric wear and, therefore, debris probably due to the smaller sliding distance of the head within the acetabular cup, thus reducing osteolysis and aseptic loosening of the prostheses (Fig. 14.1).

Since one of the major shortcomings of smaller heads is the higher dislocation rate as reported by multiple authors (Alberton et al. 2002; Berry et al. 2005; Woolson and Rahimtoola 1999), the search for bearings with the ideal "size to wear" ratio is still ongoing. Lately, the introduction of wear-resistant highly cross-linked polyethylenes (XPEs) has led to a rapid increase in the use of bigger femoral heads (Geller et al. 2006) due to their in vitro determined low wear rate.

14.3   Benefits and Constraints of Large Articulation Diameters

14.3.1 Dislocation

Dislocation is a major complication of THA and is estimated to have an incidence of 1–10 %. (Peters et al. 2007) Apart from surgical factors, the dislocation rate, though, is not only related to the diameter of the head but also to the inclination (higher inclination reduces the jump distance), anteversion and the cup design (hemispherical or sub-hemispherical). Figure 14.2 shows the different dislocation rates of 28 mm femoral heads compared to larger heads after THA procedures or revision procedures (Cuckler et al. 2004; Holubowycz et al. 2009; Peters et al. 2007). Berry et al. have also confirmed that larger heads have a lower incidence of dislocation (Berry et al. 2005).

14.3.2 Bearing Wear

Literature and register data show that osteolysis induced by wear debris is another major limiting factor for the long-term survival of THA. Therefore, it is important

Fig. 14.2 Percent of dislocations in three study groups comparing femoral heads of 28 mm vs. 36 mm diameter. *In the 616 group, the diameter of the femoral head was 38 mm. No dislocations were observed in this group

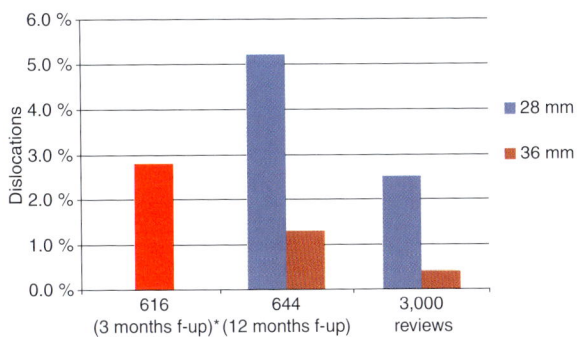

to analyse how the size of the femoral head influences this important variable. Wear rates do not only depend on the head size but also on the PE type used for the liner of the acetabular cup. Tests performed in vitro with the same femoral head, but different liners including conventional PEs, and two different types of XPEs have rendered substantially less wear for the last two types of materials (Essner et al. 2007). Tests performed by the same group with increasing head size (28, 32, 36 and 40 mm) and with liner thickness of 7.9 mm (7.4 mm for the 40 mm head) yielded excellent wear results for XPE compared to conventional PE. The wear was reduced from 47 to 1.8 mm^3/mc with a 28 mm head and to 4.3 mm^3/mc with a 40 mm head (Weir et al. 2011a, b). In another set of simulator tests, similar results were obtained. The wear rates of conventional PEs were reduced by a mean of 72 % when using XPE and heads' of 28, 32 and 36 mm (Bowhser et al. 2006). Zietz et al. compared in vitro the volumetric wear of different bearings with ceramic heads on XPE liners with 5.9 and 3.8 mm thickness and found that the volumetric wear was not detectable with 28 mm heads and only 2 and 3.1 mg/mc for 36 and 44 mm heads, respectively (Zietz et al. 2011). Clinical experience with these bearings has been recently published by Meftah et al. They have reported excellent clinical and radiographic results of 36 mm ceramic heads against XPE liners of 7.9 mm thickness at 2 years follow-up (Meftah et al. 2011). But again, these early results need to be confirmed in the clinical long-term practice.

Testing heads mounted in inverted position and modified to represent near impingement condition yielded also very good results for XPE when using heads of 36 and 44 mm and liner thickness of 3.8 and 7.9 mm compared to conventional PEs with 36 mm diameter heads (Fig. 14.3). The wear was reduced from 124 to 7 mg (−95 %) independent of the insert thickness.

Contrary, Pandorf (2007) showed that under in vitro condition the wear rate of XPE liners is doubled when increasing the head size from 28 to 36 mm, while it is decreased by almost the same amount if the 36 mm head is made from alumina instead of metal. He also reported that there is no difference in wear rate between smaller and larger diameter bearings with CoC bearings of the latest generation.

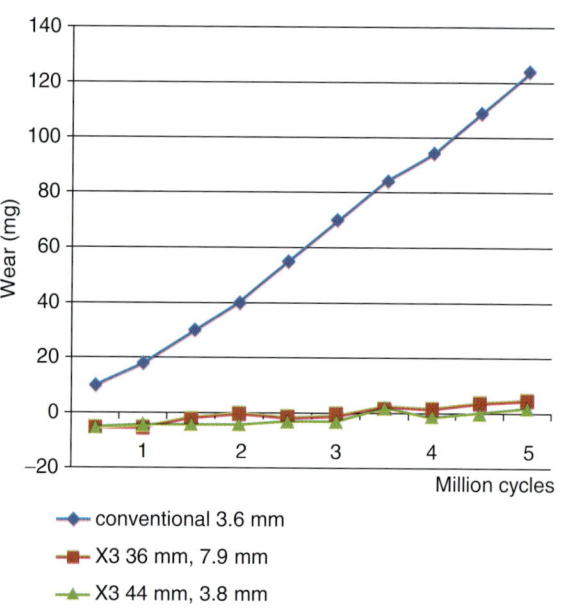

Fig 14.3 Wear characteristics in mg for 5 mc of three different linings tested under the following conditions: 12 stations, 12 soak stations, rotating test stations. Paul-type load profile with 2.000 N max and 1 Hz (Kelly et al. 2010)

14.3.3 Range of Motion and Impingement

Burroughs et al. (2005) evaluated in vitro the effect of larger heads for total hip replacement related to impingement and ROM. The dislocation and impingement tests were performed simulating pure flexion (representative of an individual sitting in chair and leaning forward). Femoral stems with cylindrical neck geometry and five different neck lengths placed in 0°, 15° and 30° of femoral anteversion were tested. All tests were repeated three times. Their results showed that 28 mm heads showed impingement in 60 % of the cases and 32 mm heads in 47 % of the cases, while 38 and 44 mm femoral heads almost eliminated component-to-component impingement. Larger heads (38 and 44 mm) also showed larger ROM. Particularly the larger heads had an advantage of 12° in pure flexion compared to the 28 mm and 7° compared to the 32 mm heads with skirt. ROM in pure flexion with different degrees of femoral anteversion was also tested with a 38 mm head. The authors observed a fully adequate ROM at external rotation with 0° anteversion and >45° of external rotation still possible with 30° of femoral anteversion. According to Kluess et al., an increased ROM and a reduced of prosthetic impingement also reduce the risk of damage of the cup rim and prosthetic neck (Kluess et al. 2007).

14.3.4 Stability and Mechanical Integrity

The size of the femoral head also plays a role in the peak contact pressure and the contact area. Different head sizes paired with XPEs inserts of different thicknesses were analysed with the finite element method and a joint compressive load of

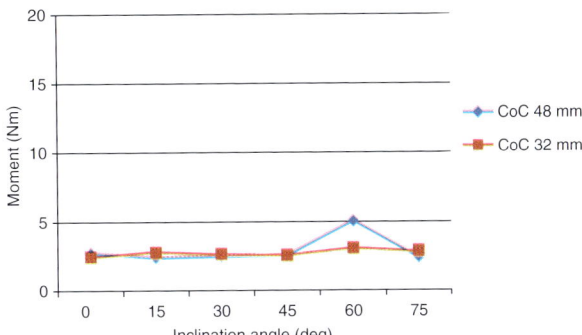

Fig. 14.4 Friction moment of ceramic-on-ceramic bearings tested with symmetric cycles ±20° at 1,700 Nm (Morlock et al. 2011)

5,338 N. The results show that for bigger heads, the minimum principal contact stress is less and the contact area larger for larger heads (Schmidt, 2007).

One of the aspects that have to be considered with particular attention is the frictional torque generated by larger heads. Schmidig et al. tested the frictional torque with different head sizes and XPE inserts of different thickness and found statistically significant differences in frictional torque, shell deformation and insert deformation, all increasing with increasing head diameter as well as liner thickness (Schmidig et al. 2009). On the other hand Morlock et al. (2011) found similar torque moments when comparing ceramic-on-ceramic (CoC) bearings of 32 and 48 mm diameter lubricated with serum and at different cup angles (Fig. 14.4).

14.3.5 Clinical Experience

Clinical experience does not always corroborate the expected results based on in vitro tests and analysis. As of today clinical studies with follow-up times of up to 8 years have been published focusing on wear and wear rate of various diameter metal heads against XPE liners. These have shown some differences between the wear rates of bearings with different head sizes. Lachiewics et al. evaluated the complete clinical and radiographic data of 90 patients (102 hips) with a minimum follow-up of 5–8 years. They found no correlation between head size and linear wear but a positive correlation between head size and volumetric wear rate. The median wear rate for all patients was 25.6 mm³/year (mean, 80.5 mm³/year), and the median of total volumetric wear was 41.0 mm³ (mean, 98.5 mm³). For 36 and 40 mm femoral heads, the total volumetric wear rate was 156.6 mm³/year (Lachiewicz et al. 2009), three times higher than the median. Nevertheless, the result for large-diameter heads is difficult to reproduce from the data provided in this publication. Bragdon et al. report comparable head penetration results and no differences of the median steady-state wear of XPE with 28 and 36 mm femoral heads in 44 patients at 3 years follow-up with different analysis methods (Bragdon et al. 2007). In a prospective study with 42 patients using cobalt chrome heads of 36, 38 or 40 mm against XPE liners, Geller et al. report no differences in head penetration for the three groups and no measurable volumetric wear at 3 years follow-up (Geller et al. 2006). Even though these are partially encouraging results that speak for the use of larger heads in combination with XPE, particularly in patients at high risk of dislocation, these studies have a limited level of evidence, and longer follow-up times and larger series of patients are required.

14.4 Discussion

In the search for the ideal bearing for THA, new bearing materials, the difficulty to simulate in vitro the clinical reality, the changing expectations of patients due to age and geographical origin, among others, play an important role on the qualitative evaluation of the bearing size and components.

Today one of the most commonly used combinations is a metal head on a polyethylene liner of the acetabular cup of 36 mm inner diameter. 22.2 mm bearings were used historically due to the confirmed fact that with smaller heads, less PE debris due to volumetric wear is released, which has been demonstrated to correlate with the aseptic loosening of the THA due to osteolysis. There are though multiple reasons to use bigger heads of 32, 36 or even 40 mm diameter as discussed before: dislocation, impingement and ROM, a major issue for revisions. Therefore, the search for materials that feature less wear despite larger bearing diameters is still ongoing.

Hope was deposited in the metal-on-metal bearing technology, but the analysis done by Smith et al. on behalf of the National Joint Registry of England and Wales, the largest THA register in the world, has demonstrated that metal-on-metal combinations should be avoided due to higher failure rates, particularly with large heads (Smith et al. 2012).

With the introduction of XPEs, larger bearings became more popular, but there are still aspects that should be investigated further, like the influence of a thinner PE liner to accommodate a larger head and the increased torque with larger heads, which result in an increase of frictional torque in in vitro tests. This could affect the fixation of the implant and also the stability of the femoral head fixation on the stem taper, since the excess of frictional torque may be transmitted to the fixation exerting higher loosening forces. The clinical significance of torque increase is still not well documented but seems to be a source of wear and corrosion at the modular interfaces with larger head diameter bearings, especially for metal head articulations.

Conclusion

Due to the multiple in vitro studies that show that an increased volumetric PE wear is expected with larger femoral heads and to the contradictory results of the few clinical studies that report no or high correlation of the volumetric wear with the bearing size, patients implanted with large metal femoral heads against XPEs should be closely monitored to appropriately identify the right indication for these prostheses and their long-term clinical outcome. While with large heads and PE articulation the friction and eventually the wear increases and may be a cause of issues on the taper fixation, CoC does not seem to be affected by this.

Taking into considerations all information from the literature, a head size over 36 mm, especially in combination with XPE, is not indicated for general use in THA, and 32 mm should be considered wherever possible.

References

Alberton GM, High WA, Morrey BF (2002) Dislocation after revision total hip arthroplasty: an analysis of risk factors and treatment options. J Bone Joint Surg Am 84-A(10):1788–1792

Berry DJ, von Knoch M, Schleck CD, Harmsen WS (2005) Effect of femoral head diameter and operative approach on risk of dislocation after primary total hip arthroplasty. J Bone Joint Surg Am 87(11):2456–2463

Bowhser JG, Williams PA, Green DD, Clarke IC, Donaldson TK (2006) Performance of mechanically enhanced crosslinked polyethylene under standard and severe wear simulator modes. Abstracts, Society of Biomaterial 2006 annual meeting, poster 544

Bragdon CR, Greene ME, Freiberg AA, Harris WH, Malchau H (2007) Radiostereometric analysis comparison of wear of highly cross-linked polyethylene against 36- vs 28-mm femoral heads. J Arthroplasty 22(6 suppl 2):125–129, 22

Burroughs BR, Hallstrom B, Golladay GJ, Hoeffel D, Harris W (2005) Range of motion and stability in total hip arthroplasty with 28-, 32-, 38-, and 44-mm femoral head sizes. J Arthroplasty 20(1):11–19

Cuckler JM, Moore KD, Lombardi AV Jr, McPherson E, Emerson R (2004) Large versus small femoral heads in metal-on-metal total hip arthroplasty. J Arthroplasty 19(8 suppl 3):41–44

Essner A, Schmidig G, Herrera L, Yau SS, Wang A, Dumbleton JH, Manley MT (2007) Hip wear performance of a next generation cross-linked and annealed polyethylene. In: Proceedings 51st ORS. Poster No: 0830 51st annual meeting of the Orthopaedic Research Society, Washington, DC

Geller JA, Malchau A, Bragdon C, Greene M, Harris WH, Freiberg AA (2006) Large diameter femoral head on highly cross-linked polyethylene: minimum 3 year results. Clin Orthop Relat Res 447:53–59

Holubowycz O, Howie DW, Middleton RG (2009) Implant-related revision after primary total hip replacement in a randomized trial of articulation size. EFORT, Podium presentation

Kelly NH, Rajadhyaksha AD, Wright TM, Maher SA, Westrich GA (2010) High stress conditions do not increase wear of thin highly crosslinked UHMWPE. Clin Orthop Relat Res. doi:10.1007/s11999-009-1154-6

Kluess D, Martin H, Mittelmeier W, Schmitz KP, Bader R (2007) Influence of femoral head size on impingement, dislocation and stress distribution in total hip replacement. Med Eng Phys 29(4): 465–471

Lachiewicz PF, Heckmann DS, Soileau ES, Mangla J, Martell JM (2009) Femoral Head Size and Wear of Highly Cross-linked Polyethylene at 5 to 8 Years. Clin Orthop Relat Res 467:3290–3296

Meftah M, Ebrahimpour PB, He C, Ranawat AS, Ranawat CS (2011) Short-term wear analysis and clinical performance of large ceramic heads on highly cross-linked polyethylene in young and active patients. Semin Arthroplasty. doi:10.1053/j.sart.2011.09.002

Morlock M, Bishop N, Perka C (2011). Keynote lecture: is bigger really better? In: 24th International Society of Technologies in Arthroplasty Annual Meeting, Bruges (Abstracts). www.istaonline.org

Pandorf T (2007) Wear of large ceramic bearings. In: Chang J-D, Billau K (eds) Bioceramics and alternative bearings in joint arthroplasty. Proceedings of the 12th BIOLOX® Symposium, Seoul, Republic of Korea, September 7–8, 2007. Steinkopf Verlag, Darmstadt. ISBN 978-3-7985-1782-0

Peters CL, McPherson E, Jackson JD, Erickson JA (2007) Reduction in early dislocation rate with large diameter femoral heads in primary total hip arthroplasty. J Arthroplasty 22(6 suppl): 140–144

Schmidig G, Patel A, Liepins I, Thakore M, Markel D (2009) Effects of acetabular shell deformation and linear thickness on frictional torque in polyethylene acetabular bearings. In: Transactions of the 53rd Annual Meeting of the Orthopedic Research Society, San Diego. Orthopedic Research Society, USA

Schmidt W, Racanelli J, Essner A, Wang A, McCarthy J (2007) The effect of thickness on contact stress in fully supported sequentially crosslinked and annealed UHMWPE acetabular inserts. In: Transactions of the 51st Annual Meeting of the Orthopedic Research Society, Washington, DC. Orthopedic Research Society, USA

Smith AJ, Dieppe P, Vernon K, Porter M, Blom AW (2012) Failure rates of stemmed metal-on-metal hip replacements: analysis of data from the national joint registry of England and Wales. Lancet 13. March, doi:10.10016/S0140-6736(12)60353-5

Weir A, Herrera L, Essner A (2011) The effect of femoral head size on the wear performance of sequentially crosslinked polyethylene. ORS annual meeting poster 1158

Weir A, Lee R, Alipit V, Essner A (2011) Differentiation between creep and wear on polyethylene. ORS annual meeting poster 1113

Woolson ST, Rahimtoola ZO (1999) Risk factors for dislocation during the first three months after primary total hip replacement. J Arthroplasty 14(6):662–668

Zietz C, Fritsche A, Mittelmeier W, Bader R (2011) In-vitro wear testing of standard vs. cross linked polyethylene liners in combination with different ceramic femoral heads. In: Proceedings of the 12th Annual Meeting of the European Federation of National Associations of Orthopaedics and Traumatology, Copenhagen (Abstract 309)

Can the Increased Loosening Rate of the Modular-Neck Hip Systems Be Attributed to Geometric Design Parameters? An Alternative Approach Using Finite Element Analysis

15

Evangelos Theodorou, Christos S. Georgiou,
Christopher Provatidis, and Panagiotis Megas

15.1 Introduction

Modular necks are a relatively new innovation in total hip arthroplasty (THA). They offer the surgeon the potential to effectively restore hip biomechanics with the ability to independently adjust offset, version, and limb length during operation. These should theoretically improve implant stability, decrease the dislocation and impingement rate, and assist in equalization of leg length (Grupp et al. 2010). Initially they were reserved for the severe torsional deformities of the developmental hip dysplasia (Umeda et al. 2003). However, due to their compelling rationale, the intraoperative flexibility and the fast learning curve, indications quickly expanded up to the younger and more active patients. To further serve the demands of these patients, several manufacturers currently combine modular necks with hard bearings, either metal on metal (MoM) or ceramic on ceramic (CoC) (Grupp et al. 2010). However, whether the advantages conferred by the neck modularity outweigh the additional complexity remains a question. Since the introduction of the modular-neck systems in the clinical practice, vulnerabilities of their application are being continuously revealed. Concerns for fretting corrosion and concomitant metal ion release from the additional MoM junction have been widely expressed

E. Theodorou, PhD • C. Provatidis, PhD
School of Mechanical Engineering, Mechanical Design & Control Systems Section,
Laboratory of Dynamics and Structures, National Technical University of Athens,
Athens, Greece
e-mail: etheod@mail.ntua.gr; cprovat@central.ntua.gr

C.S. Georgiou, MD (✉) • P. Megas, MD, PhD
Department of Orthopaedic Surgery,
University of Patras,
26504 Rion, Greece
e-mail: csgeorgiou@gmail.com; panmegas@gmail.com

K. Knahr (ed.), *Total Hip Arthroplasty*,
DOI 10.1007/978-3-642-35653-7_15, © EFORT 2013

(Gill et al. 2012; Jacobs and Hallab 2006; Grupp et al. 2010). Furthermore, corrosion, possibly influenced by the neck adapter material, may lead to fatigue component fracture at the modular site (Grupp et al. 2010). Dissociation at the stem–neck interface, even without trauma, has been also described (Kouzelis et al. 2011). The long-term success of adding a second modular junction has, therefore, yet to be established.

In fact, a latest report from the national registries has shown a significant higher revision rate for modular-neck compared to monoblock stems (Australian Orthopaedic Association 2011). Remarkably enough, not implant fracture but aseptic loosening was identified as the predominant reason for all bearing surfaces (Australian Orthopaedic Association 2011). The bioreactivity of the corrosion products at the neck–stem junction is the most plausible cause of the increased incidence of loosening (Lee et al. 1997; Cadosch et al. 2009). However, aseptic loosening is a multifactorial process, and, at present, the evidence linking osteolysis with metal hypersensitivity is circumstantial (Jacobs and Hallab 2006). Alternatively, there may be the specific design and geometric parameters of the modular necks that contribute to the failures, independently of the composition of the bearing couple or the junction corrosion (Jacobs and Hallab 2006). It is logical to presume that a deviated femoral head, at the coronal or sagittal plane, under an axial load may have different load transfer patterns than when a straight neck is used (Umeda et al. 2003). Recent stress analyses have indeed shown that the use of modular necks alters significantly the strain distribution along the femur (Umeda et al. 2003; Wik et al. 2011). This literature is particularly unfavorable with the anteverted and retroverted necks (Umeda et al. 2003; Wik et al. 2011). The changes in loading patterns raise concerns regarding adaptive hypertrophy and possible mechanical failure and loosening due to increased stress (Umeda et al. 2003). In order to investigate whether the different strain distributions of the various neck geometries play a role in the increased rate of loosening, we designed a finite element analysis (FEA) and used as reference the loading behavior of the straight-neck system. The concept and the results of this study are presented in this chapter.

15.2 Materials and Methods

15.2.1 Bone Geometry

A cadaveric femur (35 years old, male, right femur) was selected from a collection at a university anthropology department. CT scans of the femur were acquired in digital format (DICOM) on a Siemens SOMATOM Sensation4 CT Scanner. Slice thickness was set to 1 mm. Using Materialise Mimics v.8, each CT scan was individually processed providing data for the full femur geometry. The resulting three-dimensional CAD model was generated after further processing through Geomagic Studio v.9 and finally imported into SolidWorks 2008.

15.2.2 Implant

The colarless, tapered, Profemur® E stem (Wright Medical Technology Inc., Arlington, TN), made of Ti6Al4V alloy, was chosen for the investigation due to its extensive neck modularity. Eleven options of neck orientation are available from five different designs. These five neck versions include a neutral neck, an 8° angled neck for varus or valgus, an 8° angled neck for anteversion or retroversion, a 15° angled neck for anteversion or retroversion, and a neck with a combination of 4° for varus and 6° for anteversion. The latter double-angled neck can provide varus-anteversion, valgus-retroversion, varus-retroversion, and valgus-anteversion orientation, depending on the side implanted. Each of them can be in short or long configurations, so the available options are 22. To avoid the additional offset, we selected, for the study at hand, only the short neck lengths. For the same reason we used a standard 28 mm CoCr femoral head as the bearing surface.

Based on a preoperative planning for the femoral bone at hand, a size 5 was selected. The stem and the 11 short necks were scanned by a coordinate measurement machine (CMM), a Mistral 07075 by DEA–Brown and Sharpe Inc. with a Renishaw PH10M scanning head in compliance with the ISO 10360–2 standard, and were afterwards digitized. Finally the osteotomy was performed; the stem was aligned and finally inserted into the bone volume. The implementation of the 11 different modular necks and the femoral head created the final mathematical models.

15.2.3 Finite Element Analysis

The transition from the CAD environment to the FEA was accomplished through the GUI of ANSYS Workbench V.11 SP1.0, where the models were natively imported from SolidWorks 2008. Using the integrated mesh generator, a high-quality finite element mesh consisting of approximately 186,000 ten-node tetrahedral elements was generated (Fig. 15.1). The contacts between the different parts of the three-dimensional model were considered as bonded, but with the possibility to undergo minor relevant movement without separation of faces in contact, as the "no separation" option in ANSYS Workbench denotes.

15.2.4 Materials and Loading

For all materials used in the FEA, linear, elastic, isotropic properties – with homogenous distribution – were assigned. The modulus of elasticity for the bone volume was set to $EBONE,1 = 17,000$ MPa for the cortical bone (Hounsfiled units: from 3,071 to 368), $EBONE,2 = 1,000$ MPa for the cancelous (Hounsfiled units: from 368 to 741), and finally the Poisson ratio $vBONE = 0.30$. Based on technical specifications for the Profemur-E THA system, the following materials were used: Ti–alloy stem with $ESTEM = 114$ GPa, $vSTEM = 0.35$; Ti–alloy neck with $ENECK = 114$ GPa,

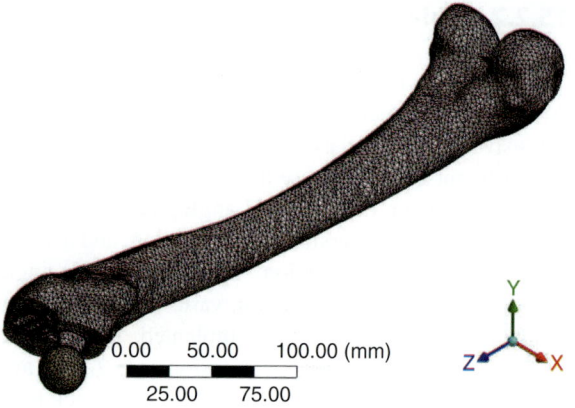

Fig. 15.1 The final finite element model

vNECK=0.35; normal femoral head ENH=200 GPa, vNH=0.3; and big femoral head with EBFH=208 GPa, vBFH=0.3.

According to previous studies the stance phase of the gait cycle was simulated, and two main forces were applied on the finite element model. The first one, with a magnitude of 2,450 N, was implemented on the modular head, on an area relevant to the corresponding cup, and represented the body weight. Forces from the main muscle groups – gluteus minimus, medius, and maximus – were applied as a single resultant force of 1,650 N, on the greater trochanter area. Both forces were applied on small areas – not on a single point – in order to avoid stress concentration phenomena. The distal part of the femur, namely, the lateral and medial condyle surface, was considered fully constrained.

15.2.5 Regions of Interest

Five three-dimensional regions of interest (ROIs), due to their clinical importance, were isolated for the result analysis (Fig. 15.2). At the anterior and posterior femoral surfaces, these were the anterior ROI (as described by the Gruen zones 8, 9, and upper half of 10) (Fig. 15.2a) and the posterior ROI (upper half of Gruen zone 12 and Gruen zones 13, 14) (Fig. 15.2b), respectively. At the medial side of the femur is the calcar ROI (Fig. 15.2c), approximately 15 mm below the osteotomy plane (Gruen zone 7 at the anteroposterior view and parts of the 8 and 14 zones at the lateral view), and at the lateral side, the lateral ROI (lower part of Gruen zone 1, Gruen zone 2 and the upper half of zone 3) (Fig. 15.2d). The final stem tip ROI is a circumferential zone around the tip of the stem (lower half of Gruen zones 3 and 5 and Gruen zone 4 at the anteroposterior view and lower half of Gruen zones 10 and 12 and Gruen zone 11 at the lateral view) (Fig. 15.2e). Strain values for each node, as well as mean values for the whole bone volume, at these ROIs were recorded. According to (Frost 1994) the modern expression of Wolff's law (1986), the nodes were divided into three categories depending on the strain absolute value (Table 15.1). To simplify the presentation of the results, the necks were named according to the Table 15.2.

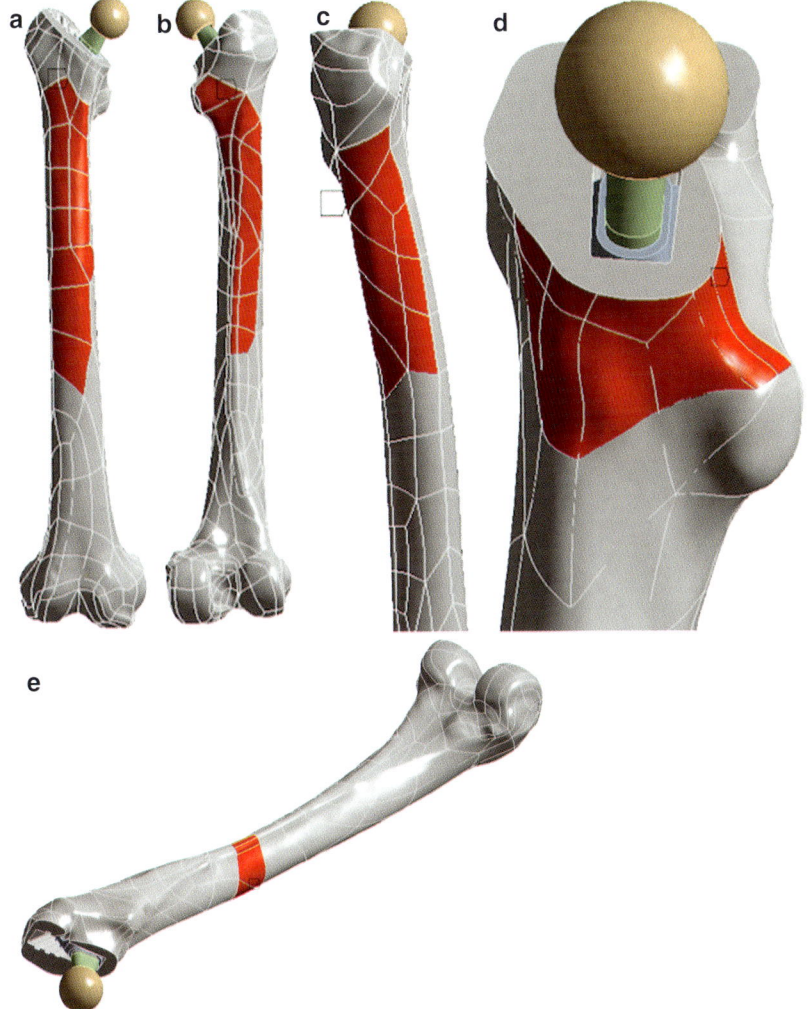

Fig. 15.2 The five regions of interest (ROIs). The anterior (**a**), posterior (**b**), lateral (**c**), calcar (**d**), and stem tip (**e**) ROIs

15.3   Results

The mean strain values recorded at the ROIs for each neck type are shown in Fig. 15.3. Compared with the straight, the anteverted (8° and 15°) necks, as well as the varus neck, present an overall increase in mean strain values. For the anteverted necks, specifically, as the version becomes greater, the anterior and posterior femoral regions are exposed to proportionally greater stresses. The 15° anteverted neck

Table 15.1 The three zones of loading according to Frost's law

Below 50 µstrains	Disuse zone	New bone is not developed normally; loss of bone occurs
50 µstrains → 1,500 µstrains	Adaptive zone	Bone conservation, tend to equal but not exceed the amount resorbed, healthy active growing
1,500 µstrains → 3,000 µstrains	Mild overload zone	Bone strengthening, changes in its architecture where and as needed to lower its strains, healthy active growing
Above 3,000 µstrains	Overload zone	Peak strains lead to bone growth, may or may not be positive

Table 15.2 Abbreviations of the neck types

Neck name	Neck type
1202-28	Short straight
1232-28	Short A: 8° anteverted P: 8° retroverted
1242-28	Short A: 15° anteverted P: 15° retroverted
1252-28	Short VAL: valgus VAR: varus
1222-28	A: varus-anteverted P: valgus-retroverted
1212-28	A: valgus-anteverted P: varus-retroverted

system showed an increase of 17 and 17.7 % in the mean strain developed at the anterior and posterior ROIs, respectively. The same neck showed the greatest strain increase also at the lateral ROI (13 %) and at the calcar ROI an increase of 6 %. At the stem tip ROI, the greatest increase was recorded with the double-angled retroverted-valgus orientation (15.4 %), while the 15° anteverted neck was the second greater (11 %). Smaller increases were recorded for the 8° anteverted neck. Interestingly enough, the retroverted necks, irrespectively of the extent of version, showed similar values to the straight-neck mean values at the calcar, lateral, and stem tip ROIs and considerable strain reduction at the anterior and posterior ROIs. For the varus neck a mild increase of 6, 8.7, 4, 4.5, and 11 % was recorded at the calcar, lateral, anterior, posterior, and stem tip ROIs, respectively. The valgus neck, on the other hand, showed an overall strain reduction. As far as the most commonly used double-angled necks, the anteverted-varus and the retroverted-valgus combinations have presented the greatest increases. At the lateral, anterior, and posterior ROIs, the values were similar for both of them (10, 5, and 10.5 %, respectively). At the calcar ROI the anteverted-varus and the retroverted-valgus orientations have shown an increase of 7.4 and 16 % and at the stem tip ROI 9 and 15.4 %, respectively.

Despite this increase in mean values, no overload at any ROI was observed for any neck type whatsoever, as shown by the distribution of nodes to Frost's law categories (Fig. 15.4).

Figures 15.5, 15.6, and 15.7 show three-dimensional images of the strain distribution in the bone volume for three neck types: the reference of the straight neck

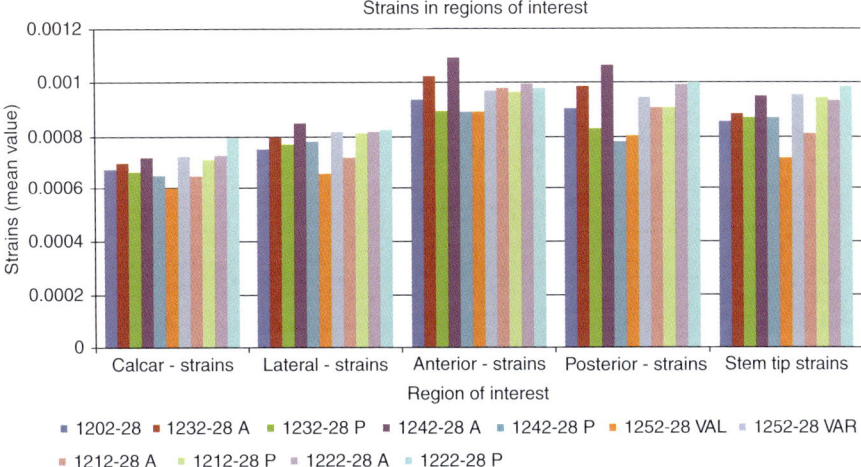

Fig. 15.3 Mean strain values at the ROIs for each neck type

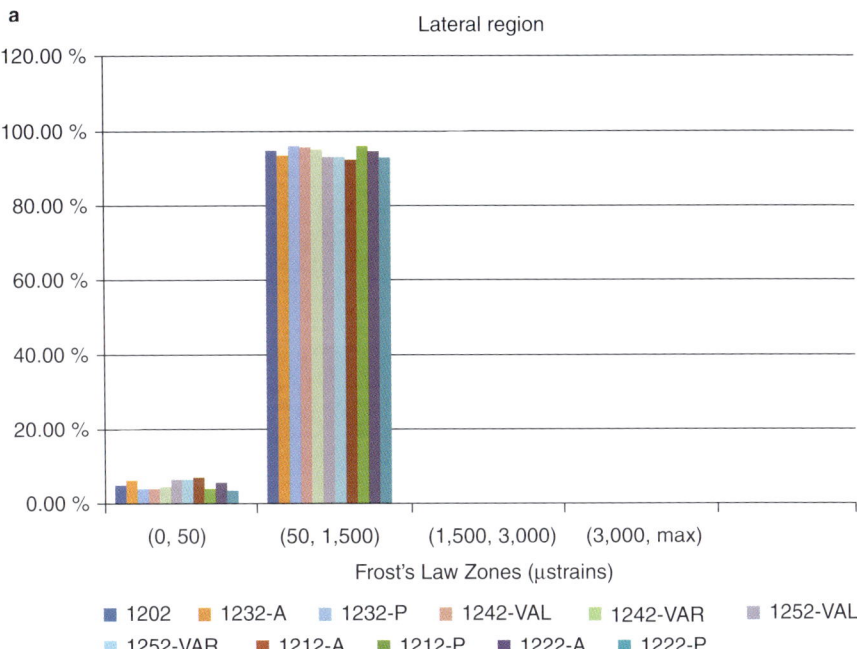

Fig. 15.4 (**a**) Distribution of the nodes to the Frost's law zone at the lateral ROI. (**b**) Distribution of the nodes to the Frost's law zone at the calcar ROI. (**c**) Distribution of the nodes to the Frost's law zone at the stem tip ROI. (**d**) Distribution of the nodes to the Frost's law zone at the anterior ROI. (**e**) Distribution of the nodes to the Frost's law zone at the posterior ROI

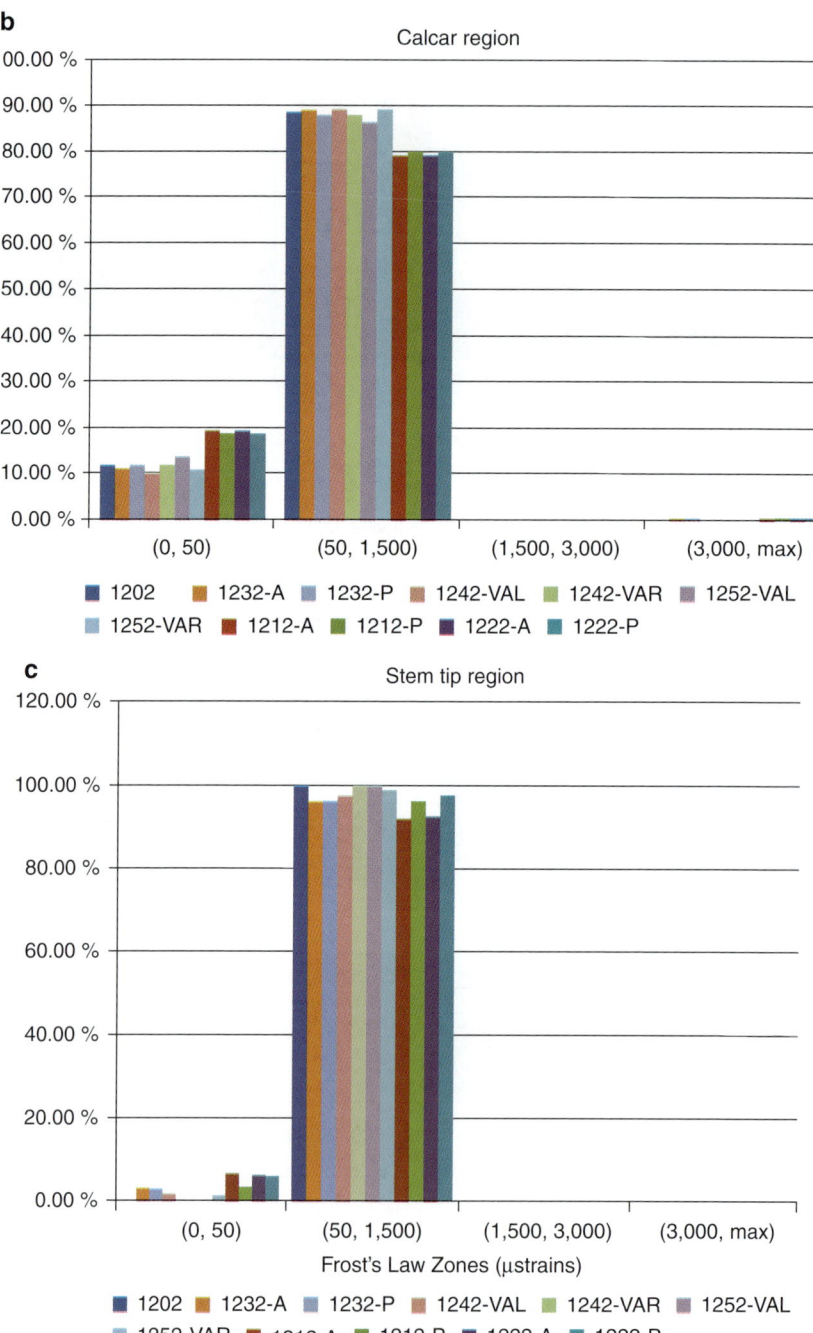

Fig. 15.4 (continued)

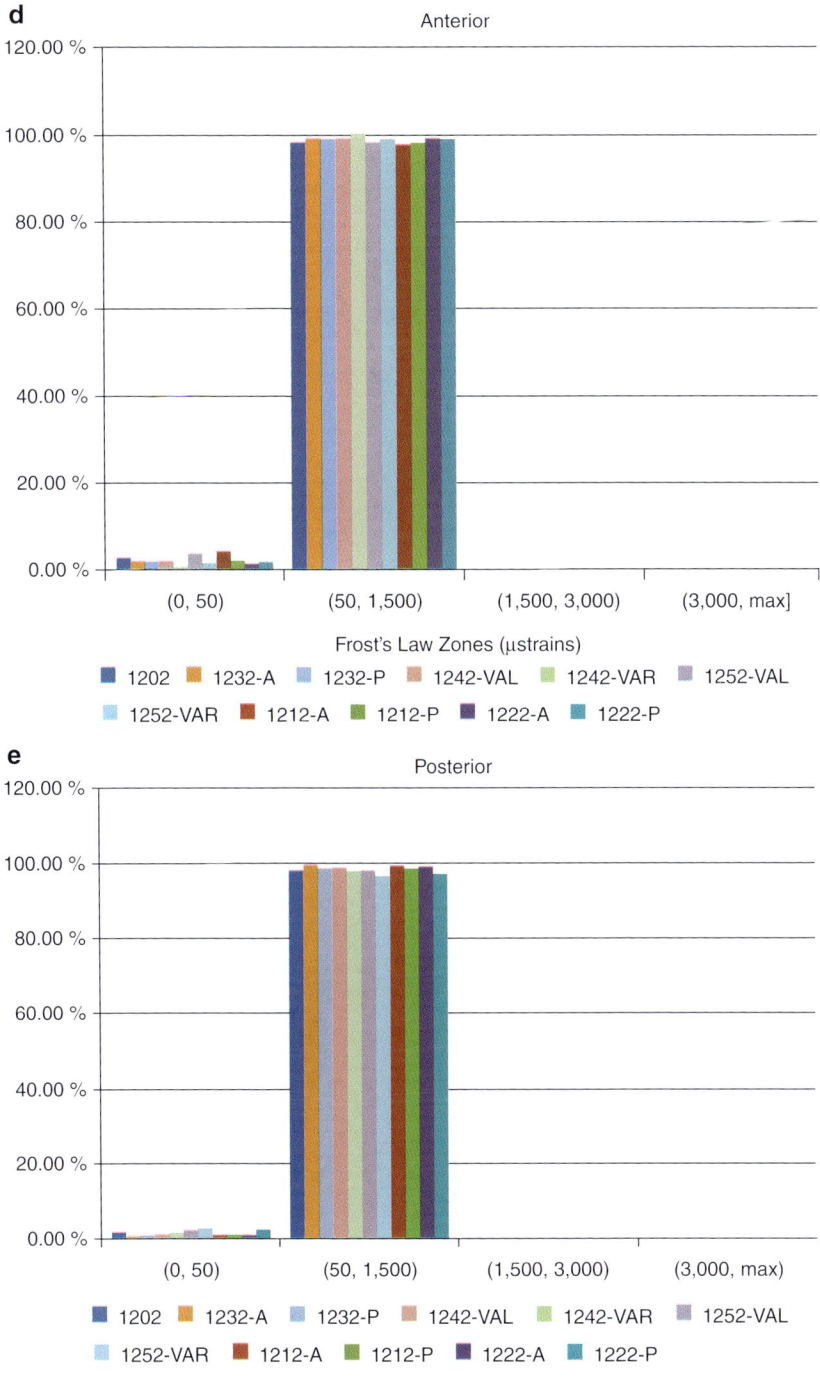

Fig. 15.4 (continued)

(Fig. 15.5) and the most incriminated in the literature, the 15° retroverted neck (Fig. 15.6) and the 15° anteverted neck (Fig. 15.7), which presented the greatest strain rise in our study. We observe that the point of maximum strain is shifted

Fig. 15.5 Three-dimensional strain distribution of the straight neck at the proximal femur

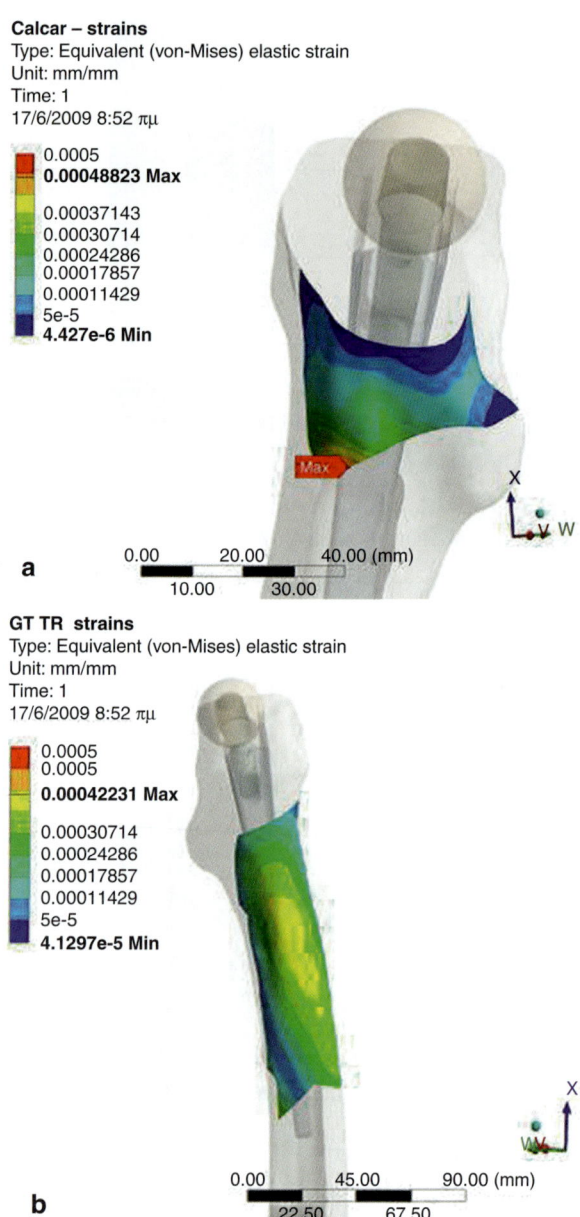

Calcar – strains
Type: Equivalent (von-Mises) elastic strain
Unit: mm/mm
Time: 1
17/6/2009 8:52 πμ

0.0005
0.00048823 Max

0.00037143
0.00030714
0.00024286
0.00017857
0.00011429
5e-5
4.427e-6 Min

Max

0.00   20.00   40.00 (mm)

10.00   30.00

a

GT TR strains
Type: Equivalent (von-Mises) elastic strain
Unit: mm/mm
Time: 1
17/6/2009 8:52 πμ

0.0005
0.0005
0.00042231 Max

0.00030714
0.00024286
0.00017857
0.00011429
5e-5
4.1297e-5 Min

0.00   45.00   90.00 (mm)

22.50   67.50

b

Fig. 15.5 (continued)

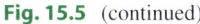

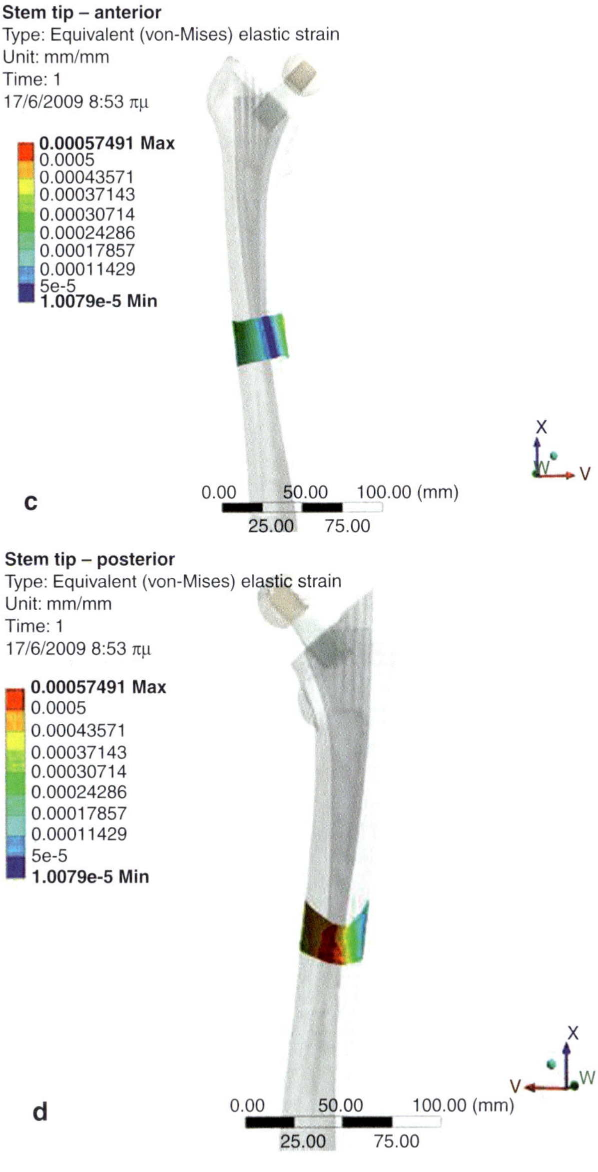

Stem tip – anterior
Type: Equivalent (von-Mises) elastic strain
Unit: mm/mm
Time: 1
17/6/2009 8:53 πμ

0.00057491 Max
0.0005
0.00043571
0.00037143
0.00030714
0.00024286
0.00017857
0.00011429
5e-5
1.0079e-5 Min

X
W → V

c

0.00   50.00   100.00 (mm)
        25.00   75.00

Stem tip – posterior
Type: Equivalent (von-Mises) elastic strain
Unit: mm/mm
Time: 1
17/6/2009 8:53 πμ

0.00057491 Max
0.0005
0.00043571
0.00037143
0.00030714
0.00024286
0.00017857
0.00011429
5e-5
1.0079e-5 Min

X
V ← W

d

0.00   50.00   100.00 (mm)
        25.00   75.00

forward with the retroverted neck and backward with the anteverted neck in relation with the straight neck. This can be explained by the direction of the neck in relation with the anterior bow of the femur. However, the anteverted neck still presents the maximum absolute strain value which is 9 % greater than that of the retroverted neck and 50 % greater than the straight neck.

Fig. 15.6 Three-dimensional strain distribution of the 15° retroverted neck at the proximal femur

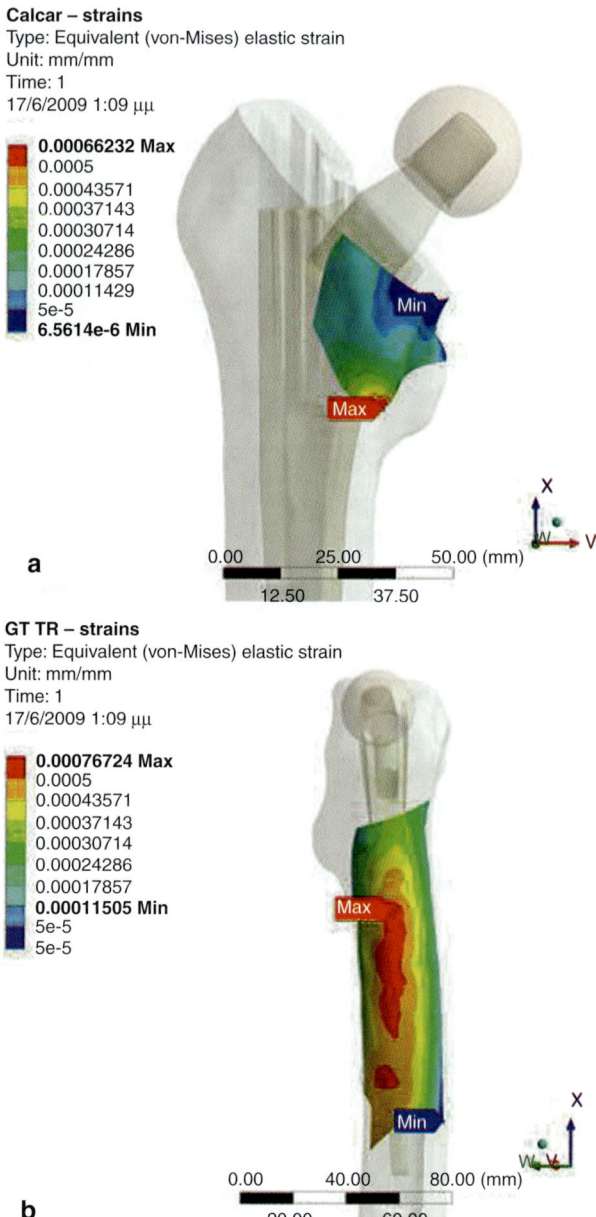

Calcar – strains
Type: Equivalent (von-Mises) elastic strain
Unit: mm/mm
Time: 1
17/6/2009 1:09 μμ

0.00066232 Max
0.0005
0.00043571
0.00037143
0.00030714
0.00024286
0.00017857
0.00011429
5e-5
6.5614e-6 Min

Min

Max

a

0.00   25.00   50.00 (mm)
      12.50   37.50

GT TR – strains
Type: Equivalent (von-Mises) elastic strain
Unit: mm/mm
Time: 1
17/6/2009 1:09 μμ

0.00076724 Max
0.0005
0.00043571
0.00037143
0.00030714
0.00024286
0.00017857
0.00011505 Min
5e-5
5e-5

Max

Min

b

0.00   40.00   80.00 (mm)
      20.00   60.00

Fig. 15.6 (continued)

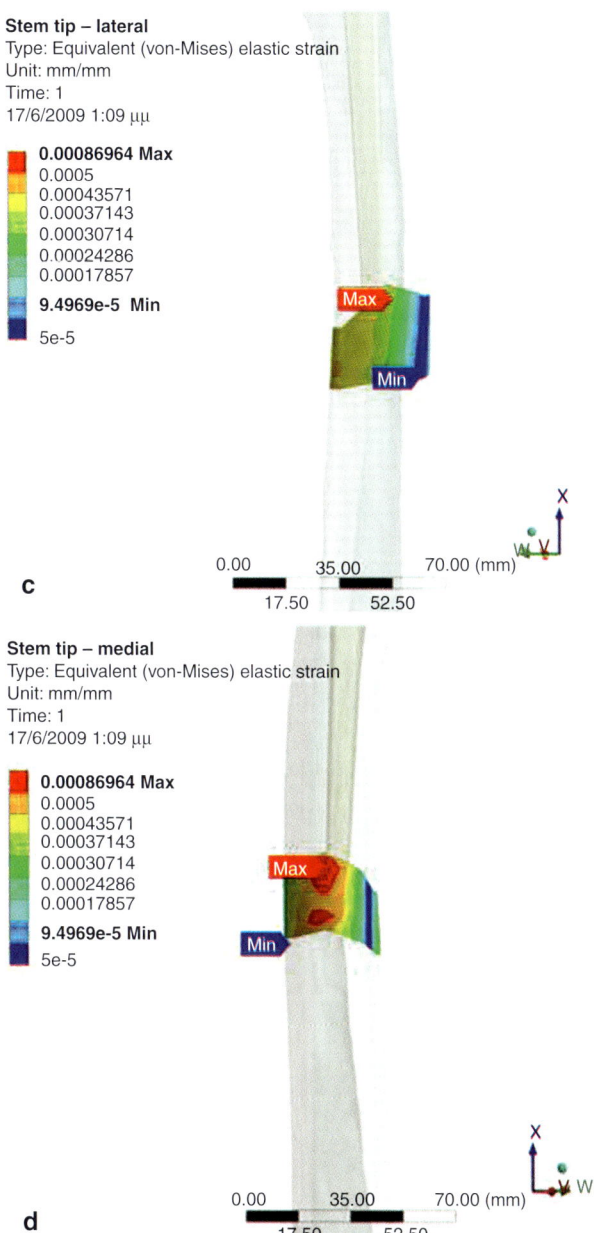

Stem tip – lateral
Type: Equivalent (von-Mises) elastic strain
Unit: mm/mm
Time: 1
17/6/2009 1:09 μμ

0.00086964 Max
0.0005
0.00043571
0.00037143
0.00030714
0.00024286
0.00017857
9.4969e-5 Min
5e-5

c

0.00   35.00   70.00 (mm)
     17.50   52.50

Stem tip – medial
Type: Equivalent (von-Mises) elastic strain
Unit: mm/mm
Time: 1
17/6/2009 1:09 μμ

0.00086964 Max
0.0005
0.00043571
0.00037143
0.00030714
0.00024286
0.00017857
9.4969e-5 Min
5e-5

d

0.00   35.00   70.00 (mm)
     17.50   52.50

Fig. 15.7 Three-dimensional strain distribution of the 15° anteverted neck at the proximal femur

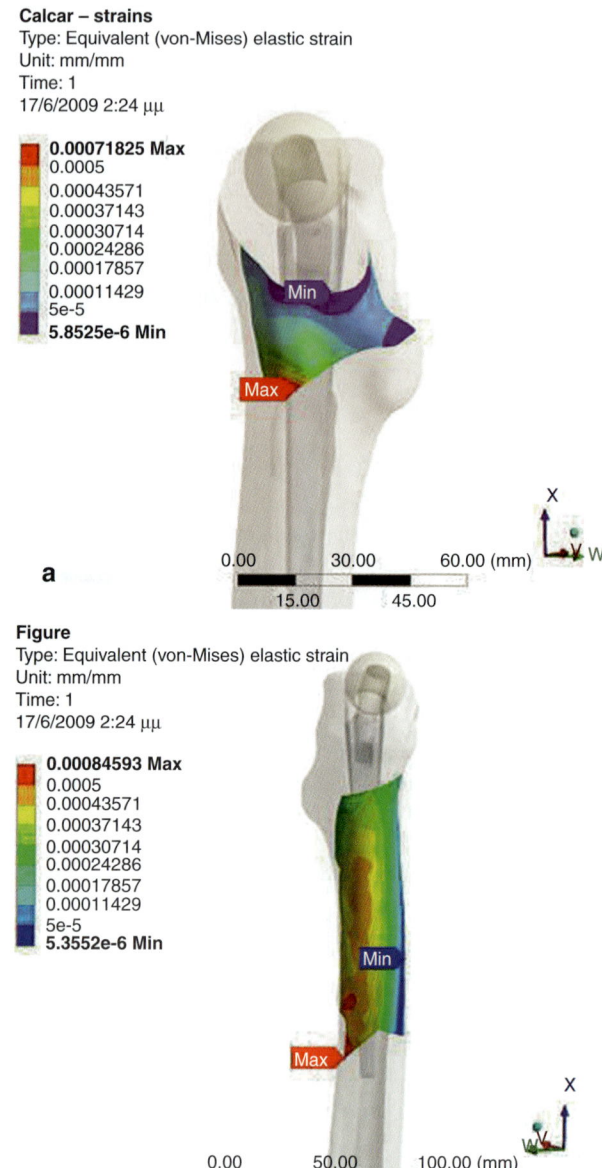

Calcar – strains
Type: Equivalent (von-Mises) elastic strain
Unit: mm/mm
Time: 1
17/6/2009 2:24 μμ

0.00071825 Max
0.0005
0.00043571
0.00037143
0.00030714
0.00024286
0.00017857
0.00011429
5e-5
5.8525e-6 Min

a

0.00   30.00   60.00 (mm)
15.00   45.00

Figure
Type: Equivalent (von-Mises) elastic strain
Unit: mm/mm
Time: 1
17/6/2009 2:24 μμ

0.00084593 Max
0.0005
0.00043571
0.00037143
0.00030714
0.00024286
0.00017857
0.00011429
5e-5
5.3552e-6 Min

b

0.00   50.00   100.00 (mm)
25.00   75.00

Fig. 15.7 (continued)

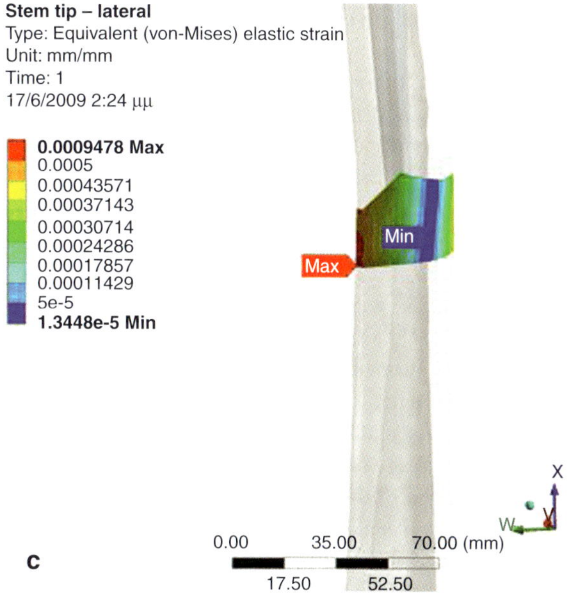
Stem tip – lateral
Type: Equivalent (von-Mises) elastic strain
Unit: mm/mm
Time: 1
17/6/2009 2:24 μμ
0.0009478 Max
0.0005
0.00043571
0.00037143
0.00030714
0.00024286
0.00017857
0.00011429
5e-5
1.3448e-5 Min
Min
Max
X
W
V
0.00
35.00
70.00 (mm)
17.50
52.50
c

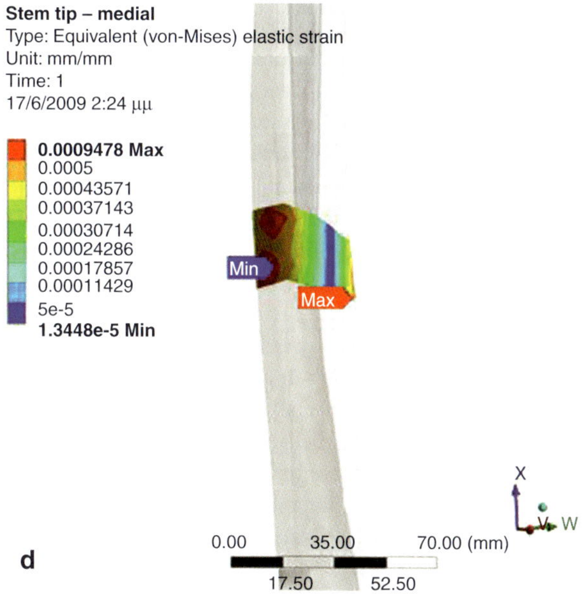
Stem tip – medial
Type: Equivalent (von-Mises) elastic strain
Unit: mm/mm
Time: 1
17/6/2009 2:24 μμ
0.0009478 Max
0.0005
0.00043571
0.00037143
0.00030714
0.00024286
0.00017857
0.00011429
5e-5
1.3448e-5 Min
Min
Max
X
V
W
0.00
35.00
70.00 (mm)
17.50
52.50
d

15.4   Discussion

THA designs incorporating modular necks have been widely implanted worldwide, since the first report on them by Toni et al. (2001). The Australian National Joint Replacement Registry, however, is the first among the national registries that performed a detailed analysis on femoral stems with exchangeable necks. At the 2011 annual report, based on 196,582 primary THA with various bearing surfaces, the cumulative percent revision at 7 years for modular-neck prostheses (total number 6,659 prostheses) was 8.9 % compared to 4.2 % for fixed femoral stems, and it was significant for all bearing surfaces with greater than 4-year follow-up (Australian Orthopaedic Association 2011). Although statistical significance was not demonstrated, the increase in revision was attributed to a higher incidence of loosening (3.2 % at 7 years compared to 1.3 % for fixed femoral neck) and not fracture (0.8 % compared to 0.6 %) (Australian Orthopaedic Association 2011). The largest case series in the literature with 5,000 modular-neck stems reports a slightly greater neck adapter failure rate of 1.2 %, but does not mention of the aseptic loosening incidence, perhaps due to the short, 2-year follow-up (Grupp et al. 2010). The explanation for the increased loosening rate should be sought in the two features of the modular necks that differentiate them from the monolithic systems: the neck–stem junction and the corrosion at this site and the various geometrical neck configurations and their biomechanical consequences.

   Corrosion at neck–stem tapers of dual modular cobalt–chrome hip prostheses has been identified as an important source of metal ion release and pseudotumor formation requiring revision surgery (Gill et al. 2012). Blood cobalt and chromium levels in patients with dual modular cobalt–chrome stems and metal-on-polyethylene articulation presented a tenfold increase compared with those of patients who had an identical prosthesis and articulation, but with a prosthesis that had no modularity at neck–stem junction (Gill et al. 2012). Retrieval studies (Kop and Swarts 2009; Gill et al. 2012; Wright et al. 2010) have further shown that the degradation of the neck–stem junction was more significant than that at the head–neck junction. This is not unexpected as the forces at the head–neck junction are transferred through a spherical bearing resulting in relatively low contact stresses, whereas there is eccentric loading at the neck–stem junction, and depending on the offset and length of the neck, these stresses can be high (Kop et al. 2012). Finite element modeling of the dual modular stem has confirmed this assumption (Gill et al. 2012). In vitro studies have also shown that the corrosion and fretting at the neck–stem junction occurs indeed eccentrically at the medial contact point between the neck and stem (Wright et al. 2010). It is further likely that increased micromovement at the neck–stem junction may occur due to the lever arm effect (Gill et al. 2012). On the other hand, the alloy used at the trunnion affects the degree of degradation. The cobalt–chromium components show crevice corrosion and fretting of the neck–stem taper, whereas the titanium components demonstrate less corrosion but higher crevice corrosion breakdown and cold welding (Kop et al. 2012). Titanium neck adapters showed significantly larger micromotions than cobalt–chromium neck adapters, and excessive micromotions at the stem–neck interface might be involved in the process of implant failure (Jauchy et al. 2011).

Metal release from modular head–neck junctions, rather than passive surface dissolution, has been already recognized to contribute to device revision (Jacobs et al. 1995). The additional taper junction corrosion, subject to higher stress levels, may be even more deleterious (Kop et al. 2012). Inflammatory mediators are released as a consequence of the cellular response to the particulate and/or ionic products of fretting and corrosion. Increased recruitment of osteoclast precursors, their subsequent differentiation into mature osteoclasts, and the increased osteoclast survival, in response to the released cytokines, may be involved in the pathomechanisms of aseptic implant loosening (Lee et al. 1997; Cadosch et al. 2009). Furthermore, investigations have demonstrated that Ti particles inhibit the expression of the osteoblastic genes that code for collagen type I and type III (Fanti et al. 1992). Other studies have revealed that nontoxic concentrations of metal ions affect the differentiation and function of osteoblastic cells in vitro (Thompson and Puleo 1995; Yao et al. 1997). Cobalt and chromium ions reduce human osteoblast activity, reduce OPG/RANKL ratio, and lead to oxidative stress (Zijlstra et al. 2012). Andrews et al. (2011) examined the effects of exposure to Co and Cr on human osteoblast and osteoclast formation and function over clinically relevant concentrations. They found that Cr(VI) reduced osteoblast survival and function, while Co(II) and Cr(III) did not affect them (Andrews et al. 2011). In contrast, osteoclasts were more sensitive to metal ions exposure. At normal serum levels, a mild stimulatory effect on developing osteoclasts was found for Co(II) and Cr(III), while at higher serum and synovial equivalent concentrations, and with Cr(VI), a reduction in cell number and bone resorption was observed (Australian Orthopaedic Association 2011). Aseptic loosening may be also mediated, at least in part by an adaptive immune response to metallic haptens (delayed-type hypersensitivity-like reaction). Metal hypersensitivity-induced osteolysis represents unappreciated and incompletely understood mechanisms of implant failure (Jacobs and Hallab 2006). However, cause and effect have not been established for aseptic loosening. Linking with local effects of metal ions and corrosion products remains circumstantial (Jacobs and Hallab 2006).

On the other hand, extended stresses at the implant–bone interface seem likely to raise the risk of implant loosening (Kleemann et al. 2003). For the monolithic implants, increased femoral anteversion alters significantly the loading patterns, while variations of offset seem to cause only minor changes (Kleemann et al. 2003). For the biomechanics of the modular-neck stems and their complex configurations, however, there are only a few reports in the literature (Umeda et al. 2003; Wik et al. 2011; Simpson et al. 2009). In a study by Umeda et al. (2003), strain gauge measurements of a modular cementless stem implanted in a synthetic femur were performed. Changing the neck from straight to anteverted or retroverted caused a large increase in strains on both, anterior and posterior, femoral surfaces, particularly at the distal part of the stem, and that increase was highly correlated with the extent of neck version. On the aspect toward which the prosthetic neck was oriented, increased compressive strains were developed, while on the opposite side increased tensile strains. Due to the anteriorly bowed femur, more bending stress was produced, especially at the stem tip area, when retroverted necks were used, as the femoral head deviates more in the sagittal plane than when an anteverted neck is used. It is worth noticing that for both anteverted and retroverted neck types, strain magnitudes on the anterior and posterior surfaces exceeded those developed on an intact femur. The highest value of strain increase, compared with the strain developed with the straight neck, was 1,195 %, and it was recorded with the extensively retroangled 22.5° neck at the anterior aspect of the femur and at the level of the stem tip (Umeda et al. 2003). Although this loading pattern of the anteverted and retroverted necks was confirmed, the extreme values of strain raise had not been reproduced in another strain gauge study on cadaveric femurs (Wik et al. 2011). In the same study, varus neck angulation was found to have a relatively small influence on strain distribution in the proximal femur (Wik et al. 2011). In contrast with these studies, an FEA reported no significant alterations in the strain distribution of a cemented stem coupled to a modular neck, positioned in anteversion and retroversion, and with two different offsets (Simpson et al. 2009).

Compared with these previous studies, our investigation has some differences. First of all, like the FEA study (Simpson et al. 2009), it evaluates the three-dimensional bone volume and not only profile lines along the femur. Furthermore, none of the aforementioned papers examine the changes in strain patterns caused by simultaneous alteration of neck–shaft angle, neck length, and version. Although we deliberately ignored the variable of neck length, our analysis included the rest variables. For these reasons we consider it a closer approximation of the real situation. However, similarly to the other FEA study, it recorded only mild changes in strain distribution. Although it is difficult to directly compare results between experimental and FEA studies, peak strain values were recorded in only one experimental study (Umeda et al. 2003) and have not been reproduced in any other investigation. This alone questions the validity of these results. On the other hand, whether the mild changes in loading patterns we have identified are solely associated with clinical problems remains uncertain. All the recorded strain values were included in the safe zones of healthy bone growth and adaptive remodeling activity, according to Frost's law, and no overload occurred. The increased strain induced by the increased offset and altered neck angles could, in fact, theoretically act beneficially in preservation of proximal bone stock in vivo, minimizing proximal femur stress shielding. However, we know that bone remodeling after implantation is proportional to the magnitude of stress applied (Weinans et al. 1993). There is a concern that long-term adaptive remodeling and subsequent changes in bone quality may have undesirable effects on the stability of the implant and, thus, may limit the life span of the THA (Wik et al. 2011).

Conclusion

Although it remains uncertain whether these changes in strain distribution patterns are clinically relevant, the anteverted and some orientations of the double-angled necks seem to be the most precarious. We believe, however, that the reported higher incidence of aseptic loosening of modular-neck stems cannot be confirmed only by the findings of this study. Instead, the explanation should be sought also in the bioreactivity and the local effects of the metal ions generated by the additional MoM junction and definitely not in the biomechanics of these systems alone.

References

Andrews RE, Shah KM, Wilkinson JM, Gartland A (2011) Effects of cobalt and chromium ions at clinically equivalent concentrations after metal-on-metal hip replacement on human osteoblasts and osteoclasts: implications for skeletal health. Bone 49(4):717–723

Australian Orthopaedic Association (2011) National joint replacement, Annual Report 2011, Australian Orthopaedic Association, Adelaide, Australia. http://www.dmac.adelaide.edu.au/aoanjirr/publications.jsp?section=reports2011. Accessed 19 June 2012

Cadosch D, Chan E, Gautschi OP, Filgueira L (2009) Metal is not inert: role of metal ions released by biocorrosion in aseptic loosening – current concepts. J Biomed Mater Res A 91(4):1252–1262

Fanti P, Kindy MS, Mohapatra S, Klein J, Colombo G, Malluche HH (1992) Dose-dependent effects of aluminum on osteocalcin synthesis in osteoblast-like ROS 17/2 cells in culture. Am J Physiol 263(6 Pt 1):E1113–E1118

Frost HM (1994) Wolff's Law and bone's structural adaptations to mechanical usage: an overview for clinicians. Angle Orthod 64(3):175–188

Gill IP, Webb J, Sloan K, Beaver RJ (2012) Corrosion at the neck-stem junction as a cause of metal ion release and pseudotumour formation. J Bone Joint Surg Br 94(7):895–900

Grupp TM, Weik T, Bloemer W, Knaebel HP (2010) Modular titanium alloy neck adapter failures in hip replacement – failure mode analysis and influence of implant material. BMC Musculoskelet Disord 11:3

Jacobs JJ, Hallab NJ (2006) Loosening and osteolysis associated with metal-on-metal bearings: a local effect of metal hypersensitivity? J Bone Joint Surg Am 88(6):1171–1172

Jacobs JJ, Urban RM, Gilbert JL et al (1995) Local and distant products from modularity. Clin Orthop Relat Res 319:94–105

Jauchy SY, Huber G, Hoenig E et al (2011) Influence of material coupling and assembly condition on the magnitude of micromotion at the stem-neck interface of a modular hip endoprosthesis. J Biomech 44(9):1747–1751

Kleemann RU, Heller MO, Stoeckle U et al (2003) THA loading arising from increased femoral anteversion and offset may lead to critical cement stresses. J Orthop Res 21(5):767–774

Kop AM, Swarts E (2009) Corrosion of a hip stem with a modular neck taper junction: a retrieval study of 16 cases. J Arthroplasty 24:1019–1023

Kop AM, Keogh C, Swarts E (2012) Proximal component modularity in THA-at what cost? An implant retrieval study. Clin Orthop Relat Res 470(7):1885–1894

Kouzelis A, Georgiou CS, Megas P (2012) Dissociation of modular total hip arthroplasty at the neck-stem interface without dislocation. J Orthop Traumatol 13(4):221–224

Lee SH, Brennan FR, Jacobs JJ et al (1997) Human monocyte/macrophage response to cobalt-chromium corrosion products and titanium particles in patients with total joint replacements. J Orthop Res 15:40–49

Simpson DJ, Little JP, Gray H et al (2009) Effect of modular neck variation on bone and cement mantle mechanics around a total hip arthroplasty stem. Clin Biomech (Bristol, Avon) 24(3):274–285

Thompson GJ, Puleo DA (1995) Effects of sublethal metal ion concentrations on osteogenic cells derived from bone marrow stromal cells. J Appl Biomater 6(4):249–258 (Winter)

Toni A, Sudanese A, Paderni S et al (2001) Cementless hip arthroplasty with a modular neck. Chir Organi Mov 86(2):73–85

Umeda N, Saito M, Sugano N et al (2003) Correlation between femoral neck version and strain on the femur after insertion of femoral prosthesis. J Orthop Sci 8(3):381–386

Weinans H, Huiskeis R, van Rietbergen B, Sumner DR, Turner TM, Galante JO (1993) Adaptive bone remodeling around bonded noncemented total hip arthroplasty: a comparison between animal experiments and computer simulations. J Orthop Res 11:500–513

Wik TS, Enoksen C, Klaksvik J et al (2011) In vitro testing of the deformation pattern and initial stability of a cementless stem coupled to an experimental femoral head, with increased offset and altered femoral neck angles. Proc Inst Mech Eng H 225(8):797–808

Wolff J (1986) The law of bone remodeling. Springer, Berlin (translation of the German 1892 edition)

Wright G, Sporer S, Urban R, Jacobs J (2010) Fracture of a modular femoral neck after total hip arthroplasty: a case report. J Bone Joint Surg Am 92(6):1518–1521

Yao J, Cs-Szabó G, Jacobs JJ, Kuettner KE, Glant TT (1997) Suppression of osteoblast function by titanium particles. J Bone Joint Surg Am 79(1):107–112

Zijlstra WP, Bulstra SK, van Raay JJ, van Leeuwen BM, Kuijer RJ (2012) Cobalt and chromium ions reduce human osteoblast-like cell activity in vitro, reduce the OPG to RANKL ratio, and induce oxidative stress. Orthop Res 30(5):740–747

Fracture of the Titanium Neck in a Modular Femoral Component

16

Tom Inglis and Bill Farrington

16.1 Introduction

The majority of uncemented femoral components used in total hip arthroplasty (THA) are of a monoblock design. This monoblock design has been around for many years and has a very low complication rate (McLaughlin and Lee 1997). Once the stem has been seated in the femur, the version of the neck cannot be altered, and the leg length and hip offset can only be changed slightly with a modular head. A modular neck-stem design (also known as a femoral stem with an exchangeable neck) has been introduced over the last few years by a number of different companies. This allows the surgeon to alter neck version, leg length and hip offset after the stem has been seated with the aim of more accurately recreating hip biomechanics to that of the native hip (Cheal et al. 1992; Ovesen et al. 2010). This should reduce the risk of impingement and dislocation after THA. This theoretical advantage has seen the modular neck-stem design grow in popularity over recent years; however, concerns are now being raised regarding their clinical results.

We report the first case of fracture of a modular neck in the modular Lima total hip replacement in Australasia. There have been approximately 5,000 of these components implanted worldwide to date. Case reports on fracture of these modular stem designs from other countries and companies do exist (Dunbar 2010; Patel et al. 2009; Wilson et al. 2010; Sporer et al. 2006) but as there are a number of different companies producing them and implanted numbers are small, it is difficult to know the true incidence of this complication. The National Joint Registry is in an ideal position in this situation to provide valuable feedback on these types of prostheses.

T. Inglis (✉) • B. Farrington
Department of Orthopaedic Surgery, North Shore Hospital,
Auckland, New Zealand
e-mail: inglistom@gmail.com

K. Knahr (ed.), *Total Hip Arthroplasty*,
DOI 10.1007/978-3-642-35653-7_16, © EFORT 2013

16.2 Case Report

A 65-year-old man underwent a primary THA of the right hip for osteoarthritis in 2009. He was 6 ft 1 in (185 cm) tall and weighed 128 kg (BMI 37.4). His past medical history included ischaemic heart disease and diabetes.

The primary procedure was performed through a posterior approach and was uneventful. The Lima modular THA system was used with a delta ceramic head articulating in a delta ceramic liner. The femoral stem and modular neck were both titanium, and an extended anteverted neck was used to provide the best stability following assessment at the time of surgery. The postoperative course was unremarkable, and the patient had been satisfied with his THA with complete pain relief and a high functional level for 18 months.

On the day of admission, he described a 'snap' in the groin following a minor twisting movement. It was painless and he was still able to weight bear. Several hours later, he felt another 'snap' in the groin, this time associated with groin pain and an inability to weight bear on the right leg. Ten days prior to this presentation, he had begun to notice an intermittent noise ('squeaking') coming from his THA.

Radiographs on admission showed a complete fracture through the base of the modular neck with the prosthetic head remaining enlocated within the acetabular component (Fig. 16.1). This was the first reported neck fracture in the Lima modular THA in Australasia.

At revision surgery we found an oblique fracture through the implant's neck, starting superiorly on the base of the neck proximal to the trunnion. The fracture exited inferiorly halfway down the trunnion (Fig. 16.2). There was no evidence of acetabular rim damage or stripe wear, which might have indicated impingement of the femoral neck on the acetabulum.

Removal of the remaining trunnion of the modular neck was challenging, with a high-speed burr used to remove it piecemeal (Fig. 16.3). The inside of the morse taper of the stem was protected as much as possible, and as there was no macroscopic damage to this taper, we decided to leave the stem in situ. We replaced the modular neck with an extended anteverted cobalt-chrome neck and long 36 mm cobalt-chrome head (Fig. 16.4). Initial recovery was uneventful.

However, 14 months after revision the patient suffered a posterior dislocation, despite the same geometry of the stem, head size and offset of the primary hip.

16.3 Discussion

The success of THA over the last 40 years has raised both patient expectation and surgical expertise. Nowadays, there is an assumption that there will be complete relief of pain and a return to near-normal hip function. One of the more common complications following THA surgery is dislocation. Dislocation of a prosthetic hip joint is disappointing for both patient and surgeon. It influences the patient's perception of their THA, causes apprehension about recurrence and affects their functional score (Chandler et al. 1982; Enocson et al. 2009; Khan et al. 2009). Recurrent

Fig. 16.1 Radiograph showing fracture at base of modular titanium neck

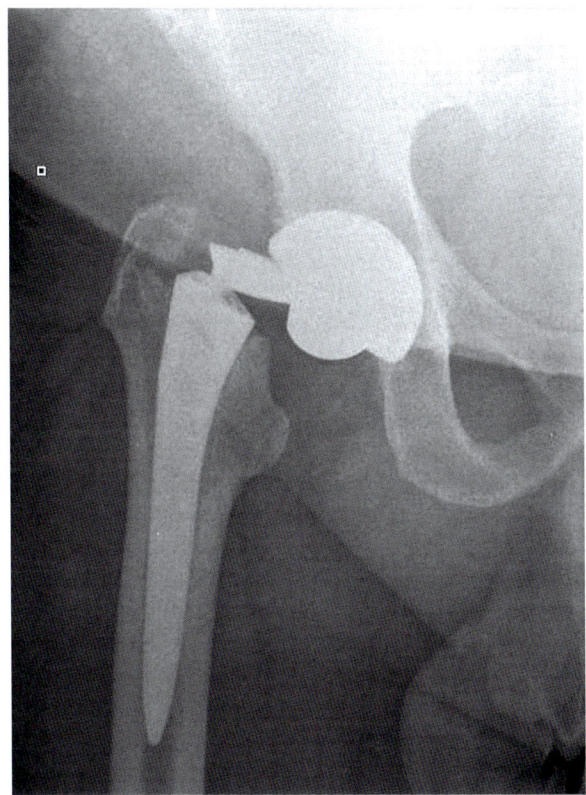

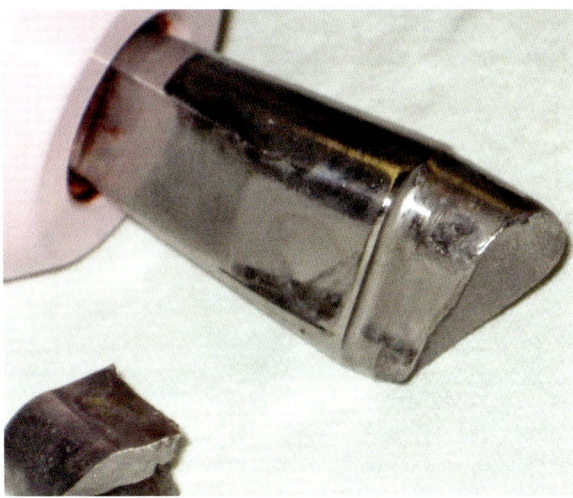

Fig. 16.2 Photograph of modular titanium neck at time of surgery

Fig. 16.3 Remnants
of fractured neck left within
morse taper requiring
removal with midas rex

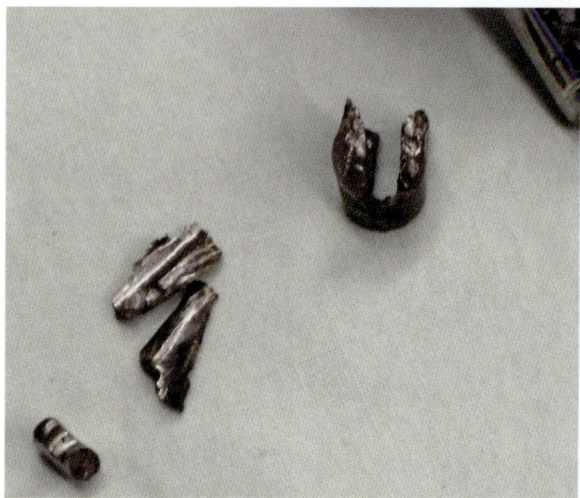

Fig. 16.4 Post operative
radiograph showing
replacement cobalt-chrome
neck

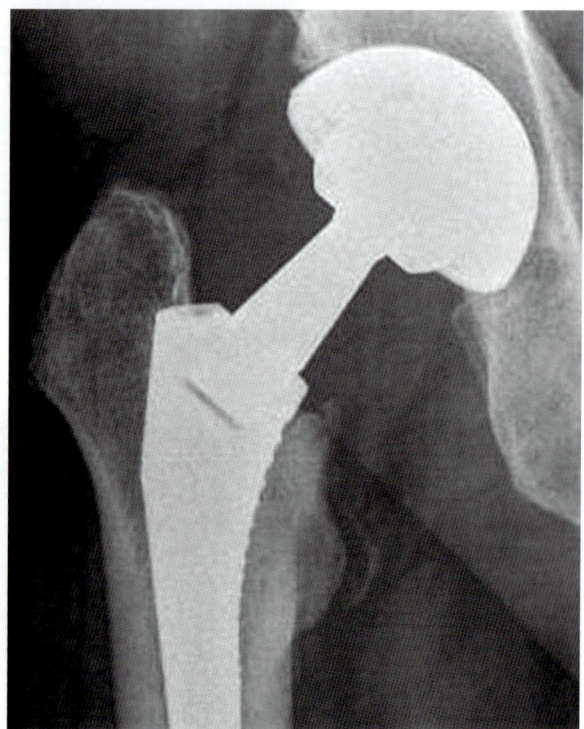

dislocation is the second most common cause of revision of a THA in most national joint registries around the world.

There have been considerable resources in both innovation and technology invested to address this issue. Many of these have aimed at increasing the size of the articulation.

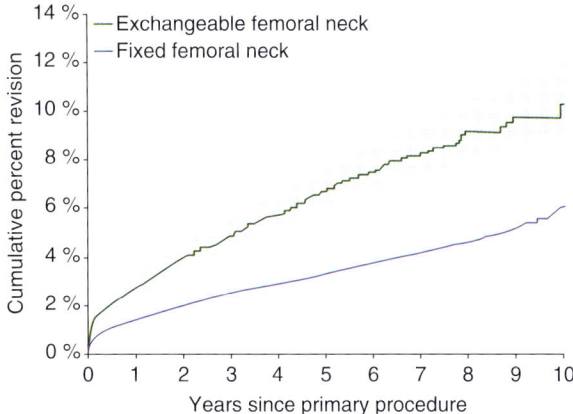

Graph 16.1 Cumulative percent revision of primary total conventional hip replacement by type of femoral neck (primary diagnosis AOA)

HR – adjusted for age and gender
Exchangeable femoral neck vs fixed femoral neck
Entire period: HR = 2.11 (1.90, 2.36), $p < 0.001$

Larger femoral heads are perceived to dislocate less frequently than smaller femoral heads, and recent data has supported this (Jameson et al. 2011). The design of a modular femoral neck and stem was also seen as an attractive proposition to reduce the risk of dislocation. This allows the surgeon intra-operatively to modify the femoral offset, anteversion and leg length after the stem has been seated (Cheal et al. 1992; Ovesen et al. 2010). This should result in a reduction in impingement and dislocation, improved hip biomechanics and fewer revisions; however, data from the Australian National Joint Registry (NJR) does not support this (Australian Othopaedic Association 2010).

In the Australian NJR modular (exchangeable neck), stems were used in 6,659 primary total conventional hip procedures undertaken for the treatment of osteoarthritis. Outcomes were compared to 166,932 procedures using fixed neck femoral stems for the same diagnosis. The cumulative percent revision at 7 years for modular stems was 8.9 % compared to 4.2 % for monoblock designs. The increased rate of revision when modular stems were used was evident for all bearing surfaces. This difference is significant for all bearing surfaces with greater than 4-year follow-up (Graph 16.1).

All modular stems (with exchangeable femoral necks) had a cumulative percent revision at least 2 times higher than monoblock (fixed neck) stems. This increase in revision was due to a higher incidence of loosening (3.2 % at 7 years compared to 1.3 % for monoblock designs), dislocation (2.0 % compared to 0.9 %) and fracture (0.8 % compared to 0.6 %) (Graph 16.2).

Modular hip systems have become increasingly popular. Modularity increases the options available at the time of surgery to modify the position of a component. On the femoral side this can affect the offset, leg length and femoral version. The ability to perform intra-operative trials with different combinations of components to determine the optimal stability is an attractive option for surgeons. Reconstruction of the femoral offset is important to obtain optimal joint function (Cheal et al. 1992) and stability (Ovesen et al. 2010) after THA.

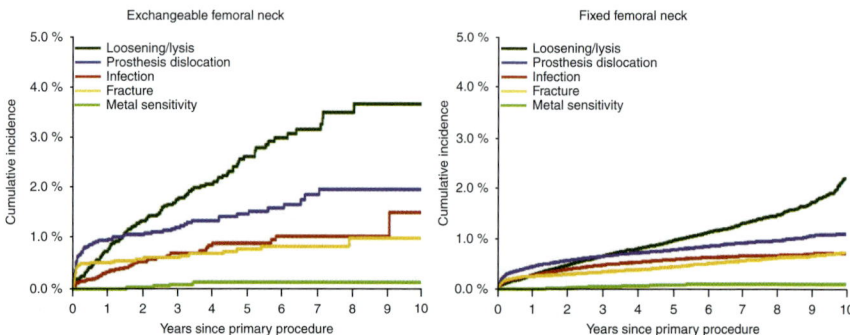

Graph 16.2 Revision diagnosis cumulative incidence of primary total conventional hip replacement by type of femoral neck (primary diagnosis AOA)

However, the introduction of a morse taper at the stem-neck junction to allow for this modularity reduces the strength of the component. This weaker construct may fail with time when compared to a monoblock system. Increased stresses are observed within femoral components with larger offsets and increased anteversion (Heller et al. 2011).

Clinical studies using modular femoral stems show only short-term results, report few complications and are generally limited to a particular brand of prosthesis. There have been a number of reports of modular connection failures (neck fractures) over recent years along with a few case reports such as ours (Dunbar 2010; Patel et al. 2009; Wilson et al. 2010; Sporer et al. 2006; Grupp et al. 2010). Most of these necks are made of titanium.

Grupp et al. (2010) reported a fracture rate of 1.4 % of titanium modular femoral necks with the Zimmer modular stem. Fractures were found to occur more frequently in men weighing over 100 kg at approximately 2 years following THA. Analysis of these necks showed a failure at the morse taper junction. They concluded that due to the location of the maximum tension on the neck and the material being titanium, the fracture was likely to be due to notch sensitivity. An increased lever arm and higher BMI would exacerbate this fatigue failure of the titanium neck, as was the case in our patient (high BMI, high neck offset and a titanium metal). Failure in this particular case was likely exacerbated by the patients' size. These patients may be the ones whose fracture occurs early, after only a few years. Time will tell whether this phenomenon occurs in all modular titanium necks.

Metal fatigue explains the process of progressive and localised structural damage that occurs when a metal is subjected to cyclical loading. If the repeated loading and unloading on the metal is above a certain threshold, microscopic cracks will form at the surface. These cracks gradually increase in size until they reach a critical point where the metal will fracture. Fatigue life is the number of stress cycles that the metal can sustain before failure. Fatigue life is influenced by a variety of factors including:

1. The type and magnitude of the cyclical stress.
2. Geometry – notches and cross-sectional shapes lead to stress concentrations where fatigue associated cracks begin.

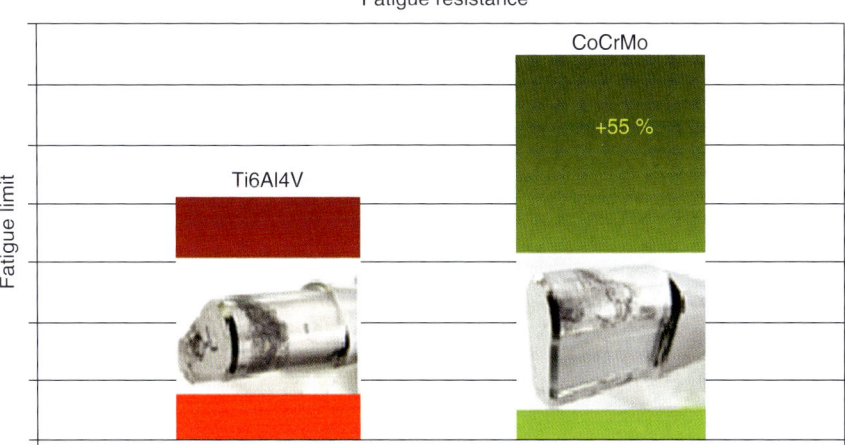

Fig. 16.5 Coupling of different materilas, i.e. CoCrMo necks on Ti alloy stems, can reduce the fretting phenomenon thus improve faitgue performance compared to Ti6AI4V on Ti6AI4V combination

3. Surface quality – roughness reduces fatigue strength.
4. Type of metal.
5. Residual stress – various manufacturing techniques (such as heating, deformation) can reduce fatigue strength by producing higher levels of tensile residual stress.
6. Corrosion – adversely affects fatigue life.
7. Grain size of the metal – smaller grains yield longer fatigue lives, although the surface finish is more critical (Stephens and Fuchs 2001).

Titanium is very notch sensitive making it susceptible to metal fatigue, and cobalt-chrome has been shown to have an increased fatigue life compared to titanium.

Since 2009, Lima has developed a cobalt-chrome neck with improved strength and fracture resistance (Fig. 16.5). Other companies have also developed this option, and it is thought that a cobalt-chrome neck is less likely to fracture (Dalla Pria 2004; Benazzo et al. 2004).

Fracture is one concern of modular necks; wear at the morse taper is another. Cobalt-chrome stems and modular necks have shown less risk of fracture than titanium necks.

However, Garbuz et al. (2010) have shown that the use of a modular taper adapter for large-head THA had 10 times the serum cobalt and 2.6 times the serum chromium levels when compared with resurfacing. The modular neck is thought to provide another interface for metal wear products with pitting corrosion and the production of metal debris. In the current climate of concern regarding ARMD (adverse reaction to metal debris), there may be more complications with this type of stem to come.

Further monitoring, especially from countries with national joint registries, is essential to evaluate modular femoral stems. Modifications to these implants may reduce potential complications, but longer-term monitoring is needed to justify their use.

References

Australian Orthopaedic Association (2010) National Joint Replacement Registry, annual report 2010. AOA

Benazzo F, Ravasi F, Dalla Pria P, Cuzzocrea F (2004) Prosthetic modularity in hip arthroplasty: from the F2L Multineck to the Modulus system. J Orthop Traumatol 5:S24–S26

Chandler RW, Dorr LD, Perry J (1982) The functional cost of dislocation following total hip arthroplasty. Clin Orthop Relat Res 168:168–172

Cheal EJ, Spector M, Hayes WC (1992) Role of loads and prosthesis material properties on the mechanics of the proximal femur after total hip arthroplasty. J Orthop Res 10:405–422

Dalla Pria P (2004) New modular system in total hip arthroplasty: the Lima Group's experience in modularity. J Orthop Traumatol 5:S20–S21

Dunbar MJ (2010) The proximal modular neck in THA: a bridge to far – affirms. Orthopaedics 33(9):640

Enocson A, Pettersson H, Ponzer S et al (2009) Quality of life after dislocation of hip arthroplasty: a prospective cohort study on 319 patients with femoral neck fractures with a one-year follow-up. Qual Life Res 18(9):1177–1184

Garbuz DS, Tanzer M, Greidanus NV, Masri BA, Duncan CP (2010) The John Charnley Award: metal-on-metal hip resurfacing versus large-diameter head metal-on-metal total hip arthroplasty: a randomized clinical trial. Clin Orthop Relat Res 468(2):318–325

Grupp TM, Weik T, Bloemer W, Knaebel H (2010) Modular titanium alloy neck adapter failures in hip replacement – failure mode analysis and influence of implant material. BMC Musculoskelet Disord 11:3

Heller MO, Mehta M, Taylor WR (2011) Influence of prosthesis design and implantation technique on implant stresses after cementless revision THR. J Orth Surg Res 6:20

Jameson SS, Lees D, James P et al (2011) Lower rates of dislocation with increased femoral head size after primary total hip replacement: a five-year analysis of NHS patients in England. J Bone Joint Surg Br 93(7):876–880

Khan RJK, Carey Smith RL, Alakeson R, Fick DP, Wood DJ (2009) Operative and non-operative treatment options for dislocation of the hip following total hip arthroplasty (Review 2006). Cochrane Database of Systematic. 4, Art. No.: CD005320. doi: 10.1002/14651858.CD005320.pub2.

McLaughlin JR, Lee KR (1997) Total hip arthroplasty with an uncemented femoral component: excellent results at ten-year follow up. J Bone Joint Surg Br 79-B(6):900–907

Ovesen O, Emmeluth C, Hofbauer C, Overgaard S (2010) Revision total hip arthroplasty using a modular tapered stem with distal fixation: good short term results in 125 revisions. J Arthroplasty 25:348–354

Patel A, Bliss J, Calfee RP, Froehlich J, Limbird R (2009) Modular femoral stem-sleeve junction failure after primary total hip arthroplasty. J Arthroplasty 24(7):1143.e1–1143.e5

Sporer SM, DellaValle C, Jacobs J, Wimmer M (2006) A case of disassociation of a modular femoral neck trunnion after total hip arthroplasty. J Arthroplasty 21(6):918–921

Stephens RI, Fuchs HO (2001) Metal fatigue in engineering, 2nd edn. Wiley, New York, p 69. ISBN 0-471-51059-9

Wilson DA, Dunbar MJ, Amirault JD, Farhat Z (2010) Early failure of a modular femoral neck total hip arthroplasty component: a case report. J Bone Joint Surg Am 92(6):1514–1517

Part V

Clinical Aspects

Wear of Hard-on-Hard Bearings in the Hip: The Influence of Loss of Conformity Under Edge Loading

17

John Fisher

17.1 Introduction

The conditions under which bearings articulate in the hip can have a significant effect on their wear performance. When the components are correctly aligned positioned and the natural hip centre is restored, then the ball and socket results in a conforming bearing for all material combinations. However, variations in positioning of components relative to the hip centre and relative to each other can cause edge loading of the head on the rim of the cup, which produces a low conforming contact and increased wear (Fisher 2011; Fisher 2012). Variations in both translational positioning and rotational positioning may lead to edge loading, but the effect on the wear rate is complex (Fisher 2012). Additionally, different bearing types and combinations react differently to edge loading. Under edge loading, a metal-on-polyethylene prosthesis produces creep and deformation to the rim of the polyethylene cup, but does not necessarily produce an increase in surface wear (Williams et al. 2003; Harris 2012). In ceramic-on-ceramic bearings, variation in translational position produces stripe wear (Nevelos et al. 2000), but variation in rotational position does not increase the wear rate (Nevelos et al. 2001a, b). In metal-on-metal bearings, variation in both translational and rotational positions can produce elevated stripe wear (Williams et al. 2008).

This review of recently published research, using novel preclinical simulation methods, presents an insight into the processes that accelerate wear and the magnitude of the increase in wear, due to different types of edge loading in hard-on-hard bearings in hip prostheses.

J. Fisher, CBE
Institute of Medical and Biological Engineering,
University of Leeds, Leeds, LS29JT, UK
e-mail: j.fisher@leeds.ac.uk

K. Knahr (ed.), *Total Hip Arthroplasty*,
DOI 10.1007/978-3-642-35653-7_17, © EFORT 2013

Fig. 17.1 Diagram showing rotational malpositioning of the cup with a steep inclination angle leading to the head contacting the rim of the cup. (**a**) Normal position of head and cup contact patch within the cup. (**b**) Rotational malposition of the cup, contact patch on the rim of the cup

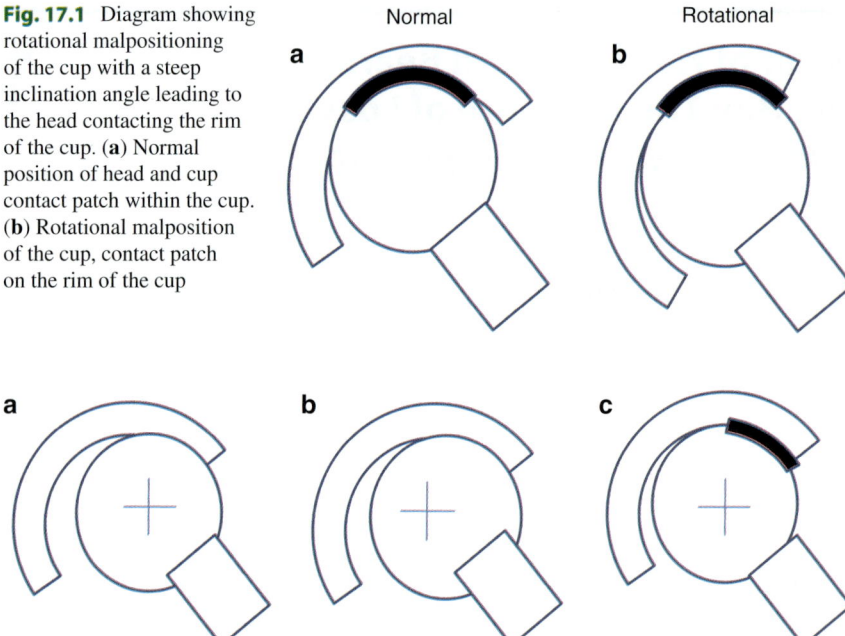

Fig. 17.2 Diagrams showing how translational malpositioning of the head or cup can lead to edge loading. (**a**) Translational malposition cup medial or head eccentric lateral. (**b**) Translational malposition head lateral deficient femoral offset. (**c**) Translational malposition leads to contact patch on the rim of the cup. However, it is too small to detect on radiographs

17.2 Methods

The variation in the rotational position of the cup (Fisher 2011), in terms of inclination, is readily identified on x-rays, and its impact on edge loading and wear has been assessed in preclinical simulation tests (Al-Hajjar et al. 2010) and is shown in Fig. 17.1. The variation in translational position, in terms of translational malposition, can occur if the cup is positioned medial of the hip centre, or if the head offset is deficient. However, in both cases the cup captures the head and on x-ray the components appear concentric, but the head remains in contact the rim of the cup (Fig. 17.2). This can result in dynamic microseparation during gait activity (Fig. 17.3) and stripe wear (Nevelos et al. 2000). While the variation in surgical translational positioning of the centres may be of the order of 1 mm or more, the dynamic microseparation of the centres during gait, which reproduces stripe wear in ceramic bearings, can be simulated in the laboratory at a level of 0.5 mm (Nevelos et al. 2000; Al-Hajjar et al. 2010), which is too small to be detected on x-ray or in fluoroscopy, but does produce edge loading, stripe wear and an increased wear rate.

A summary of the results of laboratory simulation wear studies is reported below for the simulation of variation in translational and rotational positioning of components for ceramic-on-ceramic and metal-on-metal bearings.

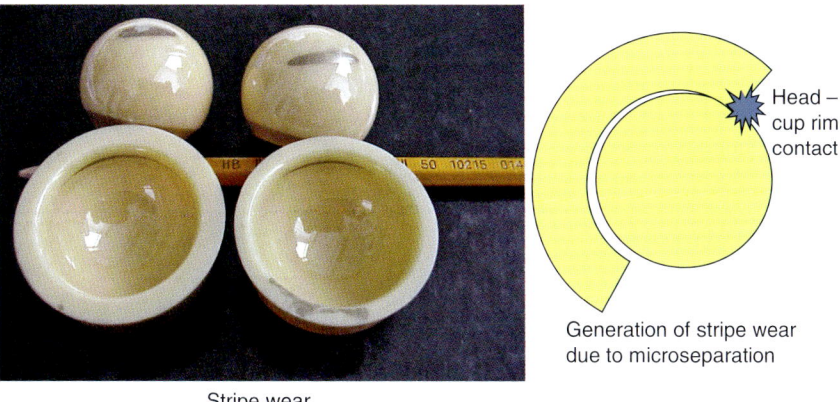

Stripe wear

Head –
cup rim
contact

Generation of stripe wear
due to microseparation

Fig. 17.3 Diagram showing how translational malpositioning can result in microseparation and stripe wear

17.3   Results

Simulator studies were undertaken under standard walking cycle conditions, with correctly positioned components, as described by ISO, as a control for the studies. For these standard conditions, the wear of the alumina ceramic-on-ceramic bearings was typically less than 0.1 mm³/million cycles and the wear of the metal-on-metal bearings typically less than 1 mm³/million cycles and less than 0.5 mm³/million cycles for larger-diameter metal-on-metal bearings (Fisher 2012). Under these standard conditions, the volumetric wear rates were substantially less than the wear rates for cross-linked and conventional polyethylene, which exceed 5 mm³/million cycles (Fisher 2012).

Rotational malpositioning of the acetabular cup in the ceramic-on-ceramic bearing, with cup inclination angles increased to 65°, did not produce an increase in wear in either Biolox Forte or Biolox Delta ceramic, with wear rates remaining less than 0.1 mm³/million cycles and no evidence of stripe wear (Nevelos et al. 2001a, b; Al-Hajjar et al. 2010).

Translational malpositioning and microseparation simulation of ceramic-on-ceramic bearings produced stripe wear and an increase in wear rates, associated with edge loading. For Biolox Forte alumina ceramic-on-ceramic bearings, the wear rates increased to between 0.5 and 1.8 mm³/million cycles (Nevelos et al. 2000; Stewart et al. 2001). These wear rates are substantially less than for cross-linked polyethylene and do not typically appear to result in adverse tissue reactions (Nevelos et al. 2001a, b). For Biolox Delta the wear rate increased, but to a much lower level of 0.1–0.25 mm³/million cycles (Al-Hajjar et al. 2010). The tougher mechanical properties of the Biolox Delta provided resistance to stripe wear under edge loading.

For 39 mm diameter metal-on-metal joint replacements rotational malposition with a cup inclination of 60° increased the wear rate to 5 mm³/million cycles (Leslie et al. 2009), with stripe wear on the femoral head and cup rim wear.

Under translational malposition and microseparation, the wear rate increased further to 9 mm³/million cycles (Leslie et al. 2009). These large increases in wear of metal-on-metal hip due to edge wear due to translational and rotational malpositioning are thought to be a cause of high clinical wear, elevated ion levels and adverse tissue reactions (Fisher 2011).

17.4   Discussion

The standard method, currently widely used to assess wear in total hip prostheses, involves simulation of a walking cycle with the components correctly positioned and aligned. In the hip this produces a conforming bearing with low wear. In the patient, there is variation in the positioning of the head and cup, both translational malpositioning and rotational malpositioning, which can result in the head articulating on the rim of the cup. It is believed that these conditions can lead to increased wear rates and contribute to the variation in clinical wear rates found in some patients (Fisher 2011). The effect of the variation in positioning and the resulting increase in wear and clinical outcome is dependent on the type of bearing.

Edge loading of metal heads on polyethylene cups has been shown not to increase surface wear in conventional polyethylene cups (Williams et al. 2003), but did cause fatigue wear and failure in gamma irradiated in air polyethylene cups, which had oxidised and had reduced mechanical properties (Harris 2012). Edge loading on highly cross-linked polyethylene cups and the potential risk of fatigue failure have not been extensively studied.

Edge loading in ceramic-on-ceramic bearings only caused stripe wear and an increase in wear with variations in translational positioning and microseparation. The increased wear rate was less than 1 mm³/million cycles, much less than the wear found with cross-linked polyethylene, and not at a level likely to cause adverse tissue reactions.

Edge loading and stripe wear in metal-on-metal bearings occurred with both translational malpositioning and also with rotational malpositioning. In both cases with large-diameter surface replacements, the wear rates increased to 9 and 5 mm³/million cycles, levels which are thought to cause elevated ion levels and adverse tissue reactions (Fisher 2011).

These studies indicate that it is now necessary to assess the wear performance of bearings in the hip, under a wider range of conditions that reflect the clinical environment. It is now recommended that a stratified approach to preclinical simulation testing is introduced which has the potential to enhance the reliability of hip prostheses (Fisher 2012).

Acknowledgments   JF is an NIHR senior investigator. His research is supported by the EPSRC, by the NIHR LMBRU Leeds Musculoskeletal Biomedical Research Unit, by the Centre of Excellence in Medical Engineering funded by the Wellcome Trust and EPSRC WT 088908/z/09/z and by the Innovation and Knowledge Centre in Medical Technologies.

References

Al-Hajjar M, Leslie IJ, Tipper J, Williams S, Fisher J, Jennings LM (2010) Effect of cup inclination angle during microseparation and rim loading on the wear of BIOLOX® delta ceramic-on-ceramic total hip replacement. J Biomed Mater Res B Appl Biomater 95:263–268

Fisher J (2011) Bioengineering reasons for the failure of metal-on-metal hip prostheses: an engineer's perspective. J Bone Joint Surg 93B:1001–1004

Fisher J (2012) A stratified approach to preclinical tribological evaluation of joint replacements. Faraday Discuss 158:59–68

Harris WH (2012) Edge loading has a paradoxical effect on wear. Clin Orthop Relat Res2330–7

Leslie IJ, Williams S, Isaac G, Ingham E, Fisher J (2009) High cup angle and microseparation increase the wear of hip surface replacements. Clin Orthop Relat Res 467:2259–2265

Nevelos J, Ingham E, Doyle C, Streicher R, Nevelos A, Walter W, Fisher J (2000) Microseparation of the centres of alumina-alumina artificial hip joints during simulator testing produces clinically relevant wear and patterns. J Arthroplasty 15:793–795

Nevelos JE, Ingham E, Doyle C, Nevelos AB, Fisher J (2001a) The influence of acetabular cup angle on the wear of "BIOLOX Forte" alumina ceramic bearing couples in a hip joint simulator. J Mater Sci Mater Med 12:141–144

Nevelos JE, Prudhommeaux F, Hamadouche M, Doyle C, Ingham E, Meunier A, Nevelos AB, Sedel L, Fisher J (2001b) Comparative analysis of two different types of alumina-alumina hip prosthesis retrieved for aseptic loosening. J Bone Joint Surg 83B:598–603

Stewart T, Tipper JL, Streicher R, Ingham E, Fisher J (2001) Long-term wear or HIPed alumina on alumina bearings for THR under microseparation conditions. J Mater Sci Mater Med 12:1053–1056

Williams S, Butterfield M, Stewart T, Ingham E, Stone MH, Fisher J (2003) Wear and deformation of ceramic-on-polyethylene total hip replacements with joint laxity and swing phase microseparation. Proc Inst Mech Eng J Eng Med 217:147–153

Williams S, Leslie I, Isaac G, Jin Z, Ingham E, Fisher J (2008) Tribology and wear of metal-on-metal hip prostheses: influence of cup angle and head position. J Bone Joint Surg Am 90 ((suppl 3)):111–117

Considerations for the Use of Bearing Partners in Total Hip Arthroplasty

18

Martin Pospischill and Karl Knahr

18.1 Introduction

Nowadays, the major limiting factor of long-term survival of total hip replacements is wear debris generated by the bearing surface (Pospischill and Knahr 2005). The debris induces osteolysis around the implant leading to subsequent aseptic loosening (Harris 2001). Due to this fact, a major effort has been made to improve the original UHMW-polyethylene introduced by Charnley in the 1960s on the one hand and to develop alternative bearing surfaces on the other hand (Santavirta et al. 2003). The surgeon can currently choose between metal-/ceramic-on-polyethylene, metal-/ceramic-on-cross-linked polyethylene, metal-on-metal, and ceramic-on-ceramic couplings. Despite the significantly reduced wear rate of all the alternative articulations, orthopedic surgeons are still faced with problems related to each single combination (MacDonald 2004; Barrack et al. 2004). Comprehensive knowledge of the characteristics of the articulating materials used by the surgeon is mandatory to avoid unexpected complications. Due to excellent long-time survivorship rates of hip replacements, the average age of a primary THA patient decreased over the last couple of years. Younger, more active patients with increasing demands on their implant are operated. For this young population, increased stability and range of motion with minimal wear of the articulations are required.

The aim of this chapter is to present our considerations on the different bearing couples and recommend an algorithm to support the surgeon for a proper choice of articulation materials.

M. Pospischill, MD (✉) • K. Knahr, MD
Orthopedic Hospital Vienna-Speising,
Speisingerstr. 109,, Vienna, A-1130, Austria
e-mail: martin.pospischill@oss.at

K. Knahr (ed.), *Total Hip Arthroplasty*,
DOI 10.1007/978-3-642-35653-7_18, © EFORT 2013

18.2   Metal-/Ceramic-on-Conventional UHMW-Polyethylene

Metal head-on ultrahigh-molecular-weight polyethylene is the original bearing couple introduced by Charnley in the 1960s. Due to its good long-term results, conventional polyethylene is still considered to be the golden standard to which wear characteristics of other articulations are compared. As the annual wear rate of metal-on-polyethylene is approx. 0.1–0.3 mm/year and the rate for ceramic-on-polyethylene is about 0.05–0.15 mm/year (Zichner and Lindenfeld 1997), the onset of visible wear and osteolysis occurs later in ceramic articulations than in metal articulations (Urban et al. 2001). The major reason for revision of these couplings is increased polyethylene wear which leads to subsequent osteolysis followed by aseptic loosening of the implant. A radiologically visible migration of the head due to polyethylene wear with clinical pain in the groin usually starts about 10 years after surgery (Pospischill and Knahr 2005).

18.3   Metal-/Ceramic-on-Cross-Linked Polyethylene

More than a decade ago, cross-linking of the polyethylene molecules by electron beams or gamma radiation became popular. Improved wear characteristics and a reduction of wear proportional to the amount of cross-linking were documented in experimental studies (Muratoglu et al. 1999; Bergstrom et al. 2003). But during the process of cross-linking, free radicals are produced which have the potential to link with an oxygen molecule. This oxidation can also happen in vivo due to diluted oxygen in the tissues leading to a reduction of durability of the poly. To address this problem, second-generation highly cross-linked polyethylenes were introduced to saturate the free radicals by sequential annealing or by infusing vitamin E into the irradiated polyethylene (Oral et al. 2006). See Fig. 18.1a, b. Long-term in vivo results of cross-linked polyethylene are still missing. The latest studies of first-generation XLPE with a follow-up up to 10 years report a significant reduction in radiological measured wear with a mean wear rate of 0.005 mm/year (Johanson et al. 2012; Thomas et al. 2011; Kuzyk et al. 2011).

18.4   Metal-on-Metal

Metal-on-metal articulations have been reintroduced by Weber in the late 1980s as an alternative to metal/ceramic-on-polyethylene bearings due to improved wear behavior of second-generation high carbon implants. Thereby a renaissance of this material combination for articulating surfaces in total hip arthroplasty started. Compared to ceramic-on-polyethylene and metal-on-polyethylene articulations, the annual wear rate is much lower (approx. 0.01 mm/year) (Greenwald and Garino 2001; Silva et al. 2005). In addition, the material properties allow the production of thinner acetabular shells to be combined with larger head diameters. For this reason,

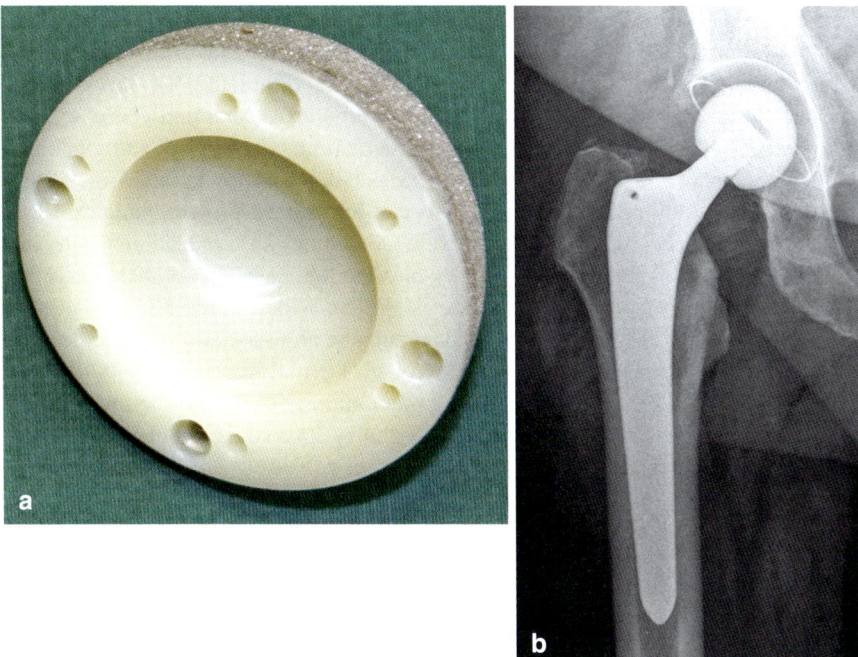

Fig. 18.1 (**a**) Vitamin E blended highly cross-linked polyethylene cup. (**b**) Vitamin E blended highly cross-linked polyethylene cup with a 36 mm ceramic head

metal-on-metal couples are mainly used for hip resurfacing. In THA larger head diameters increase the range of motion and reduce the risk of hip dislocation in younger and more active patients. Compared to ceramic, there is no risk of fracture of head or inlay due to the less sensitive mechanical characteristics of metal.

Despite these biomechanical advantages, several reports in literature showed some major disadvantages using metal-on-metal articulations. These concerns can be divided in systemic and local risks. The serum levels of cobalt and chromium ions may be significantly higher in patients with a metal-on-metal bearing compared to patients with other bearings (Jacobs and Hallab 2006), (Karamat et al. 2005). Especially in patients with a renal insufficiency, the blood levels of metal ions can accumulate and achieve very high values (Brodner et al. 2003). Nevertheless, these values are far below the limit of cytotoxicity (Allen et al. 1997). An acquired loss of efficacy of renal clearance with increasing age and comorbidities such as diabetes may lead to a further accumulation of metal ions. The long-term effect of these dissolved metal ions in vivo is still unknown. Another problem concerning the metal ion release over time is the transplacental transfer of cobalt and chromium in pregnant women with a metal-on-metal bearing (Fritzsche et al. 2012). It is reported that the mean umbilical cord blood chromium level is almost twice as high in patients with metal-on-metal bearing couples as in patients without a metal implant. The effect on the unborn child is still unknown (Ziaee et al. 2007).

In addition to these systemic reactions, several local tissue reactions are reported. Metallic wear particles can reach high levels especially in cases of impingement of the femoral and acetabular component due to incorrect implant position. As a consequence the joint capsule is exposed to a larger amount of wear particles compared to a conventional metal-on-polyethylene articulation. The typical intraoperative finding is a blackening of the joint lubricant and the synovia called metallosis (Korovessis et al. 2006). The released ions can form metal-protein complexes that are considered to act as antigens and activate the immune system leading to a hypersensitivity response (Hallab et al. 2001). This reaction leads to early osteolysis and aseptic loosening of components (Park et al. 2005; Willert et al. 2005; Baur et al. 2005; Holloway et al. 2009). Clinical data suggest an association with a delayed hypersensitivity type IV to metal, mainly cobalt. Dermal hypersensitivity to metal is found in about 10–15 % of the general population with double the incidence in patients with hip prosthesis (Dumbleton and Manley 2005). It is still unclear whether the allergy to metal alloys is preexisting preoperatively or the patients became hypersensitive secondary to metal particles. Recently several papers reported a high prevalence of pseudotumors surrounding metal-on-metal THAs and hip resurfacing prostheses. These cystic or solid tumors are sterile inflammatory lesions within the periprosthetic tissues and are thought to be a consequence of wear debris from metal-on-metal bearing couples (Hart et al. 2012). Histomorphological studies of pseudotumors show an aseptic lymphocytic vasculitis-associated lesion (ALVAL) which is characterized by the findings of massive necrosis of the periarticular tissue with infiltration of inflammatory cells (lymphocytes and plasma cells) around vessels (Willert et al. 2005). The prevalence of pseudotumors differs in the literature (Williams et al. 2011). In their case–control study of 58 hip prostheses, Hart et al. (Hart et al. 2012) found an incidence of 59 %. In the case group consisting of patients with a painful hip, a pseudotumor was diagnosed in 57 % compared to 61 % in the control group with asymptomatic patients. Pseudotumors are also common in well-positioned metal-on-metal hips (Matthies et al. 2012). The exact pathogenesis of these lesions still remains unclear.

Recent studies and data of several registries report that small heads (28 and 32 mm) are only little at risk of an adverse reaction to metal debris (ARMD) compared to conventional bearings (Malviya et al. 2010). This fact is different for large heads. Ball heads over 32 mm in diameter have a higher risk of local and systemic reactions to metal wear particles leading to higher revision rates (Smith et al. 2012). See Fig. 18.2a, b. Especially in hip resurfacing with larger head sizes, this risk is further increased.

18.5 Ceramic-on-Ceramic

Alumina ceramic is a very hard and resistant material with excellent wear characteristics. The linear wear rate is very low and described in the literature about 0.003 mm/year (Skinner 1999). The good biocompatibility of ceramic wear particles enables a significant reduction of osteolysis compared to metal-on-conventional

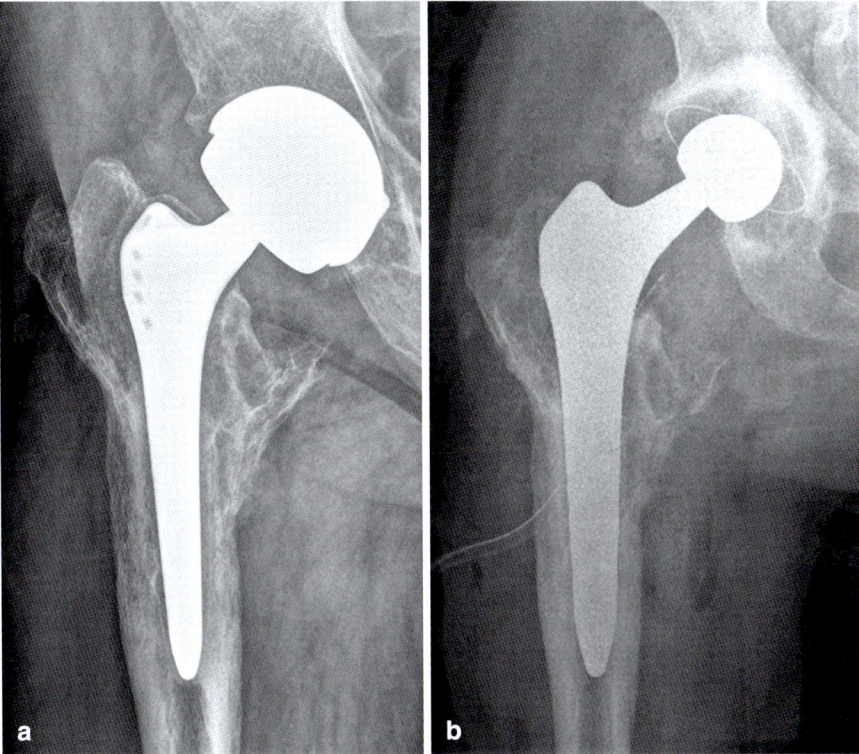

Fig. 18.2 (**a**) Early loosening of the stem due to metal wear (large-diameter head). (**b**) Exchange of cup and stem

polyethylene bearings at more than 10 years (Murphy et al. 2006). Hamadouche et al. reported a long-term study with a minimum follow-up of 18.5 years. In their study wear was unable to detect on the radiographs; the mean annual wear rate was <0.025 mm/year (Hamadouche et al. 2002).

Due to these special characteristics of the material, revisions are mainly not caused by osteolysis and secondary loosening of the implant. The most serious problems of ceramics are fracture of the material due to impingement or recurrent dislocation. Due to the low elasticity of the material, alumina ceramic bearing surfaces do not allow any deformation under load. High punctual stress can lead to fracture either of the ceramic head or the ceramic liner. Correct attachment of the ceramic ball head is mandatory to prevent possible fracture. Exact positioning of the cup is necessary to avoid edge loading by impingement at the rim of the liner (Mittelmeier and Heisel 1992). The incidence of alumina ceramic bearing fracture is low with 0.004–1.4 % for femoral heads produced after 1994 (Willmann 2000; Koo et al. 2008). Ceramic particles produced by fracture or wear may cause excessive wear on metal ball heads in metal-on-metal or metal-on-polyethylene bearings as these particles are much harder than metal. They lead to severe damage of all metal components in a very short time (= third body wear). For this reason, only ceramic-on-ceramic or ceramic-on-(cross-linked)polyethylene bearings are recommended in revision surgery.

Recently, squeaking with ceramic articulations has been reported in several studies with an incidence of 0.48–10.7 % (Restrepo et al. 2008; Walter et al. 2007; Jarrett et al. 2009). It seems to be a multifactorial problem related to microseparation, subluxation associated with impingement, implant design and cup malposition, or a combination of these factors.

New developments in ceramic bearings include the production of a toughened dispersion ceramic made of alumina and zirconia to address the problems of ceramic component fracture and squeaking (AMC alumina matrix composite). A recent paper reports no fracture with more than 100,000 AMC components (heads and liners) implanted (Masson 2009). The improved mechanical properties allow the production of thinner liners (down to 3.5 mm) and subsequently of larger head diameters, reducing the risk of impingement and increasing the range of motion with more stability (see Fig. 18.3a–c).

18.6   Recommendations

Since the beginning of modern total hip arthroplasty in the 1960s by Sir Charnley, the total number of hip replacements has increased worldwide. For many years, the standard bearing couple used in THA has been a metal head with a polyethylene liner. Nowadays, due to improvement of implant fixation and further developments of alternate and more wear-resistant bearing materials, the surgeon has a large variety of articulation partners to choose from. Especially concerning the optimal bearing surface in young patients, there is still an ongoing debate. The decision often depends on patient-related factors such as age and activity level as well as surgeons' prevalence and cost-related factors (Table 18.1).

The mean age of patients receiving a primary THA decreased during the last decade. Younger and more active patients are demanding an increased range of motion and enhanced joint stability. As a consequence larger femoral heads became more popular offering both increased range of motion and a decrease of the dislocation rate (Burroughs et al. 2005). For this reason, there is a tendency to a more frequent use of large-diameter heads. Besides these advantages, there are certain limitations. The use of a larger head diameter is only possible in combination with a thinner acetabular bearing partner using the same cup size. Conventional polyethylene thickness should not decrease below 5 mm to avoid a high failure rate due to "wear through" and cracking at the rim of the liner (Berry et al. 1994). Having in mind the latest disastrous reports on metal-on-metal bearings with large head diameters, there remain two alternative recommended options. Due to better mechanical properties and reduced wear rates by 50 % (Krushell et al. 2005), cross-linked polyethylene is said to allow the production of thinner liners (Sayeed et al. 2011). Infusing vitamin E into irradiated polyethylene seems to further improve the mechanical properties, but long-term results are still missing. In our institution

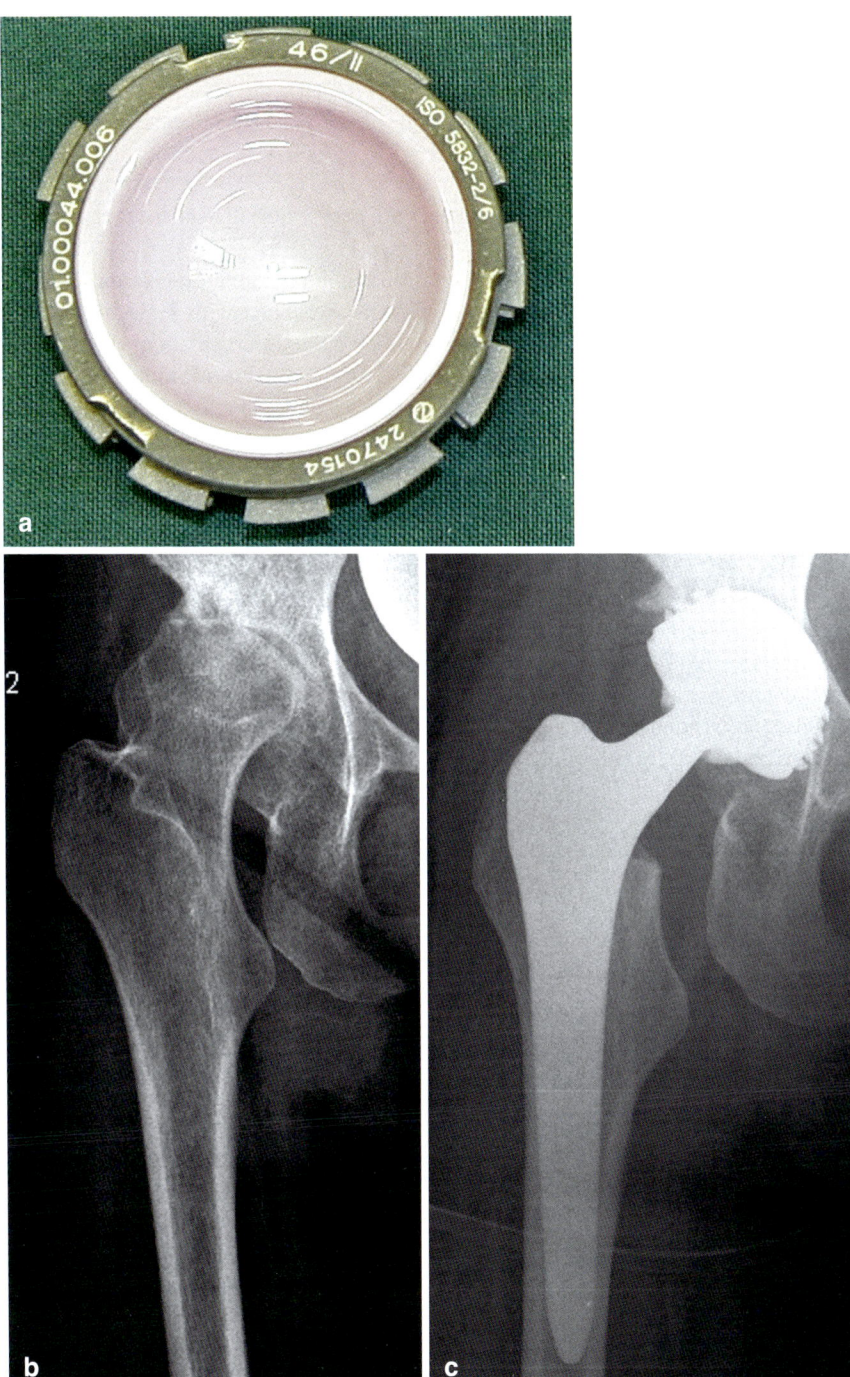

Fig. 18.3 (**a**) Alumina matrix composite ceramic liner (Biolox Delta). (**b**) Coxarthrosis after congenital hip dysplasia. (**c**) Total hip arthroplasty with a ceramic-on-ceramic articulation (cup size 46 /32 mm head)

Table 18.1 Recommendations for the use of bearing partners in THA

Young patient <60 year, activity level ↑	Ceramic-on-ceramic
Patient 60–80 year, activity level ↑	Ceramic-on-cross-linked polyethylene
Old patient >80 year, activity level ↓	Ceramic-on-conventional polyethylene

highly cross-linked polyethylene combined with a ceramic ball head is recommended for active patients between 60 and 80 years (see Fig. 18.1b).

The second option is the use of modern dispersion ceramic-on-ceramic articulations. Metal-on-metal total hip arthroplasties are associated with high failure rates using large heads >32 mm, while for ceramic-on-ceramic articulations, larger head sizes are documented with an increased survival in the registries (Smith et al. 2012). Due to their excellent wear characteristics with the lowest wear rates compared to other bearing couples, ceramic-on-ceramic articulations are our preferred material for young and active patients (Bizot et al. 2000; Hamadouche et al. 2002). We recommend the use of large-diameter ceramic-on-ceramic bearings for patients below the age of 60 years.

Recent reports on metal-on-metal bearings have shown that the benefits are not worth the risks, especially with the use of large heads >32 mm. There still exist several uncertain issues especially the long-term effects of metal wear particles and metal ions in the body. A major concern is also the lack of a method to preselect patients who could develop a local or systemic reaction to metal debris. We therefore advise against the use of large metal-on-metal articulations in THA.

Due to good long-term results and slightly lower costs, conventional polyethylene is still a favorable option for older patients with a low activity and life expectancy (>80 years).

References

Allen MJ, Myer BJ, Millett PJ, Rushton N (1997) The effects of particulate cobalt, chromium and cobalt-chromium alloy on human osteoblast-like cells in vitro. J Bone Joint Surg Br 79(3):475–482

Barrack RL, Burak C, Skinner HB (2004) Concerns about ceramics in THA. Clin Orthop Relat Res 429:73–79, 00003086-200412000-00012 [pii]

Baur W, Honle W, Willert HG, Schuh A (2005) Pathological findings in tissue surrounding revised metal/metal articulations. Orthopade 34(3):225–226. doi:10.1007/s00132-004-0761-x, 228–233

Bergstrom JS, Rimnac CM, Kurtz SM (2003) Prediction of multiaxial mechanical behavior for conventional and highly crosslinked UHMWPE using a hybrid constitutive model. Biomaterials 24(8):1365–1380, S0142961202005148 [pii]

Berry DJ, Barnes CL, Scott RD, Cabanela ME, Poss R (1994) Catastrophic failure of the polyethylene liner of uncemented acetabular components. J Bone Joint Surg Br 76(4):575–578

Bizot P, Banallec L, Sedel L, Nizard R (2000) Alumina-on-alumina total hip prostheses in patients 40 years of age or younger. Clin Orthop Relat Res 379:68–76

Brodner W, Bitzan P, Meisinger V, Kaider A, Gottsauner-Wolf F, Kotz R (2003) Serum cobalt levels after metal-on-metal total hip arthroplasty. J Bone Joint Surg Am 85-A(11):2168–2173

Burroughs BR, Hallstrom B, Golladay GJ, Hoeffel D, Harris WH (2005) Range of motion and stability in total hip arthroplasty with 28-, 32-, 38-, and 44-mm femoral head sizes. J Arthroplasty 20(1):11–19. doi:10.1016/j.arth.2004.07.008, S0883540304003924 [pii]

Dumbleton JH, Manley MT (2005) Metal-on-Metal total hip replacement: what does the literature say? J Arthroplasty 20(2):174–188

Fritzsche J, Borisch C, Schaefer C (2012) Case report: high chromium and cobalt levels in a pregnant patient with bilateral metal-on-metal hip arthroplasties. Clin Orthop Relat Res 470(8):2325–2331. doi:10.1007/s11999-012-2398-0

Greenwald AS, Garino JP (2001) Alternative bearing surfaces: The good, the bad, and the ugly. J Bone Joint Surg Am 83-A(suppl 2 Pt 2):68–72

Hallab N, Merritt K, Jacobs JJ (2001) Metal sensitivity in patients with orthopaedic implants. J Bone Joint Surg Am 83-A(3):428–436

Hamadouche M, Boutin P, Daussange J, Bolander ME, Sedel L (2002) Alumina-on-alumina total hip arthroplasty: a minimum 18.5-year follow-up study. J Bone Joint Surg Am 84-A(1):69–77

Harris WH (2001) Wear and periprosthetic osteolysis: the problem. Clin Orthop Relat Res 393:66–70

Hart AJ, Satchithananda K, Liddle AD, Sabah SA, McRobbie D, Henckel J et al (2012) Pseudotumors in association with well-functioning metal-on-metal hip prostheses: a case–control study using three-dimensional computed tomography and magnetic resonance imaging. J Bone Joint Surg Am 94(4):317–325. doi:10.2106/JBJS.J.01508

Holloway I, Walter WL, Zicat B, Walter WK (2009) Osteolysis with a cementless second generation metal-on-metal cup in total hip replacement. Int Orthop 33(6):1537–1542. doi:10.1007/s00264-008-0679-8

Jacobs JJ, Hallab NJ (2006) Loosening and osteolysis associated with metal-on-metal bearings: a local effect of metal hypersensitivity? J Bone Joint Surg Am 88(6):1171–1172. doi:10.2106/JBJS.F.00453, 88/6/1171 [pii]

Jarrett CA, Ranawat AS, Bruzzone M, Blum YC, Rodriguez JA, Ranawat CS (2009) The squeaking hip: a phenomenon of ceramic-on-ceramic total hip arthroplasty. J Bone Joint Surg Am 91(6):1344–1349. doi:10.2106/JBJS.F.00970, 91/6/1344 [pii]

Johanson PE, Digas G, Herberts P, Thanner J, Karrholm J (2012) Highly crosslinked polyethylene does not reduce aseptic loosening in cemented THA 10-year findings of a randomized study. Clin Orthop Relat Res 470(11):3083–3093. doi:10.1007/s11999-012-2400-x

Karamat L, Pinggera O, Knahr K (2005) Blood analysis for trace metals in metal-on-metal, ceramic-on-ceramic and metal-on-cross-linked PE bearings in total hip arthroplasty. Hip Int 15:136–142

Koo KH, Ha YC, Jung WH, Kim SR, Yoo JJ, Kim HJ (2008) Isolated fracture of the ceramic head after third-generation alumina-on-alumina total hip arthroplasty. J Bone Joint Surg Am 90(2):329–336. doi:10.2106/JBJS.F.01489, 90/2/329 [pii]

Korovessis P, Petsinis G, Repanti M, Repantis T (2006) Metallosis after contemporary metal-on-metal total hip arthroplasty. Five to nine-year follow-up. J Bone Joint Surg Am 88(6):1183–1191. doi:10.2106/JBJS.D.02916, 88/6/1183 [pii]

Krushell RJ, Fingeroth RJ, Cushing MC (2005) Early femoral head penetration of a highly cross-linked polyethylene liner vs a conventional polyethylene liner: a case-controlled study. J Arthroplasty 20(7 suppl 3):73–76. doi:10.1016/j.arth.2005.05.008, S0883-5403(05)00285-8 [pii]

Kuzyk PR, Saccone M, Sprague S, Simunovic N, Bhandari M, Schemitsch EH (2011) Cross-linked versus conventional polyethylene for total hip replacement: a meta-analysis of randomised controlled trials. J Bone Joint Surg Br 93(5):593–600. doi:10.1302/0301-620X.93B5.25908, 93-B/5/593 [pii]

MacDonald SJ (2004) Metal-on-metal total hip arthroplasty: the concerns. Clin Orthop Relat Res 429:86–93, 00003086-200412000-00014 [pii]

Malviya A, Ramaskandhan J, Holland JP, Lingard EA (2010) Metal-on-metal total hip arthroplasty. J Bone Joint Surg Am 92(7):1675–1683. doi:10.2106/JBJS.I.01426, 92/7/1675 [pii]

Masson B (2009) Emergence of the alumina matrix composite in total hip arthroplasty. Int Orthop 33(2):359–363. doi:10.1007/s00264-007-0484-9

Matthies AK, Skinner JA, Osmani H, Henckel J, Hart AJ (2012) Pseudotumors are common in well-positioned low-wearing metal-on-metal hips. Clin Orthop Relat Res 470(7):1895–1906. doi:10.1007/s11999-011-2201-7

Mittelmeier H, Heisel J (1992) Sixteen-years' experience with ceramic hip prostheses. Clin Orthop Relat Res 282:64–72

Muratoglu OK, Bragdon CR, O'Connor DO, Jasty M, Harris WH, Gul R et al (1999) Unified wear model for highly crosslinked ultra-high molecular weight polyethylenes (UHMWPE). Biomaterials 20(16):1463–1470, S0142-9612(99)00039-3 [pii]

Murphy SB, Ecker TM, Tannast M (2006) Two- to 9-year clinical results of alumina ceramic-on-ceramic THA. Clin Orthop Relat Res 453:97–102. doi:10.1097/01.blo.0000246532.59876.73

Oral E, Christensen SD, Malhi AS, Wannomae KK, Muratoglu OK (2006) Wear resistance and mechanical properties of highly cross-linked, ultrahigh-molecular weight polyethylene doped with vitamin E. J Arthroplasty 21(4):580–591. doi:10.1016/j.arth.2005.07.009, S0883-5403(05)00405-5 [pii]

Park YS, Moon YW, Lim SJ, Yang JM, Ahn G, Choi YL (2005) Early osteolysis following second-generation metal-on-metal hip replacement. J Bone Joint Surg Am 87(7):1515–1521. doi:10.2106/JBJS.D.02641, 87/7/1515 [pii]

Pospischill M, Knahr K (2005) Cementless total hip arthroplasty using a threaded cup and a rectangular tapered stem. Follow-up for ten to 17 years. J Bone Joint Surg Br 87(9):1210–1215. doi:10.1302/0301-620X.87B9.16107, 87-B/9/1210 [pii]

Restrepo C, Parvizi J, Kurtz SM, Sharkey PF, Hozack WJ, Rothman RH (2008) The noisy ceramic hip: is component malpositioning the cause? J Arthroplasty 23(5):643–649. doi:10.1016/j.arth.2008.04.001, S0883-5403(08)00440-3 [pii]

Santavirta S, Bohler M, Harris WH, Konttinen YT, Lappalainen R, Muratoglu O et al (2003) Alternative materials to improve total hip replacement tribology. Acta Orthop Scand 74(4):380–388. doi:10.1080/00016470310017668

Sayeed SA, Mont MA, Costa CR, Johnson AJ, Naziri Q, Bonutti PM et al (2011) Early outcomes of sequentially cross-linked thin polyethylene liners with large diameter femoral heads in total hip arthroplasty. Bull NYU Hosp Jt Dis 69(suppl 1):S90–S94

Silva M, Heisel C, Schmalzried TP (2005) Metal-on-metal total hip replacement. Clin Orthop Relat Res 430:53–61, 00003086-200501000-00007 [pii]

Skinner HB (1999) Ceramic bearing surfaces. Clin Orthop Relat Res 369:83–91

Smith AJ, Dieppe P, Vernon K, Porter M, Blom AW (2012) Failure rates of stemmed metal-on-metal hip replacements: analysis of data from the National Joint Registry of England and Wales. Lancet 379(9822):1199–1204. doi:10.1016/S0140-6736(12)60353-5, S0140-6736(12)60353-5 [pii]

Thomas GER, Simpson DJ, Mehmood S, Taylor A, McLardy-Smith P, Gill HS et al (2011) The seven-year wear of highly cross-linked polyethylene in total hip arthroplasty: a double-blind, randomized controlled trial using radiostereometric analysis. J Bone Joint Surg Am 93(8):716–722. doi:10.2106/JBJS.J.00287, 93/8/716 [pii]

Urban JA, Garvin KL, Boese CK, Bryson L, Pedersen DR, Callaghan JJ et al (2001) Ceramic-on-polyethylene bearing surfaces in total hip arthroplasty. Seventeen to twenty-one-year results. J Bone Joint Surg Am 83-A(11):1688–1694

Walter WL, O'Toole GC, Walter WK, Ellis A, Zicat BA (2007) Squeaking in ceramic-on-ceramic hips: the importance of acetabular component orientation. J Arthroplasty 22(4):496–503. doi:10.1016/j.arth.2006.06.018, S0883-5403(06)00512-2 [pii]

Willert HG, Buchhorn GH, Fayyazi A, Flury R, Windler M, Koster G et al (2005) Metal-on-metal bearings and hypersensitivity in patients with artificial hip joints. A clinical and histomorphological study. J Bone Joint Surg Am 87(1):28–36. doi:10.2106/JBJS.A.02039pp, 87/1/28 [pii]

Williams DH, Greidanus NV, Masri BA, Duncan CP, Garbuz DS (2011) Prevalence of pseudotumor in asymptomatic patients after metal-on-metal hip arthroplasty. J Bone Joint Surg Am 93(23):2164–2171. doi:10.2106/JBJS.J.01884

Willmann G (2000) Ceramic femoral head retrieval data. Clin Orthop Relat Res 379:22–28

Ziaee H, Daniel J, Datta AK, Blunt S, McMinn DJ (2007) Transplacental transfer of cobalt and chromium in patients with metal-on-metal hip arthroplasty: a controlled study. J Bone Joint Surg Br 89(3):301–305. doi:10.1302/0301-620X.89B3.18520, 89-B/3/301 [pii]

Zichner L, Lindenfeld T (1997) In-vivo wear of the slide combinations ceramics-polyethylene as opposed to metal-polyethylene. Orthopade 26(2):129–134

Total Hip Arthroplasty Using a Short, Metaphyseal-Fitting Anatomic Cementless Femoral Component in Patients with Femoral Head Osteonecrosis Who Are Less than 30 Years Old

19

Young-Hoo Kim, Jang-Won Park, and Jun-Shik Kim

19.1 Introduction

Modern cemented or cementless total hip *arthroplasty in the* patients with osteonecrosis *of femoral head is equally successful outcome as compared with patients with osteoarthrtis (Kim et al.* 2003a*; Xenakis et al.* 2001*; Mont et al.* 2001*; Babis and Soucacos* 2004*). The remaining problems in the modern cemented or cementless total hip arthroplasty are thigh pain, periprosthetic fracture, stress shielding, polyethylene wear, osteolysis, and aseptic loosening (Mallory et al.* 2001*;* Engh and Massin 1989*; Kim* 2005*).*

In an effort to reduce the periprosthetic fracture, thigh pain, and stress shielding and *to facilitate revision,* a new short, metaphyseal-fitting anatomic cementless femoral component was developed (Kim et al. 2011a, 2012). A short, metaphyseal-fitting anatomic cementless femoral component was designed to require less resection of the upper femur and/or less reaming of the femoral shaft. This serves a dual purpose of facilitating future revision while providing a postoperative state closely mimicking the originally functioning hip. The question thus arises as to whether it is possible to obtain rigid fixation of this short, metaphyseal-fitting anatomic stem without diaphyseal fixation in the highly active younger patients with osteonecrosis of femoral head.

Y.-H. Kim, MD (✉)
The Joint Replacement Center, School of Medicine,
Ewha Womans University School of Medicine, Seoul, Korea

The Joint Replacement Center, MokDong Hospital, Ewha Womans University,
911-1, MokDong, Seoul, YangCheon-Ku 158-710, Korea
e-mail: younghookim@ewha.ac.kr

J.-W. Park, MD • J.-S. Kim, MD
The Joint Replacement Center, School of Medicine,
Ewha Womans University School of Medicine, Seoul, Korea

K. Knahr (ed.), *Total Hip Arthroplasty,*
DOI 10.1007/978-3-642-35653-7_19, © EFORT 2013

The purpose of this current study was to evaluate the *midterm* clinical and radiological results of the use of the short, metaphyseal-fitting anatomic cementless femoral component in the highly active patients younger than 30 years of age who had osteonecrosis of the femoral head.

19.2 Materials and Methods

19.2.1 Patients

Between July 2005 and November 2006, the author performed consecutive primary total hip arthroplasties using a short, metaphyseal-fitting anatomic cementless femoral stem on 111 hips in 70 patients who were 30 years of age or younger; 41 patients had a bilateral arthroplasty. Patients were excluded if they were older than 30 years of age or had either a follow-up of less than 5 years after the operation. No patient died or lost to follow-up in the interim. Therefore, all patients were available for clinical and radiographic evaluation at 5.7 years (range, 5–6.5 years) after the operation. The study was approved by the institutional review board, and all patients provided informed consent.

The mean age of the patients at the time of the total hip arthroplasty was 28.8 years (range, 20–30 years). There were 52 men and 18 women. All hips with osteonecrosis had Ficat and Arlet stage III or IV changes (Ficat 1985). The presumed cause of osteonecrosis was ethanol-associated in 76 hips in 44 patients (62.8 %), steroid use in 29 hips in 20 patients (28.6 %), and idiopathic in 6 hips in 6 (8.6 %) patients.

The mean weight of the patient was 65.8 kg (range, 51–109 kg), and their mean height was 164.7 cm (range, 158–188 cm). The mean body mass index was 24.5 kg/m^2 (range, 20.4–30.9 kg/m^2).

19.2.2 Surgical Procedure

All procedures were performed by the senior author through a posterolateral approach. The index operation was using epidural anesthesia in 51 patients and general anesthesia in the remaining 19 patients. A cementless Pinnacle acetabular component (DePuy, Warsaw, Indiana) was used in all hips. These components were press-fitted after the acetabulum had been underreamed by 1 mm. One or two screws were used for additional fixation in 11 hips (10 %); the remainder did not require any screws. A 36-mm-internal diameter Biolox delta ceramic liner (CeramTec AG, Plochingen, Germany) was used in all hips regardless of the external diameter of the acetabular component which ranged from 52 to 60 mm. We aimed the acetabular component to be fixed between 40° and 45° inclination and between 20° and 30° anteversion.

All patients received a short, metaphyseal-fitting anatomic cementless femoral component (Proxima; DePuy, Leeds, United Kingdom) with a 36-mm Biolox delta ceramic modular head (Ceram Tec AG). A short, metaphyseal-fitting anatomic cementless Proxima stem is designed to have a close fit with the proximal femur with the aim of maximizing primary stability, particularly in torsion. It is manufactured using titanium alloy and is entirely porous coated with sintered titanium beads having a mean pore size of 250 μm, to which a 30-μm-thick hydroxyapatite coating is applied, except for the distal tip. The design features are a longer proximomedial portion of the stem and a highly pronounced lateral flare. A "round-the-corner" technique (Kim et al. 2011b; Santori and Santori 2010) was used for femoral broaching and insertion of the implant. The broaches and implants were inserted in a slight varus position and then rotated into the correct alignment. The size of the femoral component which was selected matched the size of the largest broach used. The dimension of the real component was 0.5 mm larger than that of the prepared metaphysis.

The patients were allowed to stand on the second postoperative day and progress to full weight bearing with crutches as tolerated. They were advised to use a pair of crutches for 6 weeks and walk with a cane thereafter if required.

19.2.3 Clinical and Radiographic Evaluation

Clinical and radiographic follow-up was undertaken at 3 months, 1 year, and yearly thereafter. The Harris hip score (Harris 1969) and the Western Ontario and McMaster Universities Osteoarthritis index (WOMAC) score (Bellamy et al. 1988) were determined before surgery and at each follow-up examination. Patients scored thigh pain on a ten-point visual analog scale (0 = no pain, 10 = severe pain). The level of activity of the patients after the total hip arthroplasty was assessed using the University of California, Los Angles (UCLA) activity score (Zahiri et al. 1998).

The occurrence of any clicking or squeaking sound emanating from the ceramic-on-ceramic bearing was recorded.

The radiographs were analyzed by a research associate who had no knowledge of the patient's identity. A supine anteroposterior radiograph of the pelvis with both hips in neutral rotation and no abduction was taken for every patient. Anteversion of the acetabular component was measured on the lateral radiograph of the hips as the angle between the horizontal line where the film cassette rested on the x-ray table and a second line marking the plane of the opening of the acetabular component. To measure inclination of the acetabular component, a line that joined the inferior margins of the teardrops was drawn in the anteroposterior pelvic radiograph. The intersection of that line with a line marking the plane of opening of the acetabular component determined the angle of inclination.

Definite loosening of the femoral component was defined when there was a progressive axial subsidence of >3 mm or a varus or a valgus shift of more than 3° (Kim et al. 2003b). Definite loosening of the acetabular component was diagnosed when there was a change in the position of the component (>2 mm vertically and/or medially or laterally) or a continuous radiolucent line >2 mm on both the anteroposterior and the lateral radiographs (Sutherland et al. 1982). Bone ingrowth into the femoral component was considered to have occurred when there was a direct contact of the trabecular bone of the femur and the femoral component. Bone ingrowth into the acetabular component was considered to have occurred when there was a direct contact of the trabecular bone of the acetabulum and the acetabular component.

The sites of any osteolysis in the acetabulum were recorded according to the system of DeLee and Charnley (1976), and those in the femur by the system of Gruen et al. (1979). Osteolysis was defined as any discretely localized radiolucency, which had been absent on radiographs taken immediately after the total hip arthroplasty.

Proximal femoral bone resorption was graded radiologically (Engh et al. 1987), with grade 1 indicating atrophy or rounding off of the calcar; grade 2, loss of density in the calcar region with preservation of the medial cortical wall to the level of the lesser trochanter; grade 3, loss of density in the calcar region with loss of the medial cortical wall to the level of the lesser trochanter; and grade 4, loss of density in the entire medial cortical wall distal to the level of the lesser trochanter.

Heterotopic ossification, if present, was graded according to the classification of Brooker et al. (1973).

19.2.4 Statistical Analysis

The change in Harris hip scores was evaluated with two-tailed Student's t-tests. The χ^2 test with Yate's correction was used to analyze complication rates and radiographic data. All statistical analyses were performed using the statistical package for social sciences, version 14.0 (SPSS Inc., Chicago, Illinois). Statistical significance was set at $p < 0.05$.

19.2.5 Source of Funding

No external funding sources were received for the purpose of this study.

19.3   Results

19.3.1 Clinical Results

19.3.1.1 Hip Score
The mean preoperative Harris hip score was 35 points (range, 11–49 points), which improved to 96 points (range, 75–100 points) at the final follow-up. The mean preoperative *total* WOMAC score was 68 points (range, 37–86 points), and the mean *total* WOMAC score at the final follow-up was 17 points (range, 5–25 points).

19.3.1.2 Functional Outcome
Dependence on walking aids and limp had decreased markedly by the final follow-up. At the latest follow-up, 61 (87 %) patients had no detectable limp, and nine patients (13 %) had a mild limp. The ability to use stairs and public transportation,

to put on footwear, and to cut toenails was improved substantially after the operation. The mean preoperative UCLA activity score was three points (range, 1–4 points), which improved to eight points (range, six to nine points) at the final follow-up.

19.3.1.3 Thigh Pain
The prevalence of transitory pain (visual analog scale, 3) in the thigh was 4 % (three of 70 patients) until 6 months after the operation. No patient had thigh pain after 1 year postoperatively.

19.3.1.4 Employment Status
Fourteen of 70 patients (20 %) changed from heavy labor work before the operation to sedentary work after the operation. The remaining 56 patients (80 %) remained in the previous occupation after the operation. No patient was allowed to participate in high-impact sports.

Clicking Squeaking Sounds
  No patient had clicking or squeaking sound.
Alumina Head or Liner Fracture
  No patient had alumina head or liner fracture.

19.3.2 Radiographic Results

19.3.2.1 Loosening
Preoperatively, the Dorr ratio (Dorr 1986) ranged from 0.33 to 0.49. Ninety-five hips (86 %) were Dorr type A, nine (8 %) were type B, and seven (6 %) were type C. As seen on the postoperative radiographs, 105 stems (95 %) were in the neutral position and six (5 %) in the varus position (<5°). The average inclination and anteversion of the acetabular component was 41° (range, 34°–47°) and 22° (range, 17°–25°), respectively. All hips had osseous integration of the acetabular and the femoral components (Fig. 19.1), and no hip exhibited any aseptic loosening of either component. At the latest evaluation, 72 hips (65 %) had grade 1 stress-shielding bone loss, 32 (29 %) had grade 2 bone loss, and 7 (6 %) had grade 3 bone loss at the calcar. No hip had grade 4 bone loss.

19.3.2.2 Osteolysis
No hip displayed femoral or acetabular osteolysis on the radiographs.

19.3.2.3 Revision
No acetabular component was revised. One femoral component was revised to a larger Proxima stem with a strut allograft and multiple cablings for a calcar fracture after a fall (Fig. 19.2). This hip healed completely and osseointegration of the prosthesis was achieved. The rate of survival of the acetabular and femoral components was 100 % at 6 years after the operation.

Fig. 19.1 Radiographs of a
29-year-old man with
osteonecrosis of both femoral
heads. (**a**) An anteroposterior
view of both hips before
surgery shows Ficat stage IV
osteonecrosis of both femoral
heads and Dorr type B
femoral bones. (**b**): An
anteroposterior view of both
hips taken 6 years after
operation shows the
acetabular and femoral
components are well fixed in
a satisfactory position in both
hips without osteolysis.
Grade 2 calcar resorption is
evident in both hips

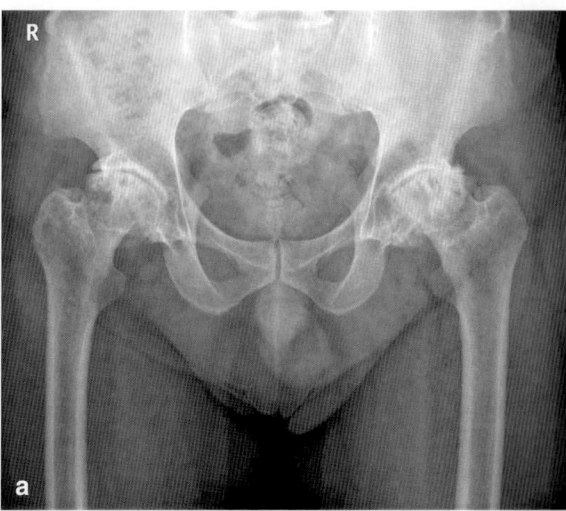

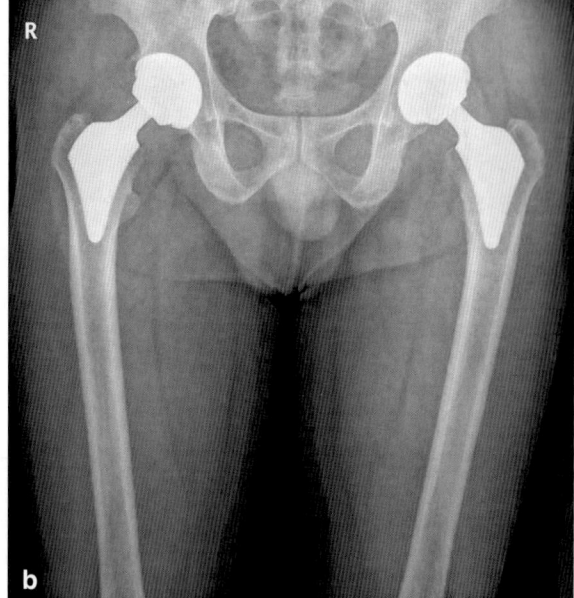

19.3.2.4 Complications

Dislocation occurred in one hip (0.9 %) at 6 months after the operation while he was
playing soccer. Dislocation was treated successfully with closed reduction and an
abduction brace for 3 months. There was no further dislocation in this hip.

One patient had a foot drop after the operation, and it resolved completely at 1
year after the operation.

No hip had a grade 3 or 4 heterotopic ossification.

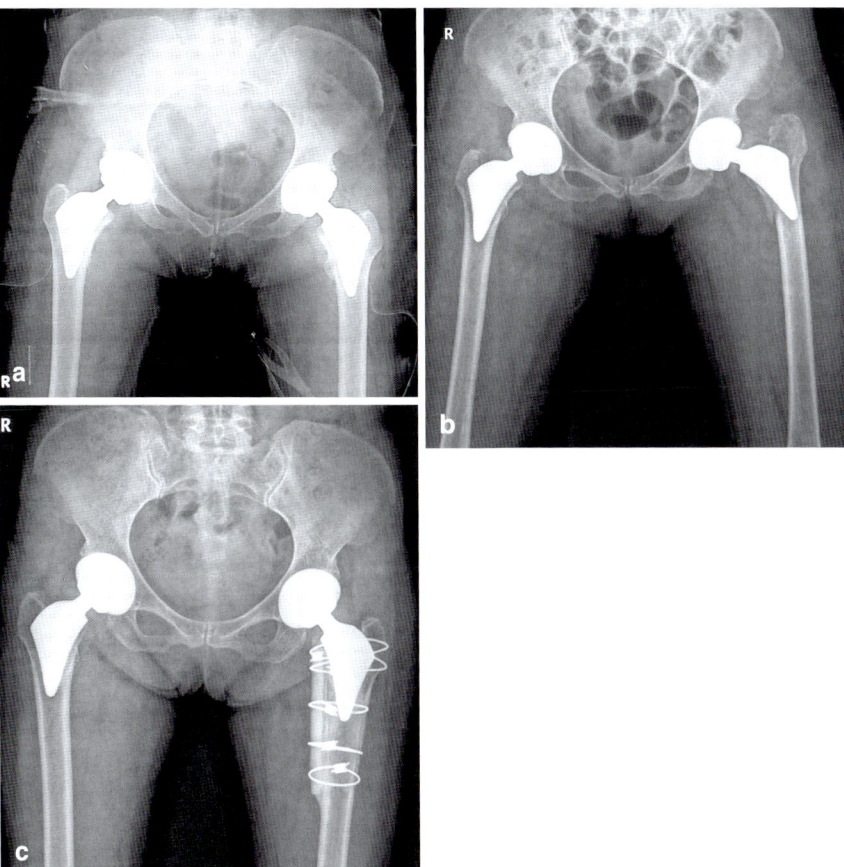

Fig. 19.2 Radiographs of a 25-year-old woman with osteonecrosis of both femoral heads. (**a**) An anteroposterior view of both hips taken immediately after the operation shows the acetabular and femoral components in both hips are embedded in a satisfactory position. (**b**) An anteroposterior view of both hips taken 7 days after the operation reveals femoral components of the left hip is displaced with calcar fracture after a fall. (**c**) An anteroposterior view of both hips taken 5 years after the reconstruction with strut allograft and multiple cablings shows the left femoral stem is fixed in a satisfactory position and strut allograft is well incorporated

19.4   Discussion

We are not aware of any other reports in the literature on the *outcome* of primary cementless total hip arthroplasty using a short, metaphyseal-fitting anatomic stem in the younger patients with osteonecrosis of the femoral head. The *midterm* results of the short, metaphyseal-fitting anatomic cementless femoral component with alumina-on-alumina bearing in our highly active patients younger than 30 years of age who had osteonecrosis of the femoral head exhibited an extremely low prevalence of thigh pain, no loosening or osteolysis, and mild stress shielding.

One major concern with the short stem was whether stable fixation of the stem can be obtained without diaphyseal fixation. Walker et al. (1999) suggested that the femoral stem below the lesser trochanter would be unnecessary for a cementless anatomic femoral stem with a lateral flare and that a short stem would suffice. Accordingly, Leali and Fetto (2004) concluded that a proximally fixed cementless femoral component with a proximal lateral flare provides significant initial stability, which had been shown to be vital to obtain long-term stability through early bone ingrowth. Biomechanical tests performed in vitro by Westphal et al. (2006) showed that stability of the proximal-fitting short metaphyseal stem was achieved when bone quality was good. Santori and Santori (2010) reported solid fixation of their custom-made short femoral stem (DePuy, Leeds, United Kingdom) similar to the Proxima stem. Their findings validated the assumption that torsional loads can be controlled without diaphyseal fixation by femoral neck preservation and lateral flare of the stem. We have shown in our study that this hip system had no mechanical failure in the younger patients who had osteonecrosis of the femoral head despite they had higher activity level. *We believe that femoral neck preservation with lateral flare of stem and the strong trabecular bone were responsible for rigid fixation of the stem without diaphyseal fixation.*

The diagnosis in this series was osteonecrosis of the femoral head in all patients. In a histological study, Calder et al. (2001) found that patients with osteonecrosis of the femoral head which also involved proximal *Gruen* zones(Gruen et al. 1979) 1, 2, 6, and 7 had evidence of extensive osteocyte death. On the contrary, Kim and Kim (2004) found that the majority of patients who had idiopathic or osteonecrosis secondary to ethanol abuse had normal or nearly normal bone in the acetabulum and in the areas of the proximal part of the femur which are crucial for fixation of the implant. The excellent results in our series are *appeared to be* attributable to the normal or nearly normal bone in the acetabulum and in the area of the proximal part of the femur.

Mallory et al. (2001) reported the survival of 120 Mallory-Head tapered cementless femoral stems (Biomet, Warsaw, Indiana) at 12.2 years' follow-up was 97.5 %. However, they observed bone resorption of the proximal femur related to stress shielding in 22 hips (18 %) and femoral osteolysis in 35 hips (29 %). The survival of the Trilock femoral component (DePuy, Warsaw, Indiana) has been reported as 95.5 % at 15 years follow-up (Teloken et al. 2002) but with associated proximal femoral resorption due to stress shielding in just under half the patients. Santori et al. (2006) reported that their custom-made femoral stem similar to our short stem had no aseptic loosening at the 5-year follow-up point. They observed mild stress shielding (calcar rounding off) in 60 % of cases (78 of 131 hips), and it was generally nonprogressive after 6 months after surgery. In our study, there was mild stress shielding, and it was nonprogressive after 1 year after surgery. We believe that absence of the distal stem minimized stress-shielding-related proximal femoral bone resorption. *However, we acknowledge that stress shielding is less in the current study compared to the other studies (i.e., Mallory-Head or Trilock stem) because of shorter follow-up.*

There are several strengths in this study. First, drawing patients from single center means there was specific coordination of surgical technique or implant used in the study. Second, a large volume of patients younger than 30 years of age had osteonecrosis of the femoral head. Third, grouping patients with high activity level to investigate the performance of the short stem. Finally, activity level data were collected in the patients and can be analyzed as a risk factor for failure.

There are several limitations in this study. First, we prospectively collected all data, but the study was not randomized and we had no control group for which we used a different component or different surgical technique to compare and contrast outcomes. Second, our migration analysis of the stem did not use the more precise methods of radiostereometric analysis (Börlin et al. 2002). Third, the duration of follow-up was short and was insufficient to allow us to draw significant conclusions, because any type of prosthesis shows good results at <5 years. However, there are strong evidences that early (less than 2 years) stability of cementless femoral stem produces good late clinical results (Engh and Massin 1989; Kim and Kim 1993). Kim and Kim (1993) reported that early migration (less than 1 year) of uncemented porous-coated anatomic femoral component was related to the aseptic loosening of the component. Engh and Massin (1989) concluded that a component was loose if there was evidence of migration of cementless femoral component at 1 year after the operation. The findings from these two studies clearly indicate that the stable femoral stem at 5.7 years after the operation can maintain the long-term stable fixation of the femoral component.

In conclusion, the short, metaphyseal-fitting anatomic cementless femoral stem provides stable fixation without diaphyseal fixation in highly active younger patients with osteonecrosis of the femoral head.

References

Babis GC, Soucacos PN (2004) Effectiveness of total hip arthroplasty in the management of hip osteonecrosis. Orthop Clin North Am 35:359–364

Bellamy N, Buchanan WW, Goldsmith CH, Campbell J, Stitt LW (1988) Validation study of WOMAC: a health status instrument for measuring clinically important patient relevant outcomes to antirheumatic drug therapy in patients with osteoarthritis of the hip or knee. J Rheumatol 15:1833–1840

Börlin N, Thien T, Kärrholm J (2002) The precision of radiostereometric measurements: manual vs. digital measurements. J Biomech 35:69–79

Brooker AF, Bowerman JW, Robinson RA, Riley LH Jr (1973) Ectopic ossification following total hip replacement: incidence and method of classification. J Bone Joint Surg Am 55: 1629–1632

Calder JD, Pearse MF, Revell PA (2001) The extent of osteocyte death in the proximal femur of patients with osteonecrosis of the femoral head. J Bone Joint Surg Br 83:419–422

DeLee JG, Charnley J (1976) Radiological demarcation of cemented sockets in total hip replacement. Clin Orthop Relat Res 121:20–32

Dorr LD (1986) Total hip replacement using APR system. Tech Orthop 1:22–34

Engh CA, Massin P (1989) Cementless total hip arthroplasty using the anatomic medullary locking stem. Results using a survivorship analysis. Clin Orthop Relat Res 249:141–158

Engh CA, Bobyn JD, Glassman AH (1987) Porous-coated hip replacement: the factors governing bone ingrowth, stress shielding, and clinical results. J Bone Joint Surg Br 69:45–55

Ficat RP (1985) Idiopathic bone necrosis of the femoral head. Early diagnosis and treatment. J Bone Joint Surg Br 67:3–9

Gruen TA, McNeice GM, Amstutz HC (1979) "Modes of failures" of cemented stem-type femoral components: a radiographic analysis of loosening. Clin Orthop Relat Res 141:17–27

Harris WH (1969) Traumatic arthritis of the hip after dislocation and acetabular fractures: treatment by mold arthroplasty: an end result study using a new method of result evaluation. J Bone Joint Surg Am 51:737–755

Kim Y-H (2005) Comparison of polyethylene wear associated with cobalt-chromium and zirconia heads after total hip replacement. A prospective, randomized study. J Bone Joint Surg Am 87:1769–1776

Kim Y-H, Kim VE (1993) Early migration of uncemented porous coated anatomic femoral component related to aseptic loosening. Clin Orthop Relat Res 295:146–155

Kim Y-H, Kim J-S (2004) Histologic analysis of acetabular and proximal femoral bone in patients with osteonecrosis of the femoral head. J Bone Joint Surg Am 86:2471–2474

Kim Y-H, Oh S-H, Kim J-S, Koo K-H (2003a) Contemporary total hip arthroplasty with and without cement in patients with osteonecrosis of the femoral head. J Bone Joint Surg Am 85:675–681

Kim Y-H, Kim J-S, Oh S-H, Kim J-M (2003b) Comparison of porous-coated titanium femoral stem with and without hydroxy apatite coating. J Bone Joint Surg Am 85:1682–1688

Kim Y-H, Choi Y-W, Kim J-S (2011a) Comparison of bone mineral density changes around short, metaphyseal-fitting and conventional cementless anatomic femoral components. J Arthroplasty 26:931–940

Kim Y-H, Kim J-S, Park J-W, Joo J-H (2011b) Total hip replacement with a short metaphyseal-fitting anatomical cementless femoral component in patients aged 70 years or older. J Bone Joint Surg Br 93:587–592

Kim Y-H, Kim J-S, Joo J-H, Park J-W (2012) A prospective short-term outcome study of a short metaphyseal fitting total hip arthroplasty. J Arthroplasty 27:88–94

Leali A, Fetto JF (2004) Preservation of femoral bone mass after total hip replacements with a lateral flare stem. Int Orthop 28:151–154

Mallory TH, Lombardi AV Jr, Leith JR, Fujita H, Hartman JF, Capps SG, Kefauver CA, Adams JB, Vorys GC (2001) Minimal 10-year results of a tapered cementless femoral component in total hip arthroplasty. J Arthroplasty 16(suppl 1):49–54

Mont MA, Rajadhyaksha AD, Hungerford DS (2001) Outcomes of limited femoral resurfacing arthroplasty compared with total hip arthroplasty for osteonecrosis of the femoral head. J Arthroplasty 16(8 suppl 1):134–139

Santori FS, Santori N (2010) Mid-term results of a custom-made short proximal loading femoral component. J Bone Joint Surg Br 92:1231–1237

Santori FS, Manili M, Fredella N, Tonci Ottieri M, Santori N (2006) Ultra-short stems with proximal load transfer: clinical and radiographic results at five-year follow-up. Hip Int 16(suppl 3): 31–39

Sutherland CJ, Wilde AH, Borden LS, Marks KE (1982) A ten-year follow-up of one hundred consecutive Müller curved-stem total hip replacement arthroplasties. J Bone Joint Surg Am 64:970–982

Teloken MA, Bissett G, Hozack WJ, Sharkey PF, Rothman RH (2002) Ten to fifteen-year follow-up after total hip arthroplasty with a tapered cobalt-chromium femoral component (tri-lock) inserted without cement. J Bone Joint Surg Am 84:2140–2144

Walker PS, Culligan S, Hua J, Muirhead-Allwood SK, Bentley G (1999) The effect of a lateral flare feature on uncemented hip stems. Hip Int 9:71–80

Westphal FM, Bishop N, Honl M, Hille E, Püschel K, Morlock MM (2006) Migration and cyclic motion of a new short-stemmed hip prosthesis – a biomechanical in vitro study. Clin Biomech (Bristol, Avon) 21:834–840

Xenakis TA, Gelalis J, Koukoubis TA, Zaharis KC, Soucacos PN (2001) Cementless hip arthroplasty in the treatment of patients with femoral head necrosis. Clin Orthop Relat Res 386:93–99

Zahiri CA, Schmalzried TP, Szuszczewicz ES, Amstutz HC (1998) Assessing activity in joint replacement patients. J Arthroplasty 13:890–895

Survival of Monoblock Acetabular Cups Versus an Uncemented Modular Cup Design: A Population-Based Study from the Swedish Hip Arthroplasty Register

20

Rüdiger J. Weiss, Johan Kärrholm, André Stark, and Nils P. Hailer

20.1 Introduction

There is an increasing use of uncemented components in total hip arthroplasty (THA) in many countries that provide population-based register data (AOA 2009; National Joint Registry of England and Wales 2010; Swedish Hip Arthroplasty Register 2010). Many of these registers report that survival of uncemented components is at best equal to cemented THA, but inferior survival rates of uncemented THA have been reported (Hailer et al. 2010). In uncemented THA, the acetabular cup appeared to be the component that was associated with an increased risk of revision, irrespective of whether revision for any reason or due to aseptic loosening was considered (Hailer et al. 2010). In a recent analysis in the Swedish Hip Arthroplasty Register, patients up to 69 years of age were found to have a reduced risk of revision due to loosening. These cups were, however, more frequently revised due to other

R.J. Weiss (✉)
Section of Orthopaedics and Sports Medicine,
Department of Molecular Medicine and Surgery,
Karolinska Institutet, Karolinska University Hospital,
Stockholm, Sweden
e-mail: rudiger.weiss@karolinska.se

J. Kärrholm
Department of Orthopaedics,
Institute of Clinical Sciences at Sahlgrenska Academy,
Gothenburg University, Gothenburg, Sweden

A. Stark
Department of Clinical Sciences,
Karolinska Institutet, Danderyd Hospital, Stockholm, Sweden

N.P. Hailer
Department of Orthopaedics,
Institute of Surgical Sciences, Uppsala University Hospital,
Uppsala, Sweden

K. Knahr (ed.), *Total Hip Arthroplasty*,
DOI 10.1007/978-3-642-35653-7_20, © EFORT 2013

reasons, and the overall revision rate did not differ between cemented and uncemented sockets (Swedish Hip Arthroplasty Register 2010).

Modularity in uncemented cup designs is popular among orthopedic surgeons. It allows visualization of dome contact when seating the cup in the acetabulum. Moreover, liner wear in modular designs can be dealt with by liner exchange alone, leaving the metal shell in place. On the other hand, modular cups allow motion to occur between the polyethylene liner and the metal shell which has been associated with backside wear and acetabular cup loosening (Young et al. 2002). The issue of backside wear led to the development of non-modular (monoblock) cup designs eliminating or at least diminishing the problem of backside wear. Early monoblock designs consisted of polyethylene molded into a titanium fiber mesh (Morscher and Masar 1988) or a solid titanium shell. More recent developments make use of polyethylene liners in a porous tantalum metal shell (Meneghini et al. 2010). The putative advantages of monoblock designs have to be weighed against drawbacks such as the inability to assess proper component seating into its bony acetabular bed due to the absence of central screw holes that are uniformly present in modular cup designs.

Our objective was to compare the survival rates of uncemented monoblock acetabular components with modular uncement cups using data from the Swedish Hip Arthroplasty Register (SHAR). Moreover, we intended to investigate whether patient- and implant-related covariates would predict an increased revision risk. Data of this study have previously been published elsewhere (Weiss et al. 2012).

20.2 Patients and Methods

20.2.1 Source of Data and Study Population

The SHAR was initiated in 1979. It collects individual-based information for hip replacement surgery on a nationwide basis in Sweden. Demographic data and details of indications for reoperation or revision, surgical technique, and the type of prosthetic components inserted are recorded. All public as well as private orthopedic units in Sweden performing THAs participate on a voluntary basis. Individual procedure registration captures between 97 and 99 % of all primary procedures.

For this study, we extracted from the SHAR all primary THAs using uncemented monoblock acetabular cups during 1999 and 2010 ($n=210$). We could identify two different cup designs: the Morscher press-fit acetabular cup (Sulzer Orthopedics Ltd., Baar, Switzerland; $n=129$ hips) (Fig. 20.1) (Morscher and Masar 1988; Morscher et al. 1997) and the trabecular metal monoblock acetabular cup system (Zimmer Inc., Warsaw, IN; $n=81$ hips) (Fig. 20.2). The modular Trilogy cup (Zimmer Inc.; $n=1,130$ hips) (Fig. 20.3) is a very commonly used uncemented cup design in Sweden and was therefore used as a control group. A previous study has suggested that hydroxyapatite (HA) coating may increase the risk of revision (Lazarinis et al. 2010). Therefore, only modular cups without HA coating were included in the reference group. Moreover, the studied monoblock cup designs did not have an HA coating.

Fig. 20.1 The uncemented Morscher press-fit cup

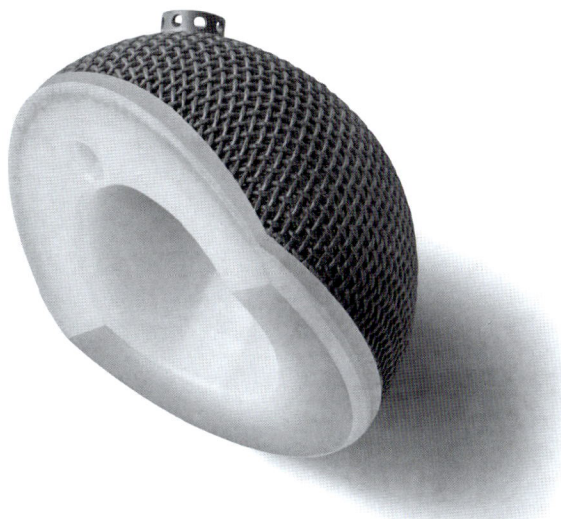

Fig. 20.2 The trabecular metal monoblock acetabular cup system

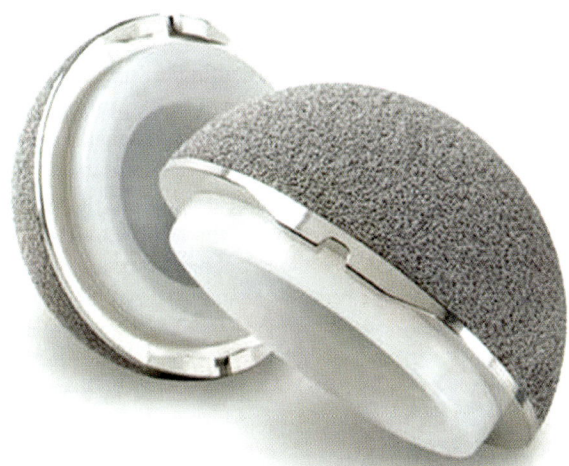

20.2.2 Statistics

Median values and standard deviations (SDs) were used as descriptive statistics. Patients were followed from the day of the primary THA and ended on the day of revision, death, emigration, or December 31, 2010. Kaplan-Meier survival analysis was performed with the type of cup as the independent factor and revision due to any reason as the endpoint. The log-rank test (Mantel-Cox) was used to investigate whether there was a statistically significant difference between the monoblock group and the controls. The endpoint for survival was defined as revision.

A Cox multiple-regression model was used to study risk factors for revision related to the patient, to the implant, and to the surgical technique. The results were expressed as hazard ratios (HRs) with corresponding 95 % confidence

Fig. 20.3 The modular
Trilogy cup

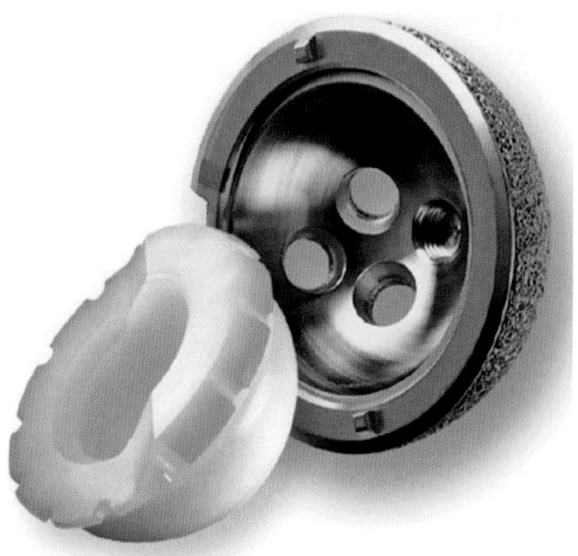

intervals (CIs). The factors studied in the simple Cox model (unadjusted) were cup design (monoblock or modular), age (<50, 50–59, 60–75, >75 years), sex, primary diagnosis before arthroplasty (primary osteoarthritis [OA], inflammatory disease [e.g., rheumatoid arthritis, Morbus Bechterew], pediatric hip disease, idiopathic femoral head necrosis, and other diagnoses), type of stem fixation (cemented or uncemented), highly cross-linked liner polyethylene (yes or no), surgical approach, and prosthesis head size. As a second step, all variables were mutually adjusted for in a multiple Cox regression analysis. After 6 years, the number of cases in the monoblock cohort was less than 50. Therefore follow-up was restricted by censoring implants still at risk beyond 6 years (Ranstam et al. 2011). In patients with bilateral THAs, both sides were included in the analysis, as other studies have shown that this had no significant effect on the risk of failure (Hailer et al. 2010; Lie et al. 2004). Differences between numerical data were analyzed using the Mann–Whitney U-test and between categorical data using the χ^2 test. The level of significance was set at $p \leq 0.05$. All analyses were performed using the PASW software (version 18.0).

20.3   Results

20.3.1 Patients

Approximately half of the patients in both the study and reference group were females. Most patients in both groups were operated due to primary osteoarthritis. At the index operation, a larger proportion of patients in the study cohort (30 %) had the diagnosis pediatric hip disease compared with the controls (14 %). In both groups, the preferred prosthesis head size was 28 mm, and an uncemented stem was

Table 20.1 Baseline characteristics

	Study group ($n=210$)	Control group ($n=1,130$)
Cup design		
Morscher press-fit cup	129 (61 %)	–
Trabecular metal monoblock cup	81 (39 %)	–
Trilogy cup	–	1,130 (100 %)
Median age at surgery, years	47 (17–83)	56 (20–90)
Sex		
Male	101 (48 %)	577 (51 %)
Female	109 (52 %)	553 (49 %)
Primary diagnosis		
Primary osteoarthritis	106 (51 %)	839 (74 %)
Inflammatory disease	21 (10 %)	34 (3 %)
Pediatric hip disease	63 (30 %)	154 (14 %)
Idiopathic femoral head necrosis	15 (7 %)	53 (5 %)
Other	5 (2 %)	50 (4 %)
Surgical approach		
Posterior	188 (90 %)	252 (22 %)
Anterior	19 (9 %)	791 (70 %)
Missing	3 (1 %)	87 (8 %)
Shell holes		
Non-holed	–	2 (0 %)
Multi-holed	–	59 (5 %)
Cluster-holed	–	1,069 (95 %)
Highly cross-linked polyethylene		
No	210 (100 %)	539 (48 %)
Yes	–	573 (51 %)
Missing	–	18 (1 %)
Head size		
22 mm	2 (1 %)	65 (6 %)
28 mm	159 (76 %)	1,036 (92 %)
≥32 mm	49 (23 %)	11 (1 %)
Missing	–	18 (1 %)
Type of stem fixation		
Uncemented	202 (96 %)	967 (86 %)
Cemented	7 (3 %)	161 (14 %)
Missing	1 (1 %)	2 (0 %)

most often used (Table 20.1). The median follow-up was 4 (0–12) years for the monoblock cups and 6 (0–12) years for the modular cup.

20.3.2 Risk of Revision (Monoblock Versus Modular Cup)

The cumulative 5-year survival with any revision as the endpoint was 95 % (95 % CI 91–98) for monoblock cups and 97 % (95 % CI 96–98) for the modular cups.

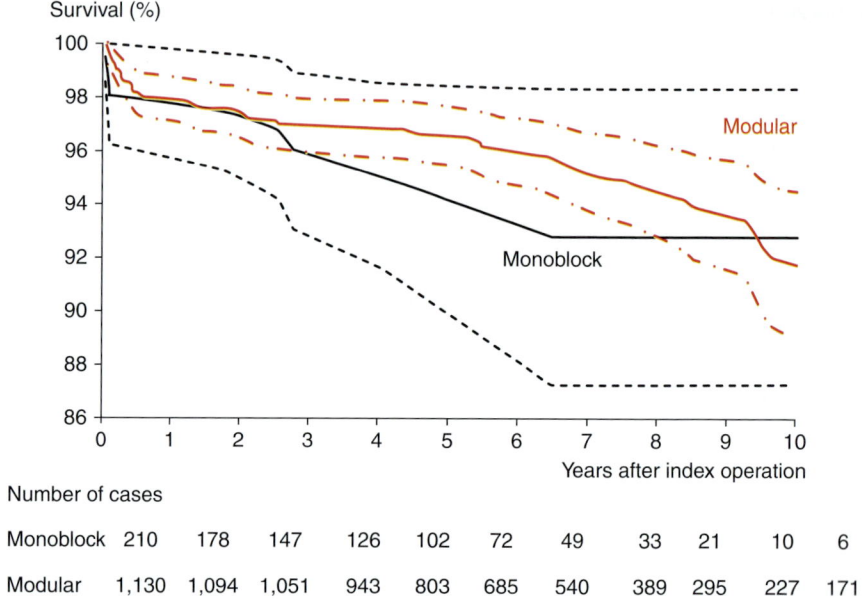

Fig. 20.4 Kaplan-Meier analysis (with 95 % confidence intervals) of monoblock and modular cups with revision for any reason as the endpoint

There was no statistically significant difference ($p=0.6$) between the two groups as shown by the Kaplan-Meier survival analysis (log-rank test) (Fig. 20.4).

We calculated the risk of revision (hazard ratios) for all covariates mentioned above. Other diagnoses compared with primary osteoarthritis were associated with an increased risk of revision (HR 5, 95 % CI 2–12). Moreover, the use of 28 mm prosthesis heads compared with 22 mm heads reduced the risk of cup revision (HR 0.3, 95 % CI 0.1–0.6) (Table 20.2). The adjusted risk of revision (multiple Cox regression analysis) did not reveal any major changes compared with the crude hazard ratios given above. There was still no statistically significant difference in revision risk comparing monoblock cups with the modular cups (HR 2, CI 0.8–6) (Table 20.2).

20.4   Discussion

The medium-term survival rates of both monoblock and modular cups were good and there was no statistically significant difference of risk of revision between the two groups. Several studies had reported excellent survival rates with the use of monoblock acetabular components. Gwynne-Jones et al. reviewed a series of 125 TJAs with the Morscher press-fit cup and presented a survival rate of 96.8 % for revision for any cause and 95.7 % for any acetabular reoperation at 13 years' follow-up (Gwynne-Jones et al. 2009).

Table 20.2 Cox regression analysis, Hazard ratios (HR) of cup revision for any reason

Covariate		No. of cases	No. of revisions	Simple Cox regression[a]			Multiple Cox regression[b]		
				HR	95 %-CI	p-value	HR	95 %-CI	p-value
Cup	Monoblock	210	8	1.3	0.6–2.7	0.6	2.2	0.8–5.8	0.1
	Modular	1,130	40	Reference			Reference		
Age	<50	415	16	Reference			Reference		
	50–59	517	15	0.7	0.4–1.5	0.4	0.9	0.4–1.9	0.7
	60–75	381	15	1.1	0.52.2	0.8	1.0	0.4–2.4	0.9
	>75	27	2	2.2	0.5–9.7	0.3	1.6	0.3–8.0	0.6
Sex	Male	678	24	1.0	0.6–1.7	0.9	1.5	0.8–2.7	0.2
	Female	662	24	Reference			Reference		
Primary diagnosis	Primary osteoarthritis	945	26	Reference			Reference		
	Inflammatory disease	55	2	1.3	0.3–5.6	0.7	1.1	0.2–4.9	0.9
	Pediatric hip disease	217	9	1.5	0.7–3.1	0.3	0.9	0.3–2.2	0.7
	Idiopathic femoral head necrosis	68	4	2.1	0.7–6.1	0.2	2.1	0.7–6.1	0.2
	Other	55	7	5.3	2.3–12	0.001	4.4	1.8–11	0.001
Surgical approach	Posterior	440	16	1.0	0.5–1.8	1.0	1.1	0.5–2.4	0.9
	Anterior	810	29	Reference			Reference		
Highly cross-linked polyethylene	Yes	573	22	1.3	0.7–2.3	0.4	1.4	0.7–3.0	0.4
	No	749	26	Reference			Reference		
Head size	22 mm	67	8	Reference			Reference		
	28 mm	1,195	40	0.3	0.1–0.6	0.001	0.2	0.1–0.5	0.001
	>32 mm	60	–	0	0–9.7	1.0	0	0–1.7	1.0
Type of stem fixation	Uncemented	1,169	42	1.4	0.6–3.5	0.5	1.1	0.4–3.1	0.9
	Cemented	168	5	Reference			Reference		

CI confidence interval

[a]Crude HR

[b]Adjusted HR (all covariates mentioned above are entered in the Cox analysis)

Garavaglia et al. documented the outcome of 335 TJAs using the same monoblock cup. There was no cup that required revision due to aseptic loosening after a mean follow-up of 10 years, and with cup revision due to any reason, the 10-year survival rate was 99 % (Garavaglia et al. 2011). Berli et al. reported the 15-year results of 280 hips implanted with the Morscher cup quoting a survival of 98 % for aseptic loosening and 95 % overall (Berli et al. 2007). Other monoblock cup designs have shown similar favorable long-term revision rates (Ali and Kumar 2003; Ihle et al. 2008).

Trabecular metal monoblock cups represent a more recent development. These cups show good survival rates: 151 hips were followed for a minimum of 8 years and no cup revision occurred during this period, and there was also no evidence of osteolytic lesions (Macheras et al. 2009). Malizos et al. followed 223 consecutive patients operated with the TMT acetabular component and documented a survival of 99 % at a mean 5-year follow-up (Malizos et al. 2008). A randomized RSA study comparing trabecular cups and titanium fiber-mesh cups in primary hip arthroplasty showed promising early results with regard to fixation of trabecular metal components to the acetabular host bone. Both cups showed excellent fixation; however, less rotation along the transverse axis was seen in trabecular metal cups (Baad-Hansen et al. 2011). Other authors confirm good early implant stability of these cups, which can be seen as an index of long-term survival and success (Kostakos et al. 2010).

Young et al. reported reduced wear and a rate of osteolysis of 2 % in monoblock cups compared with 22 % in a matched group with modular components (mean follow-up of 5 years) (Young et al. 2002). However, other authors found no difference in wear rates and prevalence of osteolysis between modular and monoblock acetabular cups (6-year follow-up). They concluded that backside wear which should be present in the modular cups did not significantly contribute to the generation of osteolysis during this intermediate observation time (Gonzalez Della Valle et al. 2004).

Potential disadvantages with monoblock cups are as follows: There are no screw or dome holes; therefore, dome contact cannot be visualized during implantation. Fixation of the monoblock cups is not rigid when the cup is inserted. If movement and failure of bony fixation is observed, the monoblock cup needs to be revised with a shell with screws (Sculco 2002).

We could show that lower prosthesis head size (22 mm compared with 28 mm) increased the risk of revision. There is evidence in the literature that small prosthesis heads increase the risk of hip dislocation (Bystrom et al. 2003). Data from the Australian Joint Replacement Registry showed that there is a significant association between small femoral head diameter and increased revision risk for dislocation in uncemented cups (Conroy et al. 2008).

Our study is limited by the lack of long-term follow-up data. Revision due to wear of polyethylene, aseptic loosening, and acetabular osteolysis may increase during subsequent follow-up. Moreover, our results should be interpreted acknowledging that highly cross-linked polyethylene was available in more than half of the modular cups but not for monoblock cups. Highly cross-linked polyethylene has been introduced to THA surgery with the aim of reducing wear particles. Several authors have shown promising results (Dorr et al. 2005; Bragdon et al. 2007).

Furthermore, a potential bias could distort our findings: In the monoblock group, median age was significantly lower, and the frequency of non-primary osteoarthritis was significantly higher than in the control group. Both of these factors are known to increase the rate of early loosening, and although we tried to correct for this potential confounder by performing multiple Cox regression analyses, a certain amount of uncertainty remains. The strength of the study is that it is based on population-based prospective observational data with an excellent compliance. Our data on survival and revisions seem to be rather complete.

In conclusion, both monoblock and modular cups showed good midterm survival rates. There was no clinically relevant difference in revision risk between the two cup designs. Further review of the current patient population is warranted to determine the long-term durability and risk of revision of monoblock cup designs.

References

Ali MS, Kumar A (2003) Hydroxyapatite-coated RM cup in primary hip arthroplasty. Int Orthop 27:90–93

AOA. Australian Orthopaedic Association National Joint Replacement Registry annual report 2009. http://www.dmac.adelaide.edu.au/aoanjrr/publications.jsp

Baad-Hansen T, Kold S, Nielsen PT, Laursen MB, Christensen PH, Soballe K (2011) Comparison of trabecular metal cups and titanium fiber-mesh cups in primary hip arthroplasty: a randomized RSA and bone mineral densitometry study of 50 hips. Acta Orthop 82:155–160

Berli BJ, Ping G, Dick W, Morscher EW (2007) Nonmodular flexible press-fit cup in primary total hip arthroplasty: 15-year followup. Clin Orthop Relat Res 461:114–121

Bragdon CR, Kwon YM, Geller JA, Greene ME, Freiberg AA, Harris WH, Malchau M (2007) Minimum 6-year followup of highly cross-linked polyethylene in THA. Clin Orthop Relat Res 465:122–127

Bystrom S, Espehaug B, Furnes O, Havelin LI (2003) Femoral head size is a risk factor for total hip luxation: a study of 42,987 primary hip arthroplasties from the Norwegian Arthroplasty Register. Acta Orthop Scand 74:514–524

Conroy JL, Whitehouse SL, Graves SE, Pratt NL, Ryan P, Crawford RW (2008) Risk factors for revision for early dislocation in total hip arthroplasty. J Arthroplasty 23:867–872

Dorr LD, Wan Z, Shahrdar C, Sirianni L, Boutary M, Yun A (2005) Clinical performance of a Durasul highly cross-linked polyethylene acetabular liner for total hip arthroplasty at five years. J Bone Joint Surg Am 87:1816–1821

Garavaglia G, Lubbeke A, Barea C, Roussos C, Peter R, Hoffmeyer P (2011) Ten-year results with the Morscher press-fit cup: an uncemented, non-modular, porous-coated cup inserted without screws. Int Orthop 35:957–963

González Della Valle A, Su E, Zoppi A, Sculco TP, Salvati EA (2004) Wear and periprosthetic osteolysis in a match-paired study of modular and nonmodular uncemented acetabular cups. J Arthroplasty 19:972–977

Gwynne-Jones DP, Garneti N, Wainwright C, Matheson JA, King R (2009) The Morscher Press Fit acetabular component: a nine- to 13-year review. J Bone Joint Surg Br 91:859–864

Hailer NP, Garellick G, Karrholm J (2010) Uncemented and cemented primary total hip arthroplasty in the Swedish Hip Arthroplasty Register. Acta Orthop 81:34–41

Ihle M, Mai S, Pfluger D, Siebert W (2008) The results of the titanium-coated RM acetabular component at 20 years: a long-term follow-up of an uncemented primary total hip replacement. J Bone Joint Surg Br 90:1284–1290

Kostakos AT, Macheras GA, Frangakis CE, Stafilas KS, Baltas D, Xenakis TA (2010 Jan) Migration of the trabecular metal monoblock acetabular cup system. J Arthroplasty 25(1):35–40

Lazarinis S, Karrholm J, Hailer NP (2010) Increased risk of revision of acetabular cups coated with hydroxyapatite. Acta Orthop 81:53–59

Lie SA, Engesaeter LB, Havelin LI, Gjessing HK, Vollset SE (2004) Dependency issues in survival analyses of 55,782 primary hip replacements from 47,355 patients. Stat Med 23:3227–3240

Macheras G, Kateros K, Kostakos A, Koutsostathis S, Danomaras D, Papagelopoulos PJ (2009) Eight- to ten-year clinical and radiographic outcome of a porous tantalum monoblock acetabular component. J Arthroplasty 24:705–709

Malizos KN, Bargiotas K, Papatheodorou L, Hantes M, Karachalios T (2008) Survivorship of monoblock trabecular metal cups in primary THA: midterm results. Clin Orthop Relat Res 466:159–166

Meneghini RM, Ford KS, McCollough CH, Hanssen AD, Lewallen DG (2010) Bone remodeling around porous metal cementless acetabular components. J Arthroplasty 25:741–747

Morscher E, Masar Z (1988) Development and first experience with an uncemented press-fit cup. Clin Orthop Relat Res 1988:96–103

Morscher E, Berli B, Jockers W, Schenk R (1997) Rationale of a flexible press fit cup in total hip replacement. 5-year followup in 280 procedures. Clin Orthop Relat Res 341:42–50

National Joint Registry (NJR) of England and Wales (2010) Seventh annual report (April 2009–March 2010). http://www.njrcentre.org.uk

Ranstam J, Karrholm J, Pulkkinen P, Makela K, Espehaug B, Pedersen AB, Mehnert F, Furnes O (2011) Statistical analysis of arthroplasty data. II. Guidelines. Acta Orthop 82:258–267

Sculco TP (2002) The acetabular component: an elliptical monoblock alternative. J Arthroplasty 17:118–120

Swedish Hip Arthroplasty Register (2010) Annual report 2010. http://www.jru.orthop.gu.se

Weiss RJ, Hailer NP, Stark A, Kärrholm J (2012 Jun) Survival of uncemented acetabular monoblock cups: evaluation of 210 hips in the Swedish Hip Arthroplasty Register. Acta Orthop 83(3):214–219

Young AM, Sychterz CJ, Hopper RH Jr, Engh CA (2002) Effect of acetabular modularity on polyethylene wear and osteolysis in total hip arthroplasty. J Bone Joint Surg Am 84-A:58–63

Index

K. Knahr (ed.), *Total Hip Arthroplasty*,
DOI 10.1007/978-3-642-35653-7, © EFORT 2013

Printing: Ten Brink, Meppel, The Netherlands
Binding: Stürtz, Würzburg, Germany